U0189498

中英双语版

中国农村之医学
我的记述

MEDICINE
IN RURAL CHINA

A PERSONAL
ACCOUNT

陈志潜　　　著

王　辰　杨维中　主　译

张孔来　主　审

郭　岩　张建新　副主审

中国协和医科大学出版社

北京

著作权合同登记：图字 01-2022-0090 号

图书在版编目（CIP）数据

中国农村之医学：我的记述 / 陈志潜著；王辰，杨维中译 . -- 北
京 : 中国协和医科大学出版社 , 2023.10
ISBN 978-7-5679-2058-3

Ⅰ . ①中… Ⅱ . ①陈… ②杨… Ⅲ . ①农村卫生 - 医疗保健事业 -
概况 - 中国 Ⅳ . ① R199.2

中国版本图书馆 CIP 数据核字（2022）第 201523 号

中国农村之医学：我的记述　Medicine in Rural China : A Personal Account

著　者：	陈志潜
主　译：	王 辰　杨维中
责任编辑：	沈冰冰　郝 莹
封面设计：	李新泉
责任校对：	张 麓
责任印制：	张 岱

出版发行：**中国协和医科大学出版社**
　　　　　（北京市东城区东单三条 9 号　邮编 100730　电话 010-65260431）
网　　址：www.pumcp.com
经　　销：新华书店总店北京发行所
印　　刷：北京联兴盛业印刷股份有限公司

开　　本：787mm×1092mm　1/16
印　　张：32.75
字　　数：520 千字
版　　次：2023 年 10 月第 1 版
印　　次：2023 年 10 月第 1 次印刷
定　　价：128.00 元

ISBN 978-7-5679-2058-3

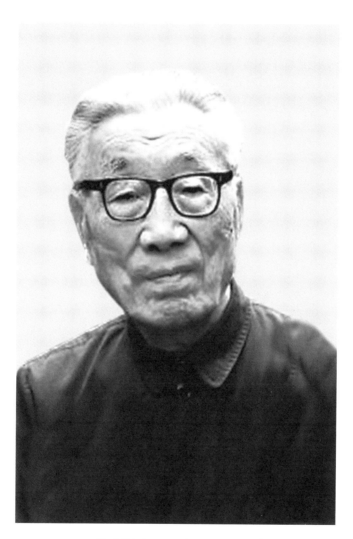

陈志潜（1903 年—2000 年）

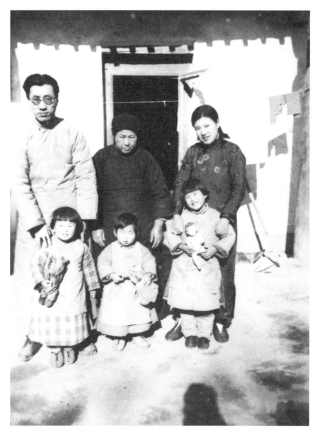

◀陈志潜博士家庭合影，摄于
1934 年河北定县。

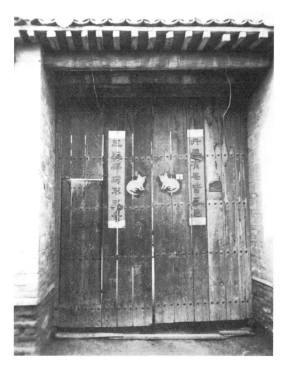

▲ 20 世纪 30 年代，农民为抵挡疾病，多用迷信的
方法。图为将一对猫的图案贴在门上，以期抵御病魔。

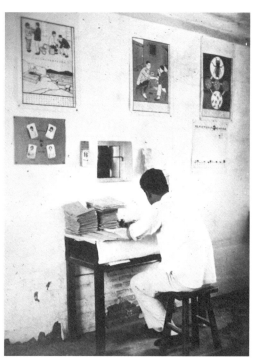

▲受过培训的卫生站医生在工作。

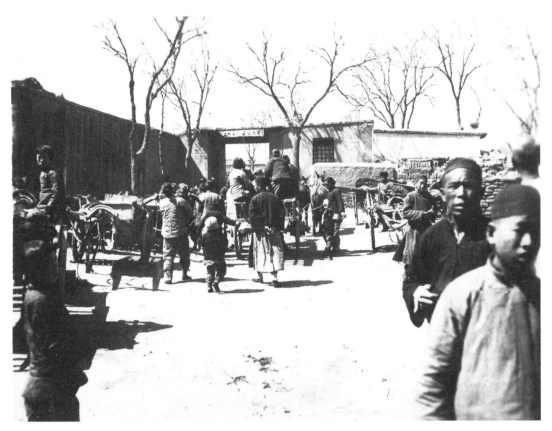

▲定县街景。

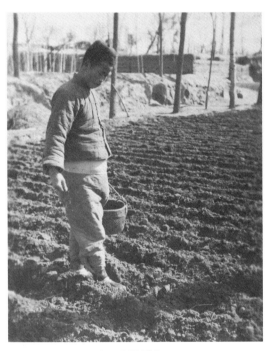

▲农民辛勤耕作。

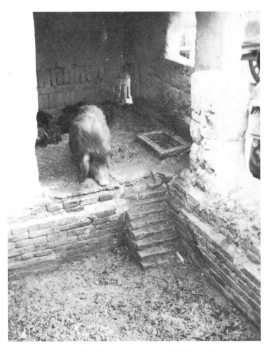

▲农村卫生状况恶劣。图为母猪进入公厕。

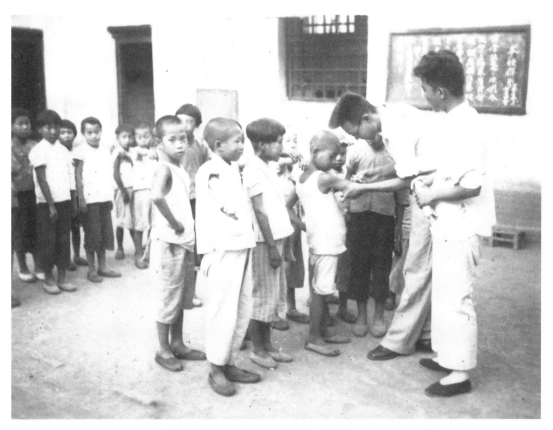

▲区卫生站的医生为学生注射伤寒疫苗。

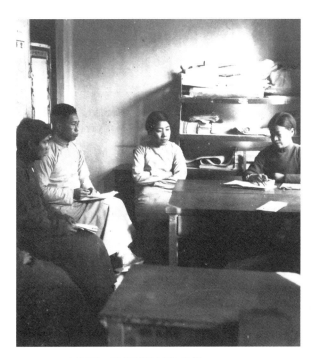

▲每周一次的学校卫生会议。

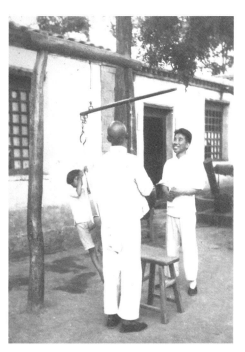

▲乡卫生站每月为儿童称体重。

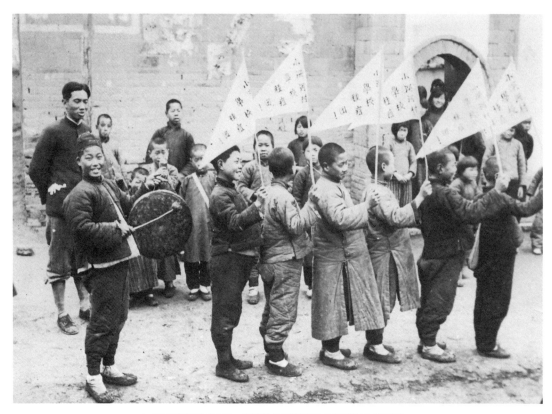

▲儿童宣传队表演，提醒村民预防免疫接种的必要性。

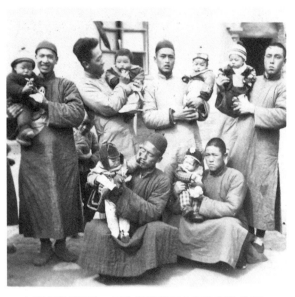

▲健康婴儿评比，图为获奖的婴儿和他们的父亲。

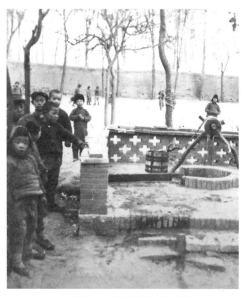

▲一口新的高质量的学校用井。

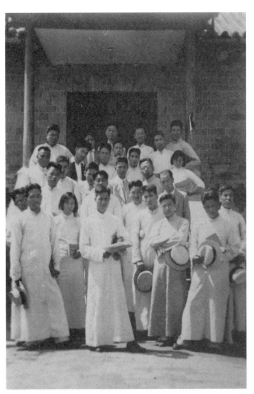

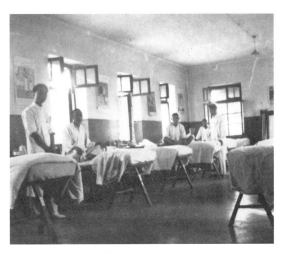

▲区医院的男性病房。

▲协和医学院学生在定县参加培训合影。

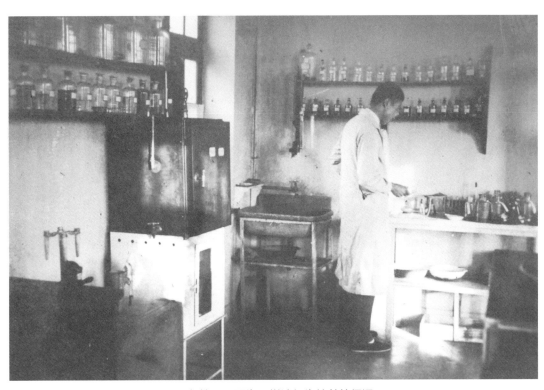

▲设备简陋，图为用煤油灯为培养箱保温。

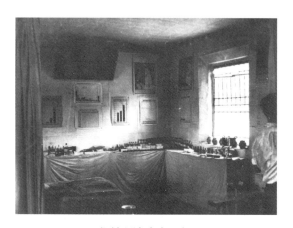

▲区保健所诊疗室一角。

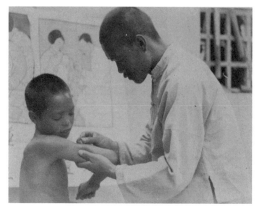

▲经过培训的乡村保健员在春秋季节给村民接种疫苗。

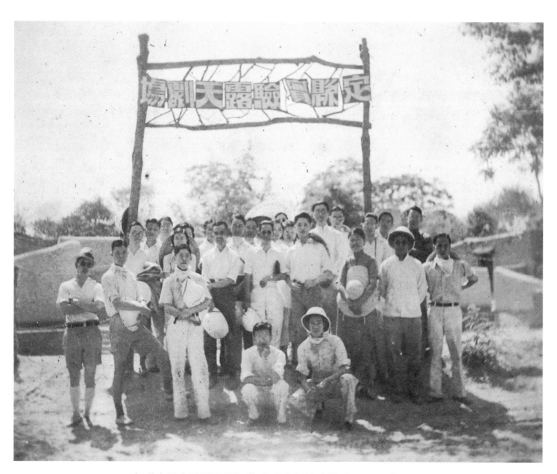

▲在"定县实验露天剧场"完成启智教育的演职人员合影。

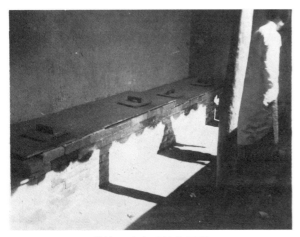

▲学校里改良后的女厕所。

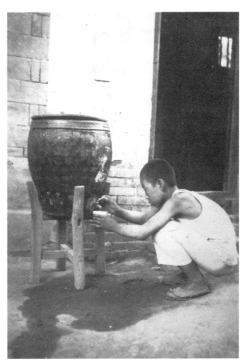

▲为学生提供消毒的清洁饮用水。

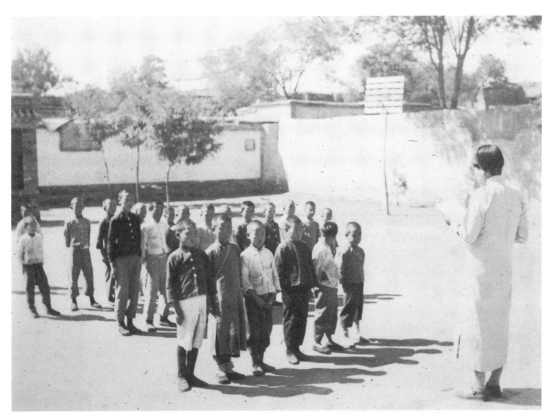

▲学生卫生护士进行健康教育。

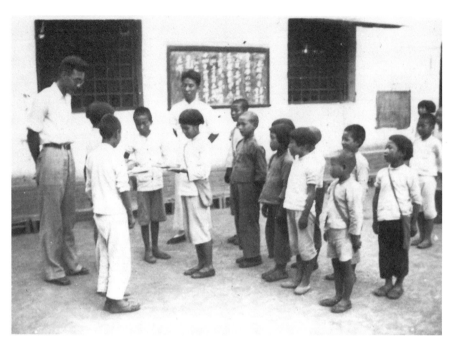

▲在学校开展学生健康晨检的工作——检查手卫生。

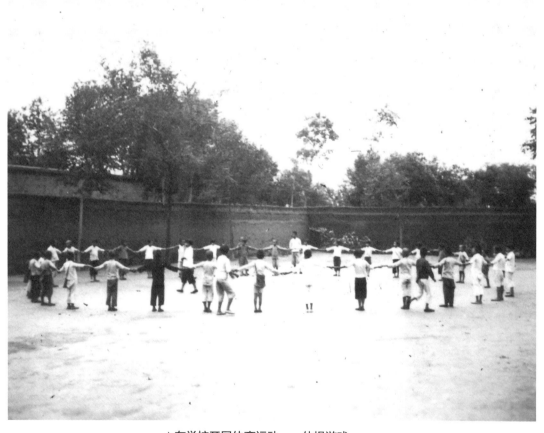

▲在学校开展体育运动——体操游戏。

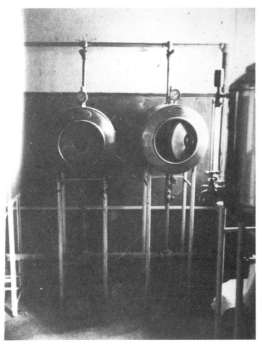

▲定县检验室的消毒锅。

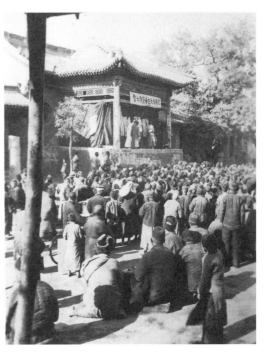

▲召开定县拒毒的群众大会。

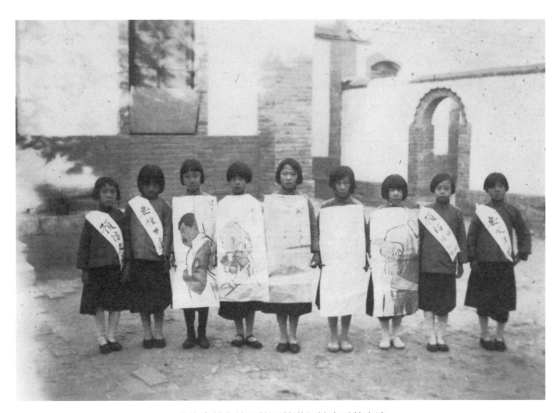

▲学生穿着有绘图的服装进行健康科普表演。

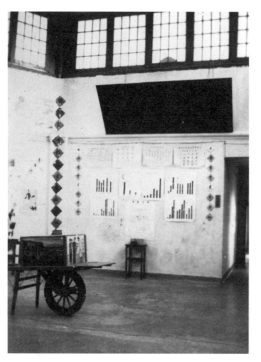

▲生命统计数据。

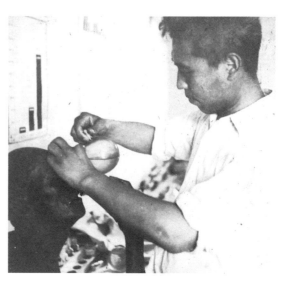

▲区保健所给村民治疗眼疾。

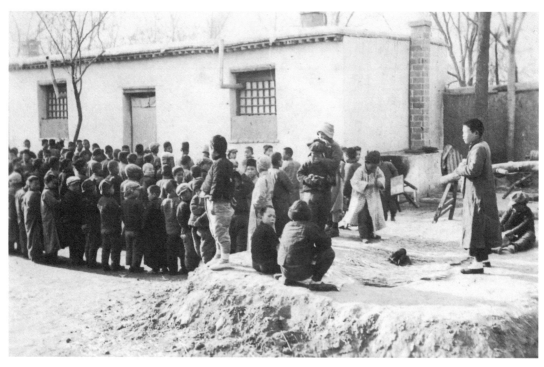

▲学生在学校浴室前集合，有序入室洗澡。

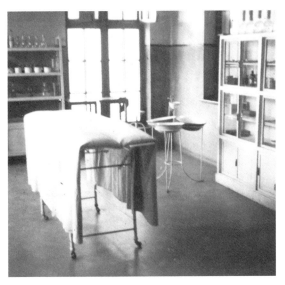

▲符合标准的手术室。

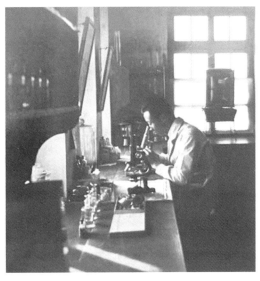

▲医院实验室。

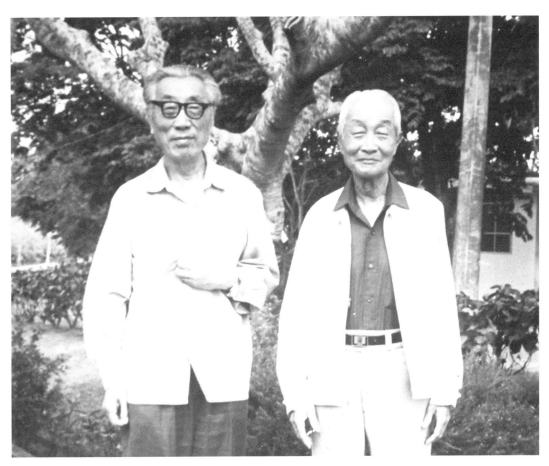

▲陈志潜博士与晏阳初博士的合影，摄于 1981 年菲律宾会面。

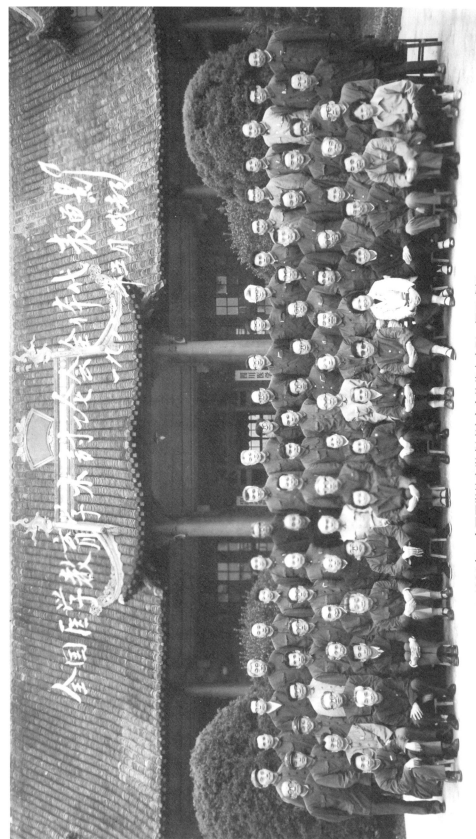

▲1981 年，全国医学教育学术讨论会全体代表合影，摄于成都。

翻译团队

主译：

王　辰　　中国医学科学院 北京协和医学院群医学及公共卫生学院
杨维中　　中国医学科学院 北京协和医学院群医学及公共卫生学院

主审：

张孔来　　中国医学科学院 北京协和医学院基础学院

副主审：

郭　岩　　北京大学公共卫生学院
张建新　　四川大学华西公共卫生学院 / 华西第四医院

译者（按姓氏拼音排序）：

丁旭虹　　中国疾病预防控制中心

冯录召　　中国医学科学院 北京协和医学院群医学及公共卫生学院

贾萌萌　　中国医学科学院 北京协和医学院群医学及公共卫生学院

冷志伟　　中国医学科学院北京协和医院

刘振谧　　四川大学华西公共卫生学院 / 华西第四医院

马礼兵　　桂林医学院附属医院

佟训靓　　北京医院

王　辰　　中国医学科学院 北京协和医学院群医学及公共卫生学院

王晓琪　　中国疾病预防控制中心

杨　阳　　四川省成都市双流区妇幼保健院

杨维中　　中国医学科学院 北京协和医学院群医学及公共卫生学院

张　婷　　中国医学科学院 北京协和医学院群医学及公共卫生学院

张建新　　四川大学华西公共卫生学院 / 华西第四医院

再译者的话

陈志潜先生是中国医生从事公共卫生的先驱与典范，是中国近现代农村公共卫生体系的创导者。

1929年陈志潜先生毕业于北京协和医学院。1932年陈志潜先生放弃做临床医生丰厚的收入和优越的北平城市生活，受学校的派遣，举家到河北定县创立了中国第一个农村卫生实验区。1984—1985年，陈志潜先生在华西医科大学公共卫生学院和美国加州大学伯克利公共卫生学院的支持下，用英文撰写了"*Medicine in Rural China-A Personal Account*"（本译本译作《中国农村之医学——我的记述》）一书，回顾了20世纪30年代他在河北定县创立农村卫生实验区的思想和工作，回顾了他后来在四川对农村医学的研究、实践和思考。在撰写过程中，陈志潜先生的助手Frederica M.Bunge女士在打字、录入、校正和编辑等方面给予了很多帮助，并为本书撰写了前言。1989年"*Medicine in Rural China-A Personal Account*"一书由美国加州大学伯克利和洛杉矶分校出版发行，在美国产生了极大的学术影响。1998年"*Medicine in Rural China-A Personal Account*"一书被国内学者翻译成《中国农村的医学——我的回忆》在四川人民出版社出版发行。

2020 年 7 月 16 日，北京协和医学院成立了群医学及公共卫生学院。学院成立伊始就把整理、挖掘协和医学院公共卫生历史，作为发扬协和优秀文化、教书育人和学科建设发展的重要工作。为了传承陈志潜先生致力于农村卫生发展的思想、理念和奉献精神，我们组织了协和医学院群医学及公共卫生学院和华西公共卫生学院的教师，对陈志潜先生的 *"Medicine in Rural China-A Personal Account"* 进行了再译。

该书是陈志潜先生在 37 年前用英文撰写的，回忆录中记载的陈志潜先生在协和医学院求学的事情，距今近百年。无论是陈志潜先生在协和学医、探索定县模式所处的时代，还是他撰写回忆录的时代，当时中国的政治、经济、文化都与当今社会已有很大的不同。对年轻的译者而言，要深入了解时间跨度大的两个时代的历史文化背景是十分困难的。然而，从历史文化的角度来看，在某些情况下译者离原作者时代越远，也许越能从历史的禁锢中跳出来，对当时的历史文化有新的认识和体会。年轻的译者们怀着对陈志潜先生景仰的心情，不仅认真研读回忆录原文，还通过其他渠道了解陈志潜先生当年在协和求学、赴美留学、在河北定县创立农村医学模式、被错划右派、在四川医学院执教、深入四川农村探索新中国的农村医学模式等情况，还努力寻求到陈志潜先生的女儿陈芙君女士、陈志潜先生的学生张孔来和张建新两位教授的悉心指导和大力帮助。

20 世纪 30 年代，中国的社会、经济十分落后，严重缺医少药，疟疾、霍乱、痢疾、伤寒、结核、寄生虫病等严重疾病肆虐，国民营养不良十分普遍。陈志潜先生根据当时的实际情况，创造性地探索出符合当时当地实际并且十分有效的农村卫生"定县模式"。今天，中国的经济社会和文化发生了巨大的变化，构建起了广覆盖的医疗卫生体系，疾病谱也发生了根本的变化，国人的平均寿命达到 78 岁。"定县模式"作为中国农村卫生史上的卓越范例很值得我们学习体会。今天，我们重新翻译陈志潜先生的回忆录，在于学习陈志潜先生"卓越为民"的思想、境界、胸怀和理念，学习他走出象牙塔投身社会，为人民、重实践、吐真言的优良品德，学习他在实践中注重思维的严谨性、方法的可操作性和结果的有效性。

陈志潜先生被誉为"农村卫生之父"，协和人和华西人都以陈志潜先生为傲。尽管我们努力想把这本书翻译得更好，但仍不免对陈先生的思想领悟不到位，甚至有翻译的错误。我们采用原文与译文对应排版的方式，以便于读者在以母语快速阅读的同时，可以对照原文更准确地领悟作者的本意，如此也更加促进译者们面对"有原文在旁可鉴"的情形，更加追求译文的"信达雅"。在此，我们特别感谢陈芙君女士和王丹红老师提供的宝贵意见。

王 辰 杨维中 张建新
2023 年 10 月

Contents

Chapter 3

Pioneering in Rural Health Development 130

Chapter 4

Medicine and Health Under Wartime Conditions 244

part 2

POSTLIBERATION CHINA

Chapter 5

The Health Experience From 1949 to 1976 270

Chapter 6

A New Era in Health Development 316

part 3

SHARING INSIGHTS

Chapter 7

Reflections on the Health Experience 394

Foreword

The sixty years spanned by these memoirs in community medicine have witnessed more progress in the health of people than the preceding 2,000 years. Worldwide infant mortality rates have been more than halved and life expectancy nearly doubled.

When Dr. C. C. Chen started his medical studies in the 1920s, few states saw the health of their citizens as a responsibility of government. By 1985, it was possible for the World Health Organization and the United Nations Children's Fund to talk seriously of universal immunization for children by 1990, of the potential for a virtual child survival revolution in many developing countries before the close of the 1990s, and of the possibility of achieving health for all by the year 2000 through primary health care.

When we explore how this transformation was possible, we see that the reasons are complex; we also see a handful of intellectual giants to whom the world community owes a deep debt of gratitude for their articulation and demonstration of the basic concepts now known as primary health care.

C. C. Chen is one of these.

His memoirs are unique, not only in the length of time they span but also in the breadth of firsthand experience with primary health care that they encompass.

社区医学回忆录所跨越的 60 年见证了人类健康方面的进步，而这 60 年取得的进步比过去 2000 年的还要多。全世界的婴儿死亡率已降低一半，人类预期寿命几乎翻了一番。

当陈志潜博士在 20 世纪 20 年代开始医学研究之时，很少有国家将公民的健康视作政府的责任。到 1985 年，世界卫生组织和联合国儿童基金会才开始认真讨论以下问题的可能性：到 1990 年普及儿童免疫；多数发展中国家在 20 世纪 90 年代末实现儿童生存革命；通过初级卫生保健，在 2000 年实现人人享有保健照护。

当我们探讨如何实现这种转变的时候，我们发现原因错综复杂；同时我们也看到少数智慧型巨人，国际社会应深深地感谢他们阐明和展示了现在被称为初级卫生保健的基本概念。

陈志潜博士就是其中之一。

他的回忆录是独一无二的，这不仅体现在回忆录的时间跨度，也体现在其所包含的初级卫生保健第一手经验的广度上。

C. C. Chen was one of the pioneers in systematically addressing the immediate social problem of overtaking the lag between modern medical knowledge and its use in a low-income community. It was in the county of Dingxian, with a largely rural population of more than 100,000, that C. C. Chen introduced the use of the scientific method to bear on addressing this lag in a low-income rural setting. In a period of a few years, he and his colleagues, working closely with Dr. James Yen and the Mass Education Movement that had come earlier to Dingxian, demonstrated dramatically successful techniques, including methods for involving villagers in improving their own health condition. The major principles they established then, described in these memoirs, have proved to be remarkably durable over the past half century and a remarkable testament to Dr. Chen and his colleagues.

One can only wish that the world community had been quicker to accept these scientific principles of sound organization so convincingly demonstrated then, including the facts that:

- The use of medical knowledge and the efficiency of health protection depend chiefly upon sound organization.
- A vertical medical system cannot stand by itself unless it is integrated with other social activities in a joint horizontal attack on the problems of social reconstruction.
- Demonstration units must take into consideration the economic practicability of extending them to the nation as a whole. This implies that the principle of self-help, or participation by the consumer, be adopted, as no low-income country can afford to make full use of available medical knowledge through tax funds alone.

As becomes apparent soon to a reader of these memoirs, C. C. Chen was first a student and later a colleague of the late Dr. John B. Grant, my father, then Professor of Public Health at the Rockefeller- endowed Peking Union Medical College. It was my privilege to accompany my

陈志潜博士是系统解决当前社会问题的先驱之一，即克服现代医学知识与其在低收入社区中使用之间的滞后。正是在定县这个拥有 10 多万农村人口的地方，陈志潜博士引入了科学方法来解决低收入农村环境中的这种滞后问题。在几年的时间里，他和他那些更早来到定县的同事一起，与晏阳初博士倡导的平民教育运动紧密合作，运用了多种切实有效的成功技术和多种方法，让村民参与到改善自身健康状况的运动中来。他们在这些回忆录中描述了当时确立的主要原则，在过去的半个世纪里被证明是长期有效的，这也彰显了陈博士和他的同事们的非凡成就。

这些规范的科学原则取得了令人信服的成果。我们希望国际社会能更快地接受它们。其基本原则如下：

- 医学知识的运用和健康保护的效率主要取决于健全的组织。
- 除非与其他社会活动相结合，对社会重建的问题进行横向联合攻克，否则垂直的医疗体系是不能独立存在的。
- 示范单位必须考虑到将其推广到全国的经济可行性。这意味着要采取自助或消费者参与的原则，因为没有一个低收入国家能够仅通过税收就充分运用现有的医学知识。

本书的读者们很快就会发现，陈志潜博士最初是我父亲兰安生博士的学生，后来成为他的同事，随后又成为洛克菲勒捐建的北京协和医学院的公共卫生学教授。1934 年我有幸陪父亲一同参观定县。我父亲是国际卫生领域以及将医学知识用于造福全民的早期先驱之一。在我父亲的指导下，陈志潜博士在定县开展了他

father on a visit to Dingxian in 1934. John Grant was one of the early pioneers in international health and in bringing medical knowledge to the benefit of populations as a whole. C. C. Chen undertook his initial work in public health at Dingxian at the urging of Dr. Grant, and Dingxian was used as an influential training ground for many of the medical students at this preeminent medical institution of the 1930s. Their visitors included men who were to leave their mark on world health in other ways. These in eluded Dr. Andrija Stampar, the Yugoslav pioneer in rural health who later was to become the first chairman of the World Health Organization (WHO), and Dr. Ludwig Rajchman, the Pole who was then Director of the Health Bureau of the League of Nations, the predecessor to WHO, and who was, after World War II, to become the founder and chairman for the first five years of the organization 1 now serve as Executive Director, the United Nations Children's Fund (UNICEF). These men all belonged to a generation who believed, to paraphrase Professor Toynbee, that theirs was the first generation for which it was possible to conceive of bringing the benefits of civilization to all humankind.

The 1937 Japanese invasion of China brought the Dingxian experiment to an untimely end. Fortunately, knowledge of this experiment was already beginning to be applied in many parts of China and was later to contribute to the extraordinary progress China has made since 1950 in improving the health of its people.

With a per capita income of probably still less than that of the United States two centuries ago, China by the 1980s has achieved a level of health in its population, when measured in terms of infant mortality rate and life expectancy, which approximates that of the United States at mid-twentieth century. If all developing countries had achieved the health conditions that China has achieved, some 8 million fewer children under the age of five years would have died (and there would have been 40 million fewer births) each year in the late 1980s. In achieving this, China has demonstrated the validity of principles first scientifically tested at Dingxian: that primary

最初的公共卫生工作。在 20 世纪 30 年代，对于北京协和医学院这所著名医学学府的医学生来说，定县是很有影响力的培训基地。在世界卫生领域留下印记的多位伟人曾拜访过那里。其中包括世界卫生组织第一任主席、南斯拉夫农村卫生工作先驱安准加·斯坦帕尔博士，以及时任国际联盟卫生局（世界卫生组织的前身）局长、波兰人路得维格·雷吉曼博士。第二次世界大战后路得维格·雷吉曼博士成为联合国儿童基金会创始人和第一任主席，我现在也供职于联合国儿童基金会。托因比教授曾说，他们都属于这样的一代人，他们相信自己是第一代能够把文明的好处带给全人类的人。

1937 年日本入侵中国，定县实验被迫终止。幸运的是，这一实验取得的成果已经开始应用于中国的许多地方，并在自 1950 年以来中国政府改善人民健康方面取得的非凡成就中做出贡献。

当时，中国的人均收入可能仍低于两个世纪前的美国，但到 20 世纪 80 年代，如果以婴儿死亡率和预期寿命来衡量，中国人口的健康水平已接近美国 20 世纪中叶的水平。如果所有发展中国家都达到 20 世纪 80 年代中国所达到的健康状况，那么在 20 世纪 80 年代末，每年五岁以下儿童死亡人数可减少 800 万（出生人数可减少 4000 万）。在实现这一目标的过程中，中国证明了这个在定县被首次科学验证的原则的有效性：初级卫生保健必须有民众的参与才能成功，否则垂直医疗体系不可能真正有效，甚至不能独立存在，除非它与其他活动相结合，共同解决发展和

health care must involve popular participation to be successful, and a vertical medical svstem cannot be truly effective, or even stand by itself, unless it is integrated with other activities in a joint attack on the problems of development and social reconstruction. Primary health care must encompass education for health, adequate food and nutrition, clean water, and shelter and clothing for protection from the environment. We have seen in China that health is not simply a "sector" but also an explicit goal to be achieved through all sectors with mass participation.

It is also notable that what John Grant and C. C. Chen learned together in China had a major impact in Europe. When John Grant went to Europe as international health advisor for the Rockefeller Foundation in the immediate postwar years, the basic principles that were hammered out in China through use of scientific methods proved to be applicable also to the more developed countries of Europe.

Many of the European countries were then in the process of revising their health systems so that the first mass applications of these principles were effective in Europe rather than China. When my father left Europe after several years, government after government honored him with decorations—from Finland in the north to France in the south—for his advice drawn from his experience with his colleagues in China and India.

Dr. C. C. Chen offers one more invaluable service to the world by sharing with us these memoirs of a lifetime dedicated to promoting the health of peoples. In reading them, one is conscious of the fact that full application of the principles developed fifty years ago at Dingxian could still bring substantial improvements in health and well-being in China as well as much larger improvements in most other developing countries. There is much to be gained even today from application of the lessons of his experience in seeking to overtake the far-too-long lag between the development of modern knowledge and its use in the setting of a low-income community.

James P. Grant

社会重建问题。初级卫生保健必须包括健康教育、充足的食物和营养、洁净的水以及免受环境影响的住所和衣物。在中国，我们看到卫生不仅仅是一个"行业"，而是一个需要通过所有行业广泛参与来实现的明确目标。

同样值得注意的是，兰安生博士和陈志潜博士在中国共同学习到的东西对欧洲产生了重大影响。在第二次世界大战后不久，当兰安生作为洛克菲勒基金会的国际健康顾问前往欧洲时，中国用科学方法制定出来的基本原则，对欧洲比较发达的国家也同样适用。

当时许多欧洲国家正在修订其卫生体系，因此这些原则的首次大规模应用在欧洲发挥了重要作用，而非在中国。当我父亲几年后离开欧洲时，从北方的芬兰到南方的法国，一个又一个政府为他颁发了勋章，以表彰他从中国和印度同事的经验中得出的建议。

陈志潜博士通过与我们分享他毕生致力于促进人民健康的回忆录，为世界提供了一项更宝贵的资源。在阅读这些内容时，读者会意识到这样一个事实：充分应用50年前在定县制定的原则，仍然可以为中国的健康和福祉带来实质性的改善，也可以为其他大多数发展中国家带来更大的改善。即使在今天，吸取他在弥补现代知识发展与其在低收入环境中应用之间过长的滞后性这一方面的经验教训，也能大有收获。

詹姆斯·P. 格兰特

译者：杨维中，贾萌萌

Preface

This book, perhaps more than most, requires a preface in order to avoid any serious misconceptions on the part of the reader. Although the book is being published by a university press, it is not a major work of research in the usual sense. It is told in the first person but is actually the product of collaboration between two individuals working at a distance from each other. Because of the specific nature of the collaboration, the reader should be warned against assuming that the attitudes and perspectives or views and interpretations expressed or implied throughout the book are unvaryingly those of its author, C. C. Chen, M.D. Emphatically, this is not the case. Material from Western sources, with its own theoretical and ideological perspectives, has been added to the draft. It is thus useful, probably even essential, for the reader to begin exploration of this volume with a clear knowledge of how the manuscript evolved and the ground it is intended to cover.

The author, a scientifically trained physician, was born in China in 1903 and lives there today with most of his family. As teacher, scholar, and administrator, he has moved repeatedly in and out of academic settings during his long career and presently holds the ranks of professor of community medicine at a key medical college.

前言

　　这本书也许比大多数书都需要一个前言，以便避免读者产生任何严重的误解。虽然这本书是由大学出版社出版的，但它并不是通常意义上的重要研究工作。本书以第一人称讲述，但实际上是年代、经历、背景等相距甚远的两个人合作的产物。由于合作的特殊性质，应提醒读者不要假定本书中所表达或暗示的所有态度、观点或看法和解释都是作者陈志潜博士的观点。显然，事实并非如此。文稿中增加了来自西方的素材，有其自身的理论和意识形态观点。因此，对于想要开始阅读此书的读者来说，清楚了解文稿的演变过程和它所想要涵盖的领域是非常有用的，甚至可能是必不可少的。

　　作者是一位受过科学训练的医生，1903 年出生于中国，目前与他的大部分家人都生活在那里。作为教师、学者和管理者，他在漫长的职业生涯中反复进出学术界，目前在一所重点医学院担任社区医学教授的职务。

During his long career, spanning some sixty years, Dr. Chen has enjoyed a number of opportunities to study and travel outside his own country. For example, he earned the degree of Master of Public Health at Harvard University in the academic year 1930/31 and has returned to the United States several times since. In 1985, after obtaining permission from Chinese authorities to come to the United States to write his memoirs, he spent several months on the campus of the University of California, Berkeley, where he devoted himself to that task. He wrote in English, a language he speaks fluently.

Dr. Chen had already completed the original draft of his text when Joyce C. Lashof, M.D., Dean of the School of Public Health, brought us together. I had just completed a master's program at the school and, before coming to Berkeley, had been chairperson of the Asia Research Team at the American University in Washington, D.C. for eight years. In that capacity I had coauthored more than a dozen multidisciplinary studies on Asian countries, including a 600-page 1980 China study. Dr. Lashof believed, therefore, that I was particularly qualified to lend editorial support to Dr. Chen's projected work.

In writing the original draft, Dr. Chen, who is first and foremost a medical scientist, had omitted almost all reference to the major historic events that provided the backdrop to the events in his life. Those who read that first version appreciated his devotion to his central topic. At the same time, they agreed that a certain amount of contextual material was necessary as the author wished to be heard internationally as well as at home. It could not be assumed that in a worldwide audience of health workers, all readers would necessarily be knowledgeable about events and conditions in China before and after liberation in 1949. So the matter was discussed with Dr. Chen, and it was agreed that some broadly descriptive material on economic and political conditions, institutions, and patterns of behavior would be included in order to provide the needed historical perspective.

在他长达 60 多年的职业生涯中，陈博士有许多出国学习和旅行的机会。例如，他于 1930—1931 学年在哈佛大学获得了公共卫生硕士的学位，此后多次前往美国。1985 年，在获得中国政府允许来美国写回忆录后，他在加州大学伯克利分校的校园里呆了几个月，全身心投入到这项工作中。他用英语写作，这是一种他能说得很流利的语言。

当公共卫生学院院长乔伊斯·拉肖夫博士邀约我们见面时，陈博士已经完成了他的初稿。当时我刚刚完成该校的硕士课程，在来伯克利之前，我曾在华盛顿特区的美国大学担任过八年的亚洲研究小组主席。在此期间，我与其他人合著了十几份关于亚洲国家的多学科研究报告，包括 1980 年一份 600 页的中国研究报告。因此，拉肖夫博士认为，我有足够的资格为陈博士的项目工作提供编辑方面的支持。

陈博士首先是一位医学家，在撰写初稿时，他几乎省略了所有的他一生经历的重大历史事件。阅读过初版的人都很欣赏他对中心话题的专注。与此同时，他们一致认为有必要增添一些历史背景，因为作者希望国内和国际上都能听到他的声音。不能假设全球的卫生工作者，所有的读者都对中国 1949 年解放前和解放后的事件及状况有所了解。因此，与陈博士讨论了这个问题后，他同意将一些关于经济和政治条件、制度和行为模式的广泛描述性材料纳入其中，以提供所需的历史视角。

Our collaboration began in December 1985 and continued over the succeeding two years. Having read the original manuscript with great care, I met with Dr. Chen in his campus office over a period of several weeks, as we discussed his personal philosophy and his goals and objectives in writing the book. The next month Dr. Chen returned to China, following lens-implant surgery. After reading the draft once again and reflecting on our taped conversations, I submitted a lengthy tentative outline for a new draft, and after he had approved that draft with some minor changes, revised and recast the existing text in accordance with it and added other major segments.

In August 1986 Dr. Chen arranged for me to spend two weeks with him at West China Union University of Medical Sciences in Chengdu, where we engaged in a fruitful exchange, going over the second draft line by line, agreeing on certain further changes as well as the addition of new material regarding important developments that had taken place in public health in early- to mid-1986. After returning to the United States, I revised the introduction and the chapters to varying degrees once again and prepared the seventh and final analytical chapter of the memoirs. By further correspondence, we worked out the details of this third and final draft, which was finalized and submitted to the publisher in January 1987. To make the work as timely as possible, we updated some points even after the book was accepted for publication late in 1987.

As to the material added to the text in the course of our collaboration, most of it is found in the historical setting components of each of the chronological chapters and in the Postliberation portion of the book as a whole. As I am not a specialist on East Asia or China, I collected the material largely from readily available English- language sources in Western libraries, particularly that of the graduate library at the University of California, Berkeley.

我们的合作始于 1985 年 12 月，并持续了两年。在仔细阅读了原稿后，我与陈博士在他校园的办公室进行了几周的会面，我们讨论了他的个人哲学观以及他写这本书的目标和目的。之后的一个月，在完成晶状体植入手术后陈博士返回了中国。在再次阅读了文稿并回顾了我们的谈话录音后，我提交了一份关于新文稿的冗长的初步大纲，在他同意了该草稿并进行了一些微小的修改之后，根据该草稿，我对现有文稿进行了修订和重新编写，并增加了其他主要部分。

1986 年 8 月，陈博士安排我在成都的华西协合医科大学与他共处两周，在那里我们进行了富有成效的交流，逐行讨论了第二稿，就某些进一步的修改以及增加一些 1986 年年初至年中在公共卫生领域重要发展的新素材达成了一致意见。回到美国后，我又对序言和各章进行了不同程度的修改，并准备了回忆录的第七章和最后的分析章。通过进一步的通信，我们制定了第三稿也是最终稿的细节，最后于 1987 年 1 月定稿后提交给出版商。为了使这本回忆录尽可能包括最新内容，我们甚至在该书于 1987 年年底即将出版时还更新了一些要点。

至于我们在合作过程中添加到书稿中的素材，大部分是每一个编年体章节的历史背景部分和解放后的部分。由于我不是研究东亚或中国的专家，我主要从西方图书馆，特别是加州大学伯克利分校的研究生图书馆，收集现成的英文资料。

The implications of that latter fact are critical to the readers' understanding and assessment of these memoirs. Western and Chinese scholars will often have widely differing interpretations of the same data, the same circumstances, and the same events; as Dr. Chen is Chinese, he presumably shares the Chinese perspective. At certain points in the text, therefore, a careful reader might want to distinguish between assertions made by the author himself and those interposed by someone else. This should not necessarily be very difficult; the assertions of the author are those of a medically informed person.

Every effort has been made to bring to Dr. Chen's attention certain passages for which he was not directly responsible; however, it cannot be said with absolute certainty that this was always the case. We had to interact through correspondence, and a process of continuing revision was being carried out. Moreover, as time passed, Dr. Chen experienced increasing visual impairment, putting him at a severe disadvantage as he was unable to read for extended periods without experiencing severe eyestrain.

Dr. Chen might have chosen to produce either a work of original research or an academic treatise on which he could engage in critical debate with other scholars in the field. Such an approach would, however, have been entirely inconsistent with the beliefs and principles to which he has adhered so strongly all his life. In fact, Dr. Chen's international renown as a physician and a pioneer in the Chinese health experience is attributable to his lifelong commitment to action and intervention, manifest especially in his experimentation with the development of a rural health system at Dingxian in North China during the 1930s.

North China constituted the northern part of so-called China proper—eighteen historic provinces within the Great Wall. Given this commitment, along with his emphasis on educational experience "in the field," it is in no way surprising that he has written a very different kind of book. Instead of speaking to an academic audience, he is addressing health activists, educators, trainers, and primary health care workers,

上述事实对读者理解和评估这些回忆录至关重要。西方学者和中国学者对相同的数据、相同的环境和相同的事件往往会有截然不同的解释；由于陈博士是中国人，他大概也有中国人的观点。因此，细心的读者可能想要区分某些内容是作者本人的主张还是其他人的想法。这或许并不困难；作者的主张是有医学背景的人才能提出来的主张。

已经尽一切努力提请陈博士关注某些他不直接负责的段落；然而我们不敢保证他对所有的内容都确实关注到了。我们不得不通信进行沟通，并进行持续的修订。此外，随着时间的推移，陈博士的视力越来越差，长时间的阅读会导致他出现严重的视疲劳，这对他非常不利。

陈博士可能会选择创作一篇原创研究著作或一篇学术论文，与该领域的其他学者进行批判性的辩论。然而，这种做法完全不符合他毕生强烈坚持的信仰和原则。事实上，陈医生作为一名医生和拥有丰富中国医疗经验的先驱而享有国际声誉，这归功于他毕生致力于医疗卫生行动和干预，尤其体现在 20 世纪 30 年代他在华北定县开展的农村卫生系统发展的实验中。

华北位于中国北方地区，包括长城以里的 18 个省份。鉴于他的奉献，以及他对"现场"教育经验的强调，他编写了一本与众不同的书也就不足为奇了。他不是在对着学术听众分享经验和观点，而是面向健康活动家、教育工作者、培训人员和初级卫生保健工作者，特别是第三世界的那些人，与他们分享一个人道主

especially those in the Third World, sharing with them the story of a humanistic attempt to find practical ways of introducing scientific medicine for people living under difficult conditions.

Sensitively aware of the limitations of his own knowledge and of the diversity of his country and its propensity for rapid change, the author has tried to confine this study to issues and problems with which he has had firsthand experience, eschewing any suggesting that what he describes in his own province or county necessarily pertains to China as a whole. As a result, we are treated to a strictly personal account of rural health development, focusing on districts and counties where Dr. Chen has lived or to which he has traveled as a public health physician. Emphasis is given to the organization, at Dingxian, of the first systematic rural health system in the nation and to the lessons drawn from that experience that may apply to the needs of village populations throughout the world today, including those of China. Dr. Chen also examines other topics on the basis of his own firsthand observation: relations between traditional and modern medicine, the quality of rural health manpower, and trends in medical and public health education.

By the same token, readers interested in subjects that are outside Dr. Chen's direct sphere of interest and activity may find their expectations unfulfilled. For examples, some readers may be disappointed that the account gives relatively little attention to family planning in China, a subject that arouses considerable interest in foreign observers. Family planning, however, is not one of the author's own areas of interest or specialization. Moreover, its policy and planning aspects are the responsibility of an agency other than the Ministry of Health, of whose activities Dr. Chen has no direct knowledge.

Denise D. Grant, also of Washington D.C., whom I came to know through the course of this study, very kindly lent selected private papers of John B. Grant used in the preparation of chapters 2 and 3.

义的故事，试图为生活在困难条件下的人们找到引入科学医学的实用方法。

作者敏锐地意识到他自己知识的局限性，以及他的国家的多样性和快速变化的倾向，试图将这项工作限定于他亲身经历过的问题，避免暗示他所描述的自己所在省份或县的情况一定能适用于整个中国。因此，从严格意义上讲，我们得到的是一份关于农村卫生发展的个人描述，聚焦在陈博士曾经居住或作为公共卫生医生去过的地区和县。重点是在定县建立的全国第一个系统的农村卫生系统，以及从这一实验中吸取的经验教训，这些经验教训可能适用于今天包括中国在内的世界各地的农村人口的需要。陈博士在其拥有第一手观察资料的基础上考察了其他问题：传统医学和现代医学的关系、农村卫生人力的素质，以及医学和公共卫生教育的发展趋势。

同样，对陈博士直接感兴趣和活动范围之外的主题感兴趣的那些读者们可能会发现本书并没有满足他们的期望。例如，因为该书对中国的计划生育给予的关注相对较少，但这一主题引起了外国观察家的极大兴趣，因此一些读者可能会感到失望。然而，计划生育并非作者本人感兴趣或擅长的领域。此外，其政策和规划方面由卫生部以外的机构负责，陈博士对其活动没有直接了解。

我通过这项工作认识的丹尼斯·D.格兰特也在华盛顿特区，她非常友好地借出了兰安生的私人论文选集，用于编写第二章和第三章。

It has been an honor to work with Dr. Chen, whom I, like countless others, hold in the highest respect. His work, I believe, is one of great importance and should contribute in an absolutely critical way to the furtherance of community medicine among rural populations throughout the world.

Berkeley, California
Frederica M. Bunge
December 1987

与陈博士合作是我的荣幸,我和其他无数人一样,对他充满了敬意。我认为他的工作非常重要,能够以绝对关键的方式为促进全世界农村人口的社区医疗做出贡献。

加利福尼亚州伯克利

弗雷德丽卡·M. 邦奇

1987 年 12 月

译者:杨维中,贾萌萌

Acknowledgments

I am indebted to the Health Science Division of the Rockefeller Foundation for a generous grant, which made it possible for me to escape from routine duties in China and to sit down quietly on the beautiful Berkeley campus of the University of California to think and write.

So many friends have extended assistance and suggestions during the course of this work that I can thank them all only by a general reference. I am especially grateful to Professor Peter Kong- Min New and to my brother, Professor Jerome Chen, who read and revised my original draft with respect to both content and language, and to Henrik L. Blum, M.D. of the School of Public Health at the University of California, Berkeley.

I wanted particularly, however, to thank Joyce C. Lashof, M.D., Dean and Professor of Public Health at the School of Public Health in Berkeley, and Kerr L. White, M.D. of the Rockefeller Foundation for their efforts to facilitate my visit to the United States and to provide support and assistance for the work. I am especially grateful for their persistence in securing the necessary provisions for the realization of a personal desire and responsibility to all those who have educated and helped me in over a half a century of my career.

致谢

　　我感谢洛克菲勒基金会健康科学处的慷慨资助，使我能够脱离中国的日常工作，安静地坐在美丽的加州大学伯克利分校校区进行思考和写作。写此书的目的之一是表达对我的恩师兰安生博士的敬意。

　　非常多的朋友在这项工作的过程中提供了帮助和建议，我谨在此统一表示感谢。特别感谢医学社会学家彼得·牛康明教授和我的弟弟、历史学家陈志让教授，他们阅读了我的原稿并针对内容和语言进行了修改。我还要感谢加州大学伯克利分校公共卫生学院的亨瑞克·布鲁姆博士。

　　然而，我想特别感谢伯克利公共卫生学院院长乔伊斯·拉肖夫教授和洛克菲勒基金会的克尔·怀特博士，感谢他们努力为我访问美国提供便利并为这项工作提供支持和帮助。我特别感谢他们持续为我提供必要条件和物质保障，以实现我的个人愿望，并使我能对在半个多世纪的事业中给予我教育和帮助的所有人尽绵薄之力。

译者：杨维中，贾萌萌

Introduction

As a scientifically trained physician, I have devoted more than five decades to the work of diffusing modern medicine in rural China, where over 80 percent of our population is to be found. The search for the best means of doing so has been the central concern of my life and provides the central thesis of these memoirs.

My interest in extending the benefits of modern health care to China's hundreds of millions of villagers stems from several strongly held beliefs, namely, that the strength of any nation lies in its common people; that the benefits offered by scientific medicine, introduced from the West, surpass those of our own traditional medicine in most respects; and that a significant impact on the national health system is produced only when the benefits of modern medicine are made available to the general population, rather than limited to a privileged few.

As a consequence of these beliefs, I have devoted my life to the development of community medicine in China. Community medicine, as I perceive it, is a scientific approach to health care based on the needs and conditions of entire populations, rather than on those of individuals alone, and on combining curative and preventive approaches, rather than relying on curative techniques alone. As I define it, it includes epidemiology,

引　言

作为一名受过科学训练的医生，我已经在中国农村推广现代医学的工作中奉献了五十多年，农村有我国 80% 以上的人口。寻找这样做的最佳方法一直是我生活中最关心的问题，也是本回忆录的中心论点。

我对让中国亿万村民享受到现代医疗保健的兴趣源于几个坚定的信念，即任何民族的力量都在于它的老百姓；从西方引进的科学医学所提供的好处，在大多数方面超过了我们自己的传统医学；只有当现代医学的好处惠及普通大众，而不是局限于少数享有特权的人，才会对国家卫生系统产生重大影响。

正是由于这些信念，我毕生致力于中国社区医学的发展。在我看来，社区医学是一种科学的保健方法，它基于整个人群而非个人的需求和条件，并结合治疗和预防方法而非仅仅依靠治疗技术。按照我的定义，它包括流行病学、生命统计和卫生管理。它

vital statistics, and health administration. It represents a more advanced approach to health care than does individualized medicine, a simple relationship between physician and patient.

The basic premises of my medical philosophy, which were established many years ago—deriving from my personal experiences as a child and as a young medical student—have provided a steadying influence, giving purpose and direction through the twists and turns of a life that has followed a rather tortuous course.

My life began, at the turn of the century, as that of an underprivileged child, in an old-style scholar's family in a remote region of China. Because of the insular environment and the unavailability of formal schooling until I reached the age of ten, my early awareness of the outside world was very slight. Offsetting this lack of sophistication, however, was the exposure, given me by my grandfather, to the rich legacy of thought underlying China's age-old civilization.

The inspiration for a life centered on improving the general welfare derived from that formative exposure to our history and culture. Confucian tradition taught that scholars are a special class, but that, with this respected status, went the responsibility, as educated men, of working for the good of the common people. An ancient Chinese teaching, roughly translated, asserts: "People are the foundation of a nation. When the foundation becomes firm, the nation becomes stabilized."

This concept, I believe, captures a principle of long standing in Chinese social philosophy, one that has influenced not only myself but countless generations of Chinese youth educated in our age- old intellectual traditions. It was, I suspect, the wellspring for the intense patriotism and political protest that surfaced in the nineteenth century, when China suffered a painful sequence of foreign invasions and military defeats. More recently, in modern times, concern for the nation and the well-being of the common people has imparted urgency to efforts for

代表了一种比医生和患者之间简单关系的个体化医疗更加先进的医疗保健方法。

我的医学哲学的基本前提是多年前建立起来的——源于我儿时和年轻医学生的个人经历——它对我产生了稳定的影响，在我经历的人生曲折中赋予了我目标和方向。

世纪之交，我出生于中国偏远地区的一个老式学者家庭中，童年时期非常贫困。由于闭塞的环境以及我 10 岁之前没有接受过正规的学校教育，我早期对外界的认识非常有限。然而，我的祖父让我接触到了中国古老文明背后的丰富思想遗产，这弥补了我修养的不足。

以改善大众福利为中心的生活灵感来自我们对历史和文化的塑造。儒家传统教导说，学者是一个特殊的阶层，但是，在这种受人尊敬的地位下，作为受过教育的人，有责任为老百姓的利益而工作。中国有句老话"民惟邦本，本固邦宁"，大致可翻译为：百姓是国家的根本，根本稳固了，国家就安宁了。

我相信，这个概念反映了中国社会哲学中一个长期存在的原则，它不仅影响了我自己，也影响了无数代在我们古老知识传统中接受教育的中国青年。我猜想，这是 19 世纪中国遭受一系列外国入侵和军事失败时，出现的强烈爱国主义和政治抗议的源泉。近代以来，对国家和百姓福祉的关注使社会改革和现代化建设迫在眉睫。我认为，缺乏这一传统的发展中国家必须特别努力培养

social reform and modernization. Developing countries that lack this tradition, I expect, must strive especially hard to develop leaders willing to sacrifice their personal ambitions for the sake of the general welfare.

To return to formative experiences in my life, probably the most consequential were the eight years spent as a young medical student at the Rockefeller Foundation-sponsored Peking Union Medical College (PUMC) in Beijing during the 1920s. There, in that center of academic excellence, I received an education in science and scientific medicine that was of lasting importance to me. It left no question in my mind of the superiority of modern medicine to our own traditional system, nor any doubt of its potential value for improving our national health, provided the people understood its principles correctly.

At the PUMCI met John B. Grant, M.D., whose influence, first as a teacher, and later as a counselor and a friend, was enduring. Grant introduced me to the concept of community medicine and led me to recognize the hazards involved in adopting foreign models in toto, rather than adapting medical practice to local needs and conditions. Equally important, he guided me toward a public health career, arguing that in so doing I could make a far more significant contribution to China than by specializing in dermatology.

As is well known, our country has undergone sweeping social and political change during the past century and a half. The millennia-old Chinese empire disintegrated in 1911, and for several decades thereafter, China suffered fragmentation and internal strife as rival groups struggled for power. Liberation in 1949, however, brought unity and stability once again under the undisputed leadership of the Chinese Communist party (CCP) and paved the way for fundamentally new forms of political, economic, and social institutions and behavior. In furthering the revolution on the scientific and technical fronts, the CCP leadership has sometimes sought, and sometimes avoided, exchange with the outside world.

愿意为了大众福祉而牺牲个人抱负的领导人。

说到我生命中的成长经历，最重要的可能是 20 世纪 20 年代在洛克菲勒基金会赞助的北京协和医学院度过的八年年轻医学生时光。在这个卓越的学术中心，我接受了科学和科学医学方面的教育，这对我的一生都有着的巨大的影响。只要人们正确理解它的原则，我毫不怀疑现代医学优于我们自己的传统体系，也不怀疑它对改善我国国民健康的潜在价值。

在北京协和医学院我遇到了兰安生博士，他先是作为我的老师，后来又作为我的顾问和朋友，对我有持久的影响。兰安生向我介绍了社区医学的概念，使我认识到全部采用外国模式而不是根据当地的需要和条件调整医疗实践的危害。同样重要的是，他引导我从事公共卫生事业，他说这样可以对中国做出比专攻皮肤病更重要的贡献。

众所周知，在过去一个半世纪里我国经历了翻天覆地的社会和政治变革。有着千年历史的中华王朝在 1911 年覆灭，此后数十年间，由于敌对集团争夺权力，中国经历了分裂和内乱。然而，1949 年在中国共产党无可争议的领导下的解放，再次给中国带来了团结和稳定，并为政治、经济和社会机构及行为的全新形式铺平了道路。在推进科技革命的过程中，中国共产党领导层在与外界交流上做到了有的放矢。

The Chinese experience in rural health development was considerably affected, both beneficially and adversely by events that unfolded against this backdrop of history. More than a century ago, Western missionaries introduced scientific medicine into our country, with all its potential for improving public health, and over the next century they established scores upon scores of modern hospitals and clinics in Chinese cities. Their efforts benefited a small segment of the population but established a pattern of individualized medicine that focused on curative treatment. This pattern was difficult to eradicate.

Meanwhile, in the 1920s, modern physicians, including Chinese nationals, inadvertently delayed the diffusion of scientific medicine probably by many decades through their demands for the abolition of traditional medicine. Fear generated by their actions caused a powerful coterie of traditional scholar-physicians in the cities to organize for collective action and to seek the intervention of high officials on their behalf. Respected by officials and the public alike, the scholar-physicians were able not only to defend what they already had but also to further extend their influence. More than fifty years later, the two systems of medicine stood on equal footing in China, each with its own schools, treatment facilities, and highly placed friends in the bureaucracy.

The Chinese health experience was also significantly influenced by the Soviet model of public health teaching after 1949 and the expansion of the rural health care infrastructure after 1958. The expansion of rural health services occurred on a scale that few might have believed possible in so short a time and was a remarkable achievement.

The solution of one problem often sets the stage for the emergence of another, however, and in this case many rural health personnel drawn into the system at that time were insufficiently trained to ensure high-quality health care in rural areas. By the mid-1980s their requirements for further training had become an issue of considerable importance.

在这一历史背景下发生的事件对中国农村卫生发展的经验产生了相当大的影响，既有有利的，也有不利的影响。一个多世纪前，西方传教士将具有改善公众健康潜力的科学医学引入我国，在接下来的一个世纪里，他们在中国城市建立了数十家现代医院和诊所。他们的努力使一小部分人群受益，但建立了以治愈性治疗为重点的个体化医疗模式。这种模式很难根除。

与此同时，在 20 世纪 20 年代，包括中国人在内的现代医生，通过要求废除传统医学，无意中将科学医学的传播推迟了可能长达几十年之久。他们的行动引起了恐惧，使得城市中实力强大的传统学者医生小团体组织集体行动，并寻求高级官员的干预。因为受到官员和公众的尊重，学者 - 医生不仅能够捍卫他们已经拥有的东西，而且还能进一步扩大他们的影响。50 多年后，两种医学体系在中国处于平等地位，各自有自己的学校、治疗设施，并在政府机构中享有很高的地位。

中国的卫生经验也受到 1949 年后苏联公共卫生教学模式和 1958 年后农村卫生保健基础设施扩张的显著影响。农村卫生服务的扩大在如此短的时间内达到了几乎无人相信的规模，这是一项了不起的成就。

然而，一个问题的解决往往会为另一个问题的出现创造条件，在这种情况下，当时许多被纳入到该系统的农村卫生人员没有得到足够的培训，无法确保在农村地区开展高质量的卫生保健。到 20 世纪 80 年代中期，他们对进一步培训的需求已经成为一个相当重要的问题。

Personal experience has taught me a great deal over this long period, and in the final chapter of these memoirs, I have tried to share insights from lessons learned. In sum, I believe that we have made memorable strides in extending health care to the common people of China. No part of our country today is without access to modern medicine, and mortality rates have been significantly lowered through mass immunizations against infectious disease. Further health benefits will derive, I believe, from any momentum we can add to a shift from hospital- and clinic-based individualized medicine to population-based medicine, combining curative and preventive approaches.

Efforts to upgrade and develop consistent standards in the training of local health personnel and to recruit medical students who are public health-minded will add to the well-being of the people. As of 1987, there was enormous variation in the depth and length of training of our rural health personnel. Improvement of quality will be realized only through the further education of these personnel. The strengthening of undergraduate medical education in public health should be given priority, with additional emphasis on fieldwork. Problem-solving specialists in public health will be most effective when rural health personnel have had a sound, well-rounded academic background before beginning their specialized training.

Experience provides other insights as well. For example, it indicates the need to support experimentation directed at finding solutions appropriate to local needs and conditions and developing innovative and idealistic leadership. Continuous progress requires constant professional exchange and, in many cases, foreign assistance.

Also in China, where scientific medicine exists side by side with a deeply entrenched and politically endorsed indigenous system of medicine, it may be particularly important that modern-trained physicians maintain the highest possible standards of practice. When scientifically trained physicians make mistakes in diagnosis, for example, popular

在这段漫长的时间里，我的个人经验教会了我很多东西，在回忆录的最后一章，我试图分享我从教训中得到的启示。总而言之，我认为我们在向中国普通民众普及医疗保健方面取得了令人难忘的进步。今天，我国任何地区都可以接触到现代医学，通过大规模预防传染病的免疫接种，我国死亡率已大大降低。我认为，如果我们能结合治疗和预防方法，促进从医院和诊所为基础的个体化医学向以人群为基础的医学转变，那么我们将获得更多的健康收益。

努力提升和发展地方卫生人员培训的统一标准，并招募具有公共卫生意识的医学生，将为人民的福祉添砖加瓦。截至 1987 年，我国农村卫生人员的培训在深度和长度上存在巨大差异。只有通过对这些人员进一步教育才能实现素质的提高。应优先加强公共卫生方面的本科医学教育，并强调现场工作。如果农村卫生人员在开始接受专业培训之前，已经有了良好的、全面的学术背景，那么公共卫生领域解决问题的专家将发挥最大的作用。

经验也提供了其他见解。例如，它表明需要支持实验，以找到适合当地需要和条件的解决办法，并发展创新和理想主义的领导力。持续的进步需要不断的专业交流，在许多情况下还需要国外的帮助。

另外，在中国，科学医学与根深蒂固、得到政治认可的本土医学体系并存，接受现代训练的医生保持尽可能高的执业标准可能尤为重要。例如，当受过科学训练的医生在诊断中犯错误时，

confidence in scientific medicine is diminished and its diffusion in society is decelerated.

In writing these memoirs, I recall that Confucius stated that "at the age of fifty one realizes what fate heaven has bestowed on him." Life expectancy has increased greatly over the millenia since Confucius lived. In present-day China a person of fifty can still look forward to what may be the crowning lifetime achievement. Even one several decades older than that can still envision ways in which he can contribute to making one's nation stronger, one's people better off.

Naturally, though, any thinking person who has already lived over eighty years, as I have, is inclined to ponder more over present and past personal achievements than future personal plans and objectives. And, in that context, most of us are apt to be surprised to realize how little we have accomplished in our lifetimes. We might have thought a lot about others; however, in terms of what we actually have been able to do to improve the well-being of others, failures usually outnumber successes.

What the eventual impact of my own work may be, perhaps only time will tell. Over the course of my lifetime, my professional influence has waxed and waned. In the mid-1980s, respect for my work was continuing to grow, and I can only hope that in time it will contribute to some degree to the social welfare of our common people, to whom I am devoted. Whatever the case, I am glad that despite many ups and downs, I have been able to keep to my original intention to serve the people.

The problems that I have faced are universal. Perhaps very few other physicians, however, have considered them over as long a period as the fifty-plus working years through which I have passed. Some physicians may have had less contact with indigenous medicine than I; others may not have lived in a period when social conditions stimulated patriotism and participation in the work of awakening the public in health matters. Some may not have had the chance of experimenting on a health system

公众对科学医学的信心就会减弱，科学医学在社会上的传播速度也会减慢。

在写回忆录的时候，我记得孔子说过："五十知天命"。自孔子诞生以来的几千年里，预期寿命已经大大增加。在今天的中国，一个人在他50岁的时候仍然可以期待获得一生中最辉煌的成就。甚至比他年长几十岁的人也能想出一些使自己的国家更强大，人民更富裕的办法。

不过，任何像我这样已经八十多岁的人，自然会更倾向于思考现在和过去的成就而不是未来个人的计划和目标。在这种情况下，我们大多数人往往会惊讶地发现，我们一生中取得的成就是多么的有限。我们可能为别人想了很多；然而，就我们实际上能够为改善他人福祉所做的事情而言，失败通常多于成功。

也许只有时间能证明我自己的工作最终会产生什么样的影响。在我的一生中，我的专业影响力时重时轻。在20世纪80年代中期，人们对我工作的尊重不断增加，我只希望有朝一日它能对我所献身的普通民众的社会福利有所贡献。无论如何，我高兴的是，尽管经历了许多起起伏伏，我仍能够保持为人民服务的初衷。

我所面临的问题是普遍存在的。然而，也许很少有其他医生像我这样考虑了这些问题五十多年。有些医生可能接触本土医学比我更少；另一些医生可能没有生活在一个社会条件刺激爱国主义和参与唤醒公众健康事务工作的时期。有些人可能没有机会在

to reach the villagers. Others may not have lived in both capitalistic and socialist societies. Still others may not have had so much to do with educational work of different types as I have. Thus, my varied personal experiences may be of interest to quite a cross section of health workers. Those who have faced similar problems may learn something, while others may find my experience irrelevant. Perhaps one inference that can be justifiably drawn from these reflections on my life in the context of rural health development in China is that it may take people a long time to realize the significance of any new, progressive, and far-reaching idea.

Community-oriented physicians are badly needed. Numerous experiences show that an integrated health delivery system, with dedicated administrators and an enthusiastic,—if only minimally trained—village-level staff, can indeed gradually bring the benefits of scientific medical knowledge to the villagers. The fundamental approach to a human endeavor of lasting value must be through education in various forms. Only when the villagers are touched with the rudiments of health information and techniques will there be hope for "health for all by the year 2000."

村民中试用卫生系统。其他人可能没有同时生活在资本主义和社会主义社会。还有一些人可能不像我那样从事不同类型的教育工作。因此，我丰富的个人经历可能会引起许多卫生工作者的兴趣。那些遇到过类似问题的人可能会有所收获，而其他人可能会觉得我的经验无关紧要。反思我在中国农村卫生发展的背景下的生活，或许可以得出一个合理的结论，那就是人们可能需要很长时间才能认识到一个新的、进步的、深远的思想的意义。

我们迫切需要以社区为导向的医生。大量的经验表明，一个综合卫生服务系统，加上敬业的管理人员和热情的村级工作人员（即使只有最低限度的培训），确实可以逐渐把科学医学知识的好处带给村民。各种形式的教育是实现人类持久价值的基本途径。只有当村民接触到基本的卫生信息和技术，"2000 年人人享有卫生保健"才有希望。

译者：杨维中，贾萌萌

Part 1

PRELIBERATION CHINA

**Medicine in Rural China
A Personal Account**

解放前的中国

中国农村之医学
——我的记述

Chapter 1

Encounter Between Two Medicines

As a child in the city of Chengdu, China in the early 1900s, I often heard people striking gongs in our neighborhood. Sometimes I would go to take a look, finding that someone was ill, usually lying in bed. The sound of gongs, together with the smell of burning incense, was supposed to drive away ghosts believed to be haunting the sick. I dimly remember that this kind of incantation has been rendered in our home—consisting of three dark rooms— during my mother's final illness. What that ritual was all about, I had no idea. I only knew that it had not saved my mother, and that she had died of some unknown disease.

The circumstances of the deaths of my mother and later my stepmother left me determined to alleviate the cycle of illness, suffering, and death besetting my family. I had seen that disease was terrible, and that indigenous Chinese medicine, formulated by respected Confucian scholars and endorsed by high-ranking officials and the emperors, had nonetheless been useless in eradicating this disease. Even as a boy, therefore, I was already convinced that our traditional methods of dealing with disease was inadequate, and that other methods must be found.

Like most Chinese, young or old, I was unaware at the time that modern medicine even existed. Imperial policies had kept China in

第 1 章

两种医学的相遇

20 世纪初，我的整个孩提时代都在成都市度过，常闻及邻居们敲锣打鼓。有时我会去凑凑热闹，目睹到有人正卧于病榻之上，人们常通过锣鼓声和焚香以驱赶致病的鬼魂。我隐约记得我母亲生病垂危时，在我们家里的三个黑暗房间里施展了念咒仪式。我并不知晓该仪式有何意义，只知道它未能够拯救我的母亲，最终，我母亲仍因未知疾病而离世。

母亲和继母相继离去，促使我决心要摆脱疾病、痛苦和死亡不断困扰我家庭的阴霾。我已经见识到疾病狰狞的面目，虽然本土的中医均由备受尊崇的儒家学者创建并且获得了达官贵人和皇权的认可，然而中医在根除疾病方面却毫无用处。因此，即使作为一个男孩，我也已经确信，仅仅依靠传统方法来治疗疾病并非可行之道，必须寻找其他方法。

和那时大多数中国人一样，无论年青人还是老年人，我也并不知道现代医学的存在。帝王政治使中国与世隔绝了数个世纪，

seclusion for centuries. Science and scientific thinking as it evolved in the West had made significant inroads only in the nineteenth century, and even then the impact was confined largely to the so-called treaty ports and other coastal cities, where foreign diplomats, business executives, missionaries, and educators plied their trades.

To be sure, "Western," or "modern," medicine had been introduced into Guangzhou (Canton), Shanghai, and other cities more than half a century before my birth. This development, however, had little or no meaning for most Chinese. For the empire's citizenry at that time was both vast—numbering well over 400 million—and overwhelmingly rural.[1] The peasantry, moreover, was scattered over an enormous expanse of territory in a myriad of tiny villages and small towns that were linked only by the most rudimentary channels of transport and communication. Among the common people, literacy was rare and news traveled slowly.

Chengdu, where I had been born and had spent my childhood, lay in interior China, about 1,000 miles southwest of Shanghai. Its inhabitants neither knew of, nor had access to, modern medical care. In sickness and suffering, they depended for help solely on indigenous Chinese medicine—a set of beliefs and practices that had been handed down over the ages and was deeply rooted in the Confucian-based cultural tradition that governed their daily lives. They trusted in it, for its worth had been vouchsafed by classical scholars and emperors and tested over countless previous generations.

Confident in this endorsement, the people of Chengdu and surrounding villages trusted traditional medicine and seldom, if ever, questioned its value—regardless of evident shortcomings. In this, they mirrored the behavior of other persons throughout rural China.

发端于西方的科学及其科学思想在 19 世纪才进入中国，即使在当时，其影响也主要限于通商口岸和其他沿海城市，外交官员、商务官员、传教士和教育家们穿梭于这些地方。

可以肯定的是，早在我出生前的半个多世纪，广州、上海以及其他城市就可循见"西方医学"或"现代医学"的足迹。然而，这样寥寥的足迹对大多数中国人而言几乎不具任何意义。因为当时帝国的人口不仅数量庞大——超过 4 亿，而且绝大多数居住在农村。此外，在广袤的土地上，农民散居于数不尽的小村庄和小乡镇里，这些小村庄和小乡镇缺乏有效的交通和通讯渠道而少有联系。在普通百姓中，识字率非常低，信息传播极为缓慢。

我出生在成都并在成都度过了我的童年时光，成都位于中国西南内陆，距上海约 1000 英里。在成都地区，人们既不知晓现代医学，也无法获得现代医疗的照护。当不幸患病或遭遇伤痛，他们只能依靠本土的中医来解除痛苦——这是一套深深扎根于儒家传统文化的信仰和实践体系，其代代相传并支配着人们的日常生活。人们对中医深信不疑，因为经典的学者们和帝王们均肯定其价值，并经历了无数代人的验证。

成都和周边乡村的人们对传统医学的不足视而不见，仍然对其充满着信心，鲜有质疑。他们像一面镜子折射出整个乡村中国民众的态度和行为。

THE LATE IMPERIAL PERIOD TO 1911

The limited diffusion of modern, or scientific, medicine in the China I knew as a child reflected the long-time imperial policy of global isolation. This policy had deprived China of the benefits of scientific discovery and industrialization over an extended period.

The attitude that foreign goods and ideas were neither needed nor wanted had evolved during the two and one-half centuries of stability under Ming rule (1368-1644) and persisted through the first two centuries of Qing rule (1644-1911) under alien Manchu overlords.[2] During the Ming and Qing dynasties, economy, art, and society had flourished.

Comparison of China's achievements in these fields with those of the less developed peoples along its land borders gave rise to the view among Chinese that their empire was the self-sufficient center of the universe. The cultural superiority of Chinese civilization had seemed indisputable. To protect this unique and cherished legacy from despoilation by foreigners, therefore, a succession of emperors had opted for safety in seclusion. As a result, over many centuries China developed as an inward-oriented, backward-looking society.[3]

The history of the high cost of this policy is well known. Chinese civilization had, indeed, enjoyed many years of stability, growth, and prosperity. Meanwhile, however, its classical Confucian scholars remained unenlightened as to the intellectual and scientific advances made in Europe during and after the Industrial Revolution. Bypassed in this way, the Chinese empire fell far behind the West in scientific and technological spheres.[4]

In the nineteenth century, the imperial government found itself gravely threatened by foreign military forces and unprepared to deal with them. A series of engagements with foreign troops armed with vastly superior weaponry inflicted defeats that the Chinese people felt as deeply

末代王朝到 1911 年

在我孩提时期，现代医学或科学医学在中国传播受限，是由于长期以来的清帝国闭关锁国的政策所致，这个政策导致中国在很长一段时间无缘受益于科学成果和工业化。

中国在明朝 (1368—1644 年) 的长达两个半世纪 (1368—1644) 形成了不需要也不接受外来物品和外来思想的固有观念，该观念一直延续至清朝 (1644—1911) 统治的前两个世纪 (1644—1911 年)。在明清时期，中国的经济、艺术、社会曾一度相当繁荣。

由于中国的经济、艺术和社会等领域的成就领先于周边不发达国家，使中国人产生了帝国是自给自足天下中心的观念。中华文明的文化优越性似乎是毋庸置疑的。因此，为了保护这一独特而珍贵的遗产不被外国人掠夺，历代帝王都选择了闭关锁国的政策以求安全。而该政策最终导致中国经历了数个世纪的飘摇，沦落为一个封闭和落后的社会。

众所周知，闭关锁国政策的代价是巨大的。中华文明的确曾有过长期稳定、增长和繁荣的辉煌。然而，当欧洲乘着工业革命之势而频频收获科学和技术累累硕果之时，中国正统的儒学者却对此一无所知。由于错失工业革命的良机，中国王朝在科学和技术领域被远远地抛在西方后面。

十九世纪，清帝国政府面临着外国军队的严重威胁，却毫无还手之力。每每与武器装备优良的外国军队交火，均连连遭遇失

humiliating. The image of the emperor and his retinue was severely damaged by these happenings, and their domestic support base was further eroded by economic difficulties, which led to widespread peasant revolts.

The dissolution of power had begun with the military defeat delivered by the British during the first Opium War (1839-1842), during the aftermath of which China was compelled to make major trade and territorial concessions to Western nations. Anti-Manchu sentiment escalated in the countryside, reflected in various plots and revolts, including the thirteen-year Taiping Rebellion (1851— 1864).[5]

Droughts, flood, and famine, disrupting economic production, brought suffering to many villagers, who depended on farming for their livelihoods. Although the villagers constituted the economic backbone of the nation, the imperial government assumed little responsibility for prevention, or alleviation, of such disasters. In life-and-death matters, the people relied on each other, and on what help they could get from practitioners of traditional medicine. With public health planning and policy nonexistent, disease was commonplace and intermittent epidemics caused many deaths.

While doing little to aid the villagers, the government in the 1860s instituted—if reluctantly—certain "self-strengthening" reforms that resulted in a modicum of industrial development. Shipyards, arsenals, and textile mills were added in places to the urban landscape. A few foreign language and technical schools were opened under official auspices. The government supported translation of a number of foreign scientific and technical publications. In all, however, the impact of the reforms was modest. They barely touched rural China.

The situation changed significantly after China's defeat by Japan in Korea (1894/95). In the final decade before its collapse, the imperial government, hoping to reassert its authority by whatever means, instituted some

败，让国人倍感羞辱。接二连三的败仗让帝王和王公贵族颜面扫地，加之国内经济不振，一时间农民起义此起彼伏。

在与英国交战的第一次鸦片战争（1839—1842 年）中，清帝国军事失败，导致清帝国权力逐步塌方，被迫在贸易和领土上向西方国家做出巨大的让步。反清情绪如燎原之火在农村蔓延，反抗和起义此起彼伏，包括持续 13 年的太平天国起义（1851—1864 年）。

干旱、洪水和饥荒破坏了农业经济和生产，给众多的以农业为生的村民带来了灾难和痛苦。虽然农民是国家的经济支撑，但清帝国政府对预防或减轻灾害却无所作为。面对生死攸关的灾害，民众只能相互依赖，从传统医学的行医者那里得到一些帮助。由于缺乏公共卫生规划和公共卫生政策，疾病肆虐，并接二连三发生各种疾病流行，造成很多死亡。

清政府几乎未采取任何措施帮助村民，与此同时，在 19 世纪 60 年代，清政府极不情愿地推行了有限的"自强"改革，发展了极少的工业，城市里出现了造船厂、兵工厂和纺织厂，官方开办了几所外语和技术学校，同时政府支持翻译了一些外国科技出版物。然而，总体而言，"自强"改革的影响甚微，几乎未惠及农村地区。

1894—1895 年的中日甲午战争期间，中国在朝鲜遭遇战败后，局势发生了显著变化。在清帝国崩溃前的最后十年里，清帝国政

important reforms, including educational and military modernization along Japanese lines. Students, sent mainly at government expense, flocked to universities abroad to expose themselves to Western learning and scientific thinking.

The belated reforms were too little and too late. Opposition gathered under republican and anti-Manchu activist Sun Yat-sen, and in October 1911, revolution broke out in South China, spreading over most of the country. On January 1, 1912, the republic of China was proclaimed, signaling the end of 2,000 years of dynastic rule.[9]

TRADITIONAL MEDICINE, EVOLUTION AND ENTRENCHMENT

Our indigenous medicine developed over a period spanning thousands of years, embedding itself in the culture as it evolved. Historians discern three overlapping stages in the process: sorcery, experimentation (mainly with herbs), and classical study and prescription.

Stages of Development

Primitive medicine practiced in ancient times was associated with witches and sorcerers. While society despised such persons, it nonetheless relied on them heavily, for they dominated the art of healing. Their methods, based on superstition, featured supplication to many gods and banishment of evil spirits.

In the next stage, beginning with the Shang period, from about 1500 to 1100 b.c, superstitious practices were gradually replaced by remedies sought from nature. Familiar with plant life, villagers looking for sources of relief from illness began to experiment with local flora and fauna. They tried grass, wood, stone, cereals, and insects, all chosen according to their shape, color, smell, and taste.[10]

府通过各种手段希望重新确立其权威，并施行了一些重要的改革，包括按照日本模式实施教育及军事现代化。主要由政府出资向国外大学派遣留学生，向西方学习并接纳科学思想。

然而，清帝国的改革力度太小并且来得太迟了。在倡导共和思想和反清活动家孙中山的领导下，反清力量不断集聚，1911 年 10 月，中国南方爆发了革命，并波及全国各地。1912 年 1 月 1 日，中华民国宣告成立，标志着两千多年封建王朝统治的结束。

传统医学及其演变和巩固

我国的本土医学发展了数千年，且已将之融入到传统文化之中不断发展。历史学家将本土医学的发展归纳为三个彼此相重叠的阶段：巫术、试验（主要是草药）和经典的研究和处方。

发展的阶段

第一个阶段是远古时期女巫和巫师主宰的原始医学，虽然社会鄙视这些人，但民众仍深信并仰赖于该体系，因为他们掌握了治病术的话语权。他们采用迷信的方法祈祷诸多神灵和驱逐邪恶的鬼魂。第二个阶段大约始于公元前 1500 到 1100 年的商代，迷信医学逐渐被自然医学所取代。熟知植物特性的村民开始寻找当地的动植物来尝试解除病痛，他们尝试使用野草、树木、矿石、谷物和昆虫，并根据其形状、颜色、气味和味道予以筛选。

Through trial and error, an increasing number of herbs were gradually identified as suitable for use, notwithstanding the intoxication that sometimes resulted from excessive dosage. Certain villagers began to specialize in collecting, preparing, and selling them, and if the patient recovered, the herb vendor and the vendor's prescription were usually given credit.

During the Chou period, as feudal rulers began to search for safe drugs for themselves, faith in witchcraft declined and respect for herbal medicine increased. Practitioners of herbal medicine were not despised, as the witches had been, but medical practice was still regarded as a somewhat dubious undertaking, and herb vendors were far from being esteemed persons. Most were, in fact, illiterate. Their lowly status was evident in a disparaging remark attributed to Confucius: "Without perseverance or hard work, one could not even become a doctor or a witch." A popular saying admonished, too, that "only medicine offered by practitioners after three generations of family practice can be trusted."

Indigenous medicine entered its third stage of development, after much of what came to constitute China Proper was unified for the first time Qin (Ch'in) emperors began to enlist scholars to study medicine and to attempt to develop theories that explained various diseases and their origins. These scholars had extensive knowledge of philosophy and other aspects of classical learning, according to which they could interpret human and social phenomena. Eventually they worked out medical classics, based in part on these sources.

For example, yin/yang theory had constituted an important strain of thought in Chinese philosophy since the Eastern Zhou (Chou) period Yin/yang theory essentially held that all cosmic forces are composed of mutually complementary opposites: yang—sun, light, hot, male, and positive; yin—moon, dark, cold, female, and negative.[11] This dualism had long been useful in explaining many phenomena in the universe, and scholar-physicians were able to correlate their ideas regarding the etiology of disease, diagnosis, and in certain instances treatment, with its postulates.

尽管过量使用这些物质偶可导致中毒，但通过反复试验，越来越多草药的特定疗效仍逐步得到确定。于是，一些村民开始专注于收集、制备和出售草药，如果患者得以康复，民众便会开始相信贩药者及其处方。

周朝年间（在时指公元前 1122 至 221 年），随着封建统治者开始为自己寻找安全的药物，民众对巫术的信任逐步下降，反之，对草药的尊崇则逐步增加。草药行医者并没有像女巫那样广受诟病，但其医疗实践仍然受到质疑，且草药行医者并非受人尊崇。事实上，大多数草药行医者是文盲，孔子也贬低他们的社会地位："人而无恒，不可为医，乃至巫医。"。中国也有俗话说："医不三世，不服其药"。

公元前 221 年，中国首次统一江山之后，本土医学进入第三个发展阶段，秦帝王开始招募学者学习医学，并试图构建解释各种疾病及其原因的理论。这些学者依赖其熟稔于心的哲学和经典学说，并将之用于人体和社会现象的解释。最终，基于部分理论的支撑，创立了经典医学著作。

例如，自公元前 771—221 年东周以来，阴阳学说成为了中国哲学中重要的思想体系之一。阴阳学说的基本思想是认为世间一切均由相辅相成并相互对立的二元结构组成：太阳、光亮、炽热、雄性和正面等属阳，月亮、黑暗、寒冷、女性和背面等属阴。长期以来，二元论被用来解释世间的诸多现象，儒医们也将阴阳学说运用于对病因、诊断以及特定的治疗实例的阐述。

Working out their ideas in this way, through a combination of their own experience and an analysis of classical literature, the scholar-physicians (ru-yi) were able to offer theoretical explanations of medical phenomena that scholars in other fields accepted as legitimate. The two groups spoke from a basis of common understanding in language and learning. Equally important, the explanations of the scholar-physicians were credible to ordinary Chinese because they were consistent with what people had already accepted on faith as part of their cultural tradition.

In the unity and prosperity of the Han period medicine made unprecedented strides, and scholar-physicians solidified their new exalted position at the court. Emperor Wu-di coined the title "Scholar of Prescriptions" for the scholar-physicians who served the court. Emperor He-di established an imperial medical bureau—the first government medical organization, and appointed Guoyu, a highly respected scholar, as its chief. Imperial physicians began to feel that the pulse was an index for the objective detection of ill health. They developed acupuncture, a medical technique based on a traditional Taoist theory that maintenance of health depends on free circulation of T'chi (life-force energy, controlled by yin/yang balance). One of the best known acupuncture practitioners was HuaTuo, who also performed surgical operations under alcohol-induced anesthesia and, stressing prevention, emphasized the importance of physical exercise in health promotion and maintenance. He encouraged people to imitate the bird, monkey, deer, bear, tiger, and horse in motion. He indicated that the limbs and torso could become supple and strong, blood could circulate regularly, and diseases of the extremities could be prevented.

The scholar-physicians of the Jin (Chin) dynasty contributed significantly to the formulation of medical classics, collectively producing 256 medical treatises. Their broad-based knowledge rarely benefited the general public, however, as they served chiefly the emperor and court officials. Practitioners dealing with the needs of the general public relied for the most part on a single reference work, Zhou Hou Fang. The emperor rarely, if ever, personally assumed responsibility for unmet health needs.

结合自身经验和对古籍文献的解读，再加之阴阳学说的运用，儒医们得以对多种医学现象进行理论阐释，且其他领域的学者也认为这样的理论解释合理可信。基于共同的语言和认知体系，这两个群体的话语是合拍的。同样重要的是，对于普通百姓而言，儒医们的解释是可信的，因为儒医们的解释符合其业已信仰的传统文化。

汉朝（公元前 206—220 年）年间，由于国家的统一和繁荣，医学取得了前所未有的进步，儒医们在朝野巩固了其尊贵地位。汉武帝授予御医们"处方学者"的称号。汉和帝设立了第一个皇家医疗机构——御医局，并任命备受尊敬的学者郭玉为主管。御医们开始意识到诊脉是检测健康状况的客观指标。基于道教理论中维持健康状况需真气（阴阳平衡维持的生命力）自由循环的学说，他们发展出了针灸治疗方法。华陀（公元 110—207 年）是最著名的针灸医生之一，他利用酒精诱导麻醉施行外科手术。他还重视预防，强调在促进和维持健康中身体锻炼的重要性。华佗鼓励人们模仿鸟、猴、鹿、熊、虎、马的动作进行锻炼，他指出，模仿动物的动作可使肢体和躯干灵活而强壮，可确保血脉通畅并可预防四肢疾病。

晋朝（公元 265—420 年）的儒医们对古典医学作出了巨大贡献，他们收集编撰了 256 册医学著作。由于他们主要为帝王和达官贵人服务，故普通百姓鲜有从其广博的知识中受益。民间行医者承担起解除民众疾病的需求，然而他们大多数仅有《肘后方》作为参考书籍。帝王几乎未承担民众的健康需求，即使偶尔有，也是寥寥无几。

Despite the gratifying nature of their new position, some scholar-physicians were uncomfortably aware of the shortcomings of medical practice at that time. One wrote: 'The practitioners of today merely inherit ideas from their predecessors and prescribe drugs without much thought; they are quite unable to cure difficult cases."

In the millennium between the start of the Song dynasty and the close of the imperial period in 1911, Chinese society wholly embraced indigenous medicine. In various periods, medical institutions were established to serve the imperial household, to regulate medical practice, and to stimulate medical thought. For example, the Song emperors founded an imperial medical college whose scholars ultimately produced an extensive body of medical literature. Yuan rulers organized an imperial college of physicians. The reputation of Chinese medicine spread to Japan, and during two centuries of Ming rule, a number of Japanese medical students were permitted to come to China to gain an appreciation of Chinese medical principles.

Death and morbidity rates from communicable and infectious diseases were extremely high. Few Chinese at the time accepted the general concept that the environment influences the incidence of disease, or that many diseases are contagious; thus, prevention was given little consideration. Curative, rather than preventive, medicine was seen as the essential component of health care.

Scholar-physicians served the wealthy elite of urban China; undereducated and largely self-taught traditional practitioners provided medical relief for other urban dwellers and to rural China. In both cases, herbalists represented the majority of practitioners; demand for their services far exceeded that for acupuncturists and surgeons.

Qing officialdom assumed no responsibility for oversight of the medical field. Medical education was informal and practice was wholly unregulated. It was a free-for-all. Much of what transpired between patient

尽管儒医们对其社会地位甚为满意，但仍有一些儒医意识到医学实践的缺乏而惴惴不安。有人写道"今日开诊治病者仅仅是囫囵吞枣地继承先辈观点和开具处方而已，而对疑难病例则束手无策。"

从宋朝（公元 960—1279 年）开始到 1911 年清帝国结束的1000 年间，中国社会完全接纳了传统医学。不同时期均建立了为皇室服务、规范医疗实践和鼓励医学探索的御医局。例如，宋朝帝王建立了皇家御医局，御医局的学者得以出版了大量医学文献。元朝统治者（公元 1279—1368 年）组建了皇家医学堂。在明朝统治的两个多世纪里，中国医学的成就蜚声日本，日本许多医学生前来中国研习中国医学的原理。

传染性疾病和感染性疾病所致的死亡人数和死亡率非常高。当时几乎没有国人具备环境可影响疾病发生的观念，或未意识到诸多疾病具有传染性，故重视疾病预防一事则无从谈起。治疗而非预防被视为健康照护的核心要素。

儒医只为中国城市中的达官贵人服务。未受良好教育和主要靠自学的传统医学行医者则为城市和农村的平民提供医疗救济，这两种传统行医者均以草药医生为主，这类医生的需求量远远超过针灸医生和外科医生。

清朝官员未承担对医学领域进行监督的职能。既缺乏正规的医学教育，医学实践也全然不规范，处于自由竞争状态。患者和

and physician, moreover, was enveloped in an aura of secrecy. Sharing of experience among practitioners was uncommon. In fact, successful treatments were often kept from the knowledge of competing physicians.

Consolidation of the Position of Traditional Medicine

If indigenous medicine had been left entirely in the hands of village practitioners and if its approach to treatment had continued to be based on superstition and empirical experience alone, public confidence in it would probably have gradually declined. In rural areas traditional practitioners were typically no different from their urban counterparts. They were simple, peasant farmers, unable to read and write. What they knew about healing arts had been self-taught or learned through apprenticeship. Herbal remedies and superstitious practices were all they could recommend for medical relief.

Once imperial interest had focused the attention of urban-based classical scholars on the study of medicine, however, the perpetuity of traditional medicine was assured. Scholar-officials turned to ancient Chinese classics for insight, assembling a body of literature to validate the methods of treatment that were thereafter applied. Later generations of scholar-physicians, concentrated in the cities, had access to a growing library of medical texts and learned through empirical trials as well as through reading and study. The substance of traditional medicine as practiced in urban China eventually differed quite markedly from its rural variant. In many cases treatment was very likely more efficacious, and in any event, patient confidence in this form of traditional practice was reinforced by prevailing respect for ancient classical learning. In the process, the principles of medicine formulated by the scholar-physicians were legitimized by ancient classical thought, and in time, an attack on traditional medicine came to be regarded as an attack on the cherished national cultural heritage itself.

The perpetuation of traditional medicine was further assured by the broadening

医生之间的诊疗过程也被蒙上了神秘的色彩。行医者之间鲜有经验交流，事实上，成功的治疗方法在彼此竞争的行医者间也常常讳莫如深。

巩固传统医学的地位

如果本土医学完全掌握在乡村行医者的手中，且仅延用迷信和经验的方法来治疗，则民众对本土医学的信心可能会逐渐下降。在农村地区，传统行医者通常与城市的行医者相差无几，他们就是纯朴的农民，不会读书和写字。他们通过自学或跟师学艺而掌握治病技能，草药和迷信是他们悬壶济世的全部资本。

帝王一度对城市里的经典学者所进行的医学学说感兴趣，传统医学的亘古传承便得以保证。儒医官员专注于研究中国古代经典医学著作，从大量文献中发掘认可的治疗方法并采纳之。聚集在城市的后代儒医们（准官员）能够进入存放越来越多医学书籍的皇家书库，并通过阅读和研究，以及实际经验的方法来学习医学。长此以往，中国城市开展的传统医学与农村开展的传统医学产生了本质的区别。大多数情况下，中国城市传统医学的治疗可能疗效更优，无论如何，因对古典著作研习甚为尊崇，故病人更信任这种源于传统的实践形式。在这个过程中，儒医构建的医学原理借助于古典思想而得以转为正统权威的医学体系，从此之后，任何对传统医学的抨击均被视为对珍贵的民族文化遗产本身的抨击。

由于此类医疗实践的形式有着广泛的政治基础，使得传统医

political base of this form of medical practice. Over the centuries, quite naturally, scholar-physicians developed a vested interest in the viability of their vocation, while, in their professional capacity, they acquired high social standing and important connections. As educated men, they had many friends in high places. They spoke the same language and shared the same background as scholar-officials. In fact, some were scholar-officials themselves or were related to them through kinship ties. By 1911 scholar-physicians had so solidified their position that traditional medicine not only survived the collapse of the old feudal order under which it had become so entrenched but also expanded and prospered. Persons interested in health and medical in China today would learn a great deal by studying that entrenchment process.

CHRISTIAN MISSIONARIES AND THE
ADVENT OF MODERN MEDICINE

Modern medicine, introduced by Christian missionaries from the West, mainly the United States, initially offered little or no challenge to the preeminence of traditional medicine. Although some work was done in outlying rural centers, missionary medical practice was confined largely to urban hospitals and clinics. Then, as now, however, only a small minority of Chinese lived in the cities, and the patient load of even these urban facilities was small relative to the total urban population. As for the rural majority, it had almost no knowledge of, or experience with, modern medicine whatsoever.

Limited penetration was not the only reason for the relative unimportance of scientific medicine as of 1911. Modern medicine had evolved out of an alien civilization, with whose institutions and patterns of behavior it was difficult for the Chinese to identify. Modern medicine had been borrowed whole, in no way adapted to fit Chinese resources or conditions. It was part of a foreign way of thinking, in an era when

学具备了亘古传承的保障。几个世纪以来，儒医非常自然地获得了职业的生存权力，同时，职业能力又使他们获得较高的社会地位并建立了重要的社会关系网。作为受过教育的人群，他们拥有庙堂之上的诸多朋友。儒医与文官之间有着共同的话语体系和共同的出身背景。事实上，一些儒医本身就属于文官，或与文官有着裙带关系。儒医的地位非常牢固，以至于在 1911 年封建王朝崩塌之时，传统医学不仅得以保留，且进一步扩展和昌盛。如今，对中国卫生和医学发展历程感兴趣的人们，通过对传统医学的巩固过程进行研究，必然受益匪浅。

基督教传教士与现代医学的传入

现代医学（或科学医学）由基督教传教士从西方（主要是从美国）传入我国。传入之初，面对传统医学所具有的压倒性优势，现代医学毫无挑战之力。虽然传教士也在边远农村的中心开展了少许医疗实践，但大量医疗实践仍主要限于在城市的医院和诊所。和现在一样，当时仅少数中国人居住在城市中，且城里的医疗设施能够承载的患者数量相对于整个城市的人口而言也极度匮乏。对于大多数农村人口而言，则几乎没有任何现代医学的知识或经验。

到 1911 年为止，民众对科学医学体系知之甚浅，并非导致科学医学发展局限的唯一原因。由于现代医学起源于外国文明，其制度体系和行为模式难以为国人所接受。全盘照搬现代医学，也根本不符合中国现有的资源和条件。当外来思想被严重质疑且

foreign ideas were highly suspect or unwelcome. Traditional medicine, by contrast, was anchored in the Chinese world view and was suited to Chinese-perceived realities.

Missionary Medicine

Missionary medical activity began in China in the early 1830s but rapidly expanded in the latter part of the nineteenth century, seemingly as sponsors in the West became convinced of its potential as a channel for Christian proselytization. Medical work by missionary physicians was generally associated with the dissemination of Christian beliefs and the message of conversion, although the para-mountcy of the medical versus the evangelical goal varied from time to time and place to place.[12]

The first missionary fully trained as a physician was Peter Parker, who established a clinic in Guangzhou in 1835. There, despite his unfamiliarity with antisepsis or anesthesia, Parker treated a variety of simple ailments and performed various surgical procedures with a degree of success that won him many patients.[13] That small beginning heralded what in the late nineteenth century became a substantial medical missionary effort, as sponsors in the United States and Canada grew increasingly enthusiastic about evangelist prospects. A Western chronicle notes that the number of missionary hospitals increased from 10 to 61 between 1850 and 1889, and that within another fifteen years or so the number of missionary hospitals had risen to 362. In addition, there were 244 ambulatory-care facilities.[14]

Missionaries also established many teaching hospitals and medical colleges as well, including Hunan-Yale Medical College in Changsha, Hunan Province; Saint John's College in Shanghai; Lingnan University in Guangzhou; Union Medical College in Beijing; and West China Union University schools of dentistry and medicine in Chengdu, Sichuan Province. There was also a French- sponsored Roman Catholic school in Shanghai. In addition to the missionary schools, there was a German

广受诟病的时代，现代医学也被视为外来思想的组成部分之一。相比之下，传统医学根深蒂固植入国人的世界观中，而且符合国人所能感知到的现实情况。

教会医学

在中国，教会医学的活动始于 1830 年代，并于 19 世纪后半叶迅速扩展，由于这类活动均由西方国家赞助，故民众认为这类活动表面上是教会医学活动，实则是以基督教传教为目的。尽管传教士活动目的因时因地而异，偶以行医为主，偶以传播福音为主，但是传教士医生的医疗工作一般都与传播基督教信仰和皈依基督教的信息多有联系。

第一个接受全面培养并成为医生的传教士是彼得·帕克，他于 1835 年在广州建立了一家诊所。尽管他不熟悉消毒或麻醉，但帕克成功治疗了多种普通疾病并开展了各种外科手术，从而吸引了许多患者慕名而来。十九世纪末，这个良好的小开端预示着医学传道将获得巨大的成就，美国和加拿大的赞助者对传道前景的热情与日俱增。一份西方编年史的记录显示，1850 年至 1889 年期间，教会医院的数量从 10 家增至 61 家，其后的 15 年间，教会医院的数量进一步急速增加至 362 家。此外，还有 244 家流动的诊疗机构。

教会还建立了许多教学医院和医学院，包括湖南省长沙市的湖南湘雅医学院、上海的圣约翰学院、广州的岭南大学、北京的协和医学院，以及四川成都的华西协合口腔学院和医学院。教会

medical college under secular administration.

The content and method of teaching in these institutions were patterned mainly on the basis of Anglo-American models. After completing what in most cases was a six-year curriculum, graduates usually went to work in a missionary hospital or entered private practice.

This was consistent with the basic missionary approach to health care, in which the central frame of reference was the hospital or the clinic, providing treatment for individual patients. Missionaries began by building facilities for patient care, and although they undertook some immunization efforts and did some health education work, their main thrust while in China was on curative medicine.

Returned Students

Meanwhile, among the urban educated elite, many young persons were beginning to see that their ambitions might be just as well satisfied by studying modern medicine as by reading the Chinese classics in the hope of becoming scholar-officials. Some enrolled in missionary colleges; however, foreign schools—a few in Britain and the United States, but especially those in Japan—drew larger numbers. By 1910 the number of students, including medical students, enrolled in Western institutions exceeded 10,000. After returning home, those who had studied abroad were commonly referred to as "returned students."[15]

Graduates in medicine among this foreign-educated group were interested in keeping abreast of developments in their field through contact and discussion with other modern physicians. A logical forum would have been the medical association that missionary physicians had organized and to which many belonged, notwithstanding the fact that the functions of that group had become largely social. To their disillusionment, however, the returned students found themselves barred from membership in the missionary organization. Accordingly, in 1915

还在上海创建了一所由法国赞助的罗马天主教学校。除了教会学校外，还有一所非教会管理的德国医学院。

这些院校的教学内容和方法主要以英美模式为基础。大多数情况下，在完成六年制课程后，毕业生通常就职于教会医院或成为私人开业医生。

这与教会提供健康照护的路径本质上是一致的：即以医院或诊所为中心对个体患者进行治疗。传教士首先通过建立医疗设施为患者提供照护，尽管他们也开展了少许免疫接种和健康教育工作，但其在中国的主要精力还是限于治疗医学。

归国留学生

与此同时，在城市中诸多受过良好教育的优秀青年开始意识到他们可以通过学习现代医学实现自己的抱负，就像中国古代的御医们通过研读经典著作实现其成为文官的抱负一样。这类青年中，有的就读于在中国的教会学校，有的前往外国的院校留学，英国和美国较少，而日本学校则吸引了大量的留学生。截至 1910 年，前往西方学校入学的人数（包括医科学生在内）超过一万人。这些学习归国的学生通常被称为"归国学生"。

这些受过外国教育的医学毕业生通过与其他现代医生的交流和讨论而紧跟医学领域的进展。教会医生们成立了医学协会以进行逻辑讨论，许多教会医生则顺理成章地加入了医学协会。虽然这一团体的作用已经很社会化了，然而，令留学生们倍感失望的是，他们发现自己被排挤在教会的医学协会的之外，于是，留学

they founded their own group, which in time absorbed the missionary-established group.

Relations with Scholar-Physicians

At that time relations between the two groups of Chinese physicians—modern and traditional—were no more productive or extensive than those between the two groups of modern physicians. In fact, like missionary physicians, modern Chinese physicians were generally disdainful of traditional medicine, displaying little respect for it as a discipline or for its practitioners as individuals. For the most part, their attitude was nonchalant at best and at times frankly contemptuous.

Centuries of trial and error had produced a large body of experience as well as a pharmacopoeia that warranted at least some degree of scientific investigation. Yet returned students and medical missionaries paid no attention to it. Quite to the contrary, they ignored any possibilities for collaboration in either research or practice. Modern physicians were totally complacent in their belief in the superiority of European achievement in medicine, and the merits or demerits of traditional medicine were a matter of indifference to them.

One or two modern medical scientists were exceptions to the prevailing attitude, expressing respect for traditional practitioners and acknowledging that some traditional remedies might be worthy of scientific observation. One of these persons was Dr. Edward H. Hume, a medical missionary at Hunan-Yale Medical College. Another was Wu Lien-teh, a returned student from Britain and a modern physician of national stature. Wu's positive attitude toward traditional medicine was particularly significant, insofar as it had been he who, through the use of a scientifically based immunization campaign, had finally contained a nation-threatening plague outbreak in Manchuria, against which traditional practitioners had been totally helpless.

生群体于 1915 年他们成立了自己的医学协会，并及时吸收了教会医生参与。

儒医与现代医生的关系

当时，像中国现代医生和传统医生之间并未建立联系的情况一样，同属现代医生的教会派和留学生派之间也没有形成富有创造力的或更广泛的联系。事实上，与教会医生一样，中国的现代医生也普遍对传统医学不屑一顾，无论是对作为一门学问的传统医学还是作为传统医学的个人行医者，都缺乏对他们的尊重。漠不关心已经是他们抱持的最佳态度了，有时露骨地地表现出轻蔑。

经过数百年无数试验和失败，传统医学总结出了丰富的经验和药典，并一定程度能为科学研究提供了线索。然而，归国留学生和教会医生则对此视而不见。恰恰相反，他们忽视了在研究或实践中进行合作的任何可能性。现代医生全都自信满满地相信欧洲医学成就的优越性，而对传统医学的功过则完全漠不关心。

有两位现代医学科学家则与普遍漠视之态度持截然相反的态度，其对传统行医者表现出充分的尊重并认为一些传统疗法可能值得采用科学方法予以深入研究。其中一人是湖南湘雅医学院的医学传教士爱德华·休姆博士。另一位是英国留学归国的学生，也是一位全国著名的现代医生伍连德。伍连德对传统医学的积极态度颇具重要意义，正是因为他，才得以通过推广科学的免疫接种运动，最终遏制了满洲里爆发的鼠疫疫情，解除了鼠疫对全国的威胁，而传统行医者则对此完全束手无策。

In fact, containment of the Manchurian plague by means of a massive scientifically based immunization campaign had been a watershed event in the history of modern medicine in our country, disposing many Chinese more favorably to a system previously rejected for its foreign origin. Wu's success in halting the tide of death was to many persons a telling demonstration of the value of scientific procedures. Government officials, ordinary people, and even some traditional practitioners came to see this medicine from the West in a new light, thinking it might after all have some value for China.

Aside from this episode, however, traditional scholar-physicians in those days were as unimpressed by modern physicians as modern physicians were by them. Far from feeling themselves threatened by the new medicine from the West, they knew the extent of their support and recognized that most Chinese regarded modern medicine as "foreign" and not to be trusted except perhaps with respect to surgery. At that time, it was commonplace to hear someone assert that missionary physicians and Western medicine were competent in surgical cases, but that one should still rely on indigenous medicine for treatment of disease. This attitude was understandable for the groundwork for a generalized appreciation of science, and scientific principles had not yet been laid in our country.

A LIFETIME RESOLVE TAKES SHAPE

Chengdu, of course, was far away from China's capital, Beijing, where a minority of persons were coming to regard science and scientific thinking as a force that could bring great benefit to our society. It was far, too, from Manchuria, where Wu had so dramatically demonstrated the efficacy of modern medical procedures. Word—even of climactic events in other parts of the empire— reached us belatedly, if at all.

事实上，通过大规模的科学免疫运动遏制满洲里的瘟疫，是我国现代医学史上的一个分水岭，该事件使得许多之前排斥源于国外的医学体系的国人更加赞成现代医学。伍连德阻止死亡潮的成功案例，足以向许多人证明科学措施的价值。政府官员、普通百姓，甚至一些传统行医者，都以全新的眼光来审视来自西方的医学，并认为该体系对中国具有一定价值。

然而，除了该事件之外，传统的儒医和现代医生仍然彼此漠然。儒医们完全没有感到自己受到了起源于西方的、现代的新医学之威胁，他们深知自己备受国人尊崇，并知道大多数国人除认可现代医学的外科之外，将其余现代医学均视为"外国的"，不值得信任。那时，民众们普遍认为教会医生和西医在外科手术方面更胜一筹，但内科疾病的治疗还得依靠本土医学。这一态度是完全可理解的，因为在民众中尚未建立起鉴赏科学和理解科学原理的基础。

做出毕生的决定

成都远离中国的首都北京，在北京，已有少数人开始认识到科学和科学思维作为一种力量，可以给我们的社会带来巨大的收益。成都也远离满洲里，在满洲里，伍连德已经充分地证明了现代医学方法的有效性。各类新闻，即使是全国热议的事件，传播至成都时也为时很晚。

In that isolated part of China (highways and rail transportation came only much later) we were dependent on ourselves and on traditional resources. When herbal remedies failed, we occasionally even resorted to practices based on superstition. For example, when I was twelve years of age, 1 contracted malaria, for which there was no effective treatment. In a desperate attempt to save my life, however, my family subjected me to having my legs whipped and forced me to run around in a courtyard with firecrackers exploding under my knees. The hope was that the noise would drive away the evil spirits that might be causing my illness.

It was not my own experiences, however, but the lingering illnesses and deaths of other family members that made me feel so keenly the need for another way to cope with disease. I had never seen my paternal grandparents; they died very early. After my mother's death, which I learned much later was caused by tuberculosis of the spine, and before my father's remarriage, I had gone to live briefly with my maternal grandparents. My grandfather, who had been educated in the Chinese classics, tutored me at home.

At one time or another, my father's household in Chengdu included, besides myself, my mother, my younger brother, my elder sister, and my father's brother and sister. My uncle disappeared one day, never to be seen again. Like most Chinese youth of his day, he had had no education and, unable to support himself, and being reluctant to add to the burdens of the family, he chose to fade into oblivion. Apart from my father and his brother, everyone in the household died during my childhood. My father's sister, possibly like my mother, succumbed to tuberculosis and my brother, to typhoid fever. What illness took my sister's life we never knew.

My father remarried, and then, just as I was able to attend a formal school for the first time, my stepmother contracted a serious illness. We did not know what she was suffering from at the time, either, although later I was able to deduce that she had contracted pulmonary tuberculosis.

在这个偏僻的土地上（很晚才有公路和铁路运输），我们依靠自己和传统资源开展诊疗。当草药疗法无效时，甚至偶尔会采用迷信的做法。例如，我十二岁时曾罹患疟疾，那时尚无有效的治疗办法，为了挽救我的生命，家人用尽力气鞭打我的腿部，强迫我在燃放着爆竹的院子里奔跑，并寄希望于膝盖下的爆竹声可以赶走导致我患病的恶魔。

然而，使我强烈感受到迫切需要另外一种方法来对抗疾病的想法并非源于我的自身经历，而是家庭成员接二连三的疾病和离世。我从来没有见过我的曾祖父母，他们英年早逝。在我母亲去世之后很久，我才得知她是因为脊椎结核而离世。父亲再婚之前，我曾经和外祖父母生活了一段时间，我外祖父曾在中国的私塾里接受过教育，他在家里指导我学习。

在成都的家里，除了我与我父亲之外，还有我的母亲、弟弟、姐姐和我父亲的弟弟和妹妹。有一天，我叔叔突然失踪，从此杳无音讯。和当时大多数中国年青人一样，叔叔因未受教育而不能维持生计，也不愿增加家庭的负担，于是选择了离家消失。幼年时期，除了我父亲和他弟弟以外，家庭成员均因病相继离世。我父亲的妹妹可能和我母亲一样死于肺结核，我弟弟则死于伤寒，我们甚至无从知晓我姐姐是什么疾病让她离世的。

我父亲随后再婚，然而，就在我第一次进入正规学校上学时，我的继母罹患重病，但我们当时并不知晓其罹患何种疾病，后来我推断她罹患肺结核。

Her illness was distressing, as she had been very good to me in many ways, always treating me kindly, and encouraging me to obtain as much education as possible.

Fearing that traditional medicine would fail her, as it had so utterly failed my own mother, 1 subconsciously vowed to try to find something to help her. Because of this childhood experience with suffering, disease, and death, from an early age I was determined to find another, better system of medicine and to make that medicine available throughout urban and rural China.

疾病持续折磨着她，但继母仍一直悉心照料着我生活，并鼓励我尽可能接受更多的教育。

我感到传统医学无法有效治疗她的病，就如传统医学完全不能挽救我自己的母亲一样，我下意识地发誓要设法探寻能够帮助她的可行之道。由于童年时遭受的痛苦、疾病和死亡经历，使我从小就决心寻找另一种更好的医学体系，并使中国城乡能够获得这个医学体系的照护。

译者：张建新，杨阳

Chapter 2

Ideas and Ideals: Medical Students and Social Change

At the age of fourteen in 1917, I accompanied my stepmother to the French consulate in Chengdu, where she went as a last resort seeking treatment for her illness. The attending physician examined her, using a thermometer, a stethoscope, and, to take her blood pressure, a sphygmomanometer. I was impressed by the status and prestige the physician seemed to enjoy, and more so by the scientific instruments at his disposal. Then and there, I determined to become a modern physician myself. I had no idea how this could be accomplished, of course, and much less any notion that it would require years of formal study.

Nonetheless, aided by a chance event or two, considerable determination, and the boyhood conviction that no dream, however distant, is impossible to fulfill, I managed to achieve my ambition within little more than a decade. In 1921 I was admitted to an elite medical college, newly established in Beijing by an American philanthropic organization, and in 1929 I graduated from that institution as a fully qualified physician. Academic, geographic, and economic obstacles, not to mention a linguistic barrier, had stood in the way of reaching that milestone. Such were the difficulties, however, that confronted many young people who aspired to higher education in our country at that time.

理念和理想:
医学生和社会变革

1917 年,14 岁的我陪同继母到法国驻成都领事馆,为她的病最后一次寻医求治。医生用温度计、听诊器对她进行了检查,并用血压计测量了她的血压。这位医生看起来享有很高的地位和声望,他所使用的科学仪器更是令我印象深刻。从那时起,我就下决心自己要成为一名现代医生。当然,我不知道怎样才能实现这个梦想,更不知道这需要多年的正式学习。

尽管如此,由于我在孩提时代就坚信没有什么梦想是不可能实现的,借助一两次机遇,又凭借着坚定的决心,我在十年多的时间里成功地实现了我的抱负。1921 年,我被一所美国慈善组织在北京新建的知名医学院——协和医学院录取,1929 年我从协和毕业,成为一名完全合格的医生。且不说语言上的障碍,学术上、地理上和经济上的种种障碍,都阻碍着我完成这一里程碑式的目标。然而,这就是当时我国许多有志于接受高等教育的年轻人所面临的困境。

The world that I knew as a student at the Peking Union Medical College (PUMC) from 1921 to 1929 was far removed from that of my boyhood in Chengdu. I had exchanged the isolated intellectual realm of traditional society for the expansive world of science and scientific thinking. Beijing in North China was a huge city, pulsating with life. It was China's capital and the 1920s was a turbulent era of growing national consciousness, as recurrent antiimperialist and antigovernment protest merged with reformist intellectual currents to forge a national cultural awakening.

Intellectuals and students were calling for wholesale national renewal, and, in that process, science was seen to be the key. In fact, to many influential persons in public life, the potentialities of science and scientific thinking for the betterment of human life seemed almost boundless. Science became, in effect, a philosophical doctrine whose precepts could be applied to issues and problems in all realms of life.

At the PUMC I was deeply absorbed in my scientific studies. Nonetheless, beginning in 1925, I became increasingly caught up in the fervor of the national awakening and engrossed in the academic and social issues it engendered. My intensifying patriotism made me more determined than ever to find some way to improve the health of our common people. The appeals of science and social conscience were competing for my time and attention.

Resolution of this dilemma came after I began public health studies in 1926 under John B. Grant, M.D. Grant, the Far Eastern representative of the International Health Divison of the Rockefeller Foundation, had been detailed to establish a department of public health at the college. Grant was concerned with the whole spectrum of social medicine, and unlike many of his peers, was less interested in the pursuit of scientific knowledge for its own sake than for its applications for the betterment of human life. His medical philosophy was multifaceted, emphasizing community- based planning and a combination of curative and preventive services.

1921 年至 1929 年，我就读于北京协和医学院，那期间我所认识的世界与我在成都时的童年印象相去甚远。我的思想已经从闭锁的传统社会知识领域转换到了科学和科学思维的广阔世界。北京位于中国北部，是一个充满活力的大城市。20 世纪 20 年代是一个民族意识不断增强的动荡时代，反复出现的反帝和反政府抗议与改革主义的思想潮流相结合，形成了民族文化的觉醒。

知识分子和学生奋起疾呼全面的民族复兴，在这个过程中，人们认为科学是关键。事实上，对当时在社会上具有影响力的人来说，科学和科学思维似乎拥有改善人类生活的无限潜力。科学实际上成为一种哲学教义，其教条可以适用于生活中所有领域的问题和难题。

在北京协和医学院，我全身心地投入到系统的学习中。然而，从 1925 年开始，我渐渐被卷入到民族觉醒的热潮中，并埋头研究由此而产生的学术和社会问题。日益强烈的爱国主义精神驱使我比以往任何时候都决心要寻找改善大众健康的途径。我的时间和精力同时被科学研究和社会责任感所占据，难以平衡。

这一困境在 1926 年得到了解决，因为我在兰安生的指导下开始进行公共卫生研究。兰安生是洛克菲勒基金会国际卫生部的远东代表，他在北京协和医学院建立了公共卫生系。兰安生关注整个社会医学领域，与他的许多同行不同，他不只是追求医学知识本身，而对其应用于改善人类生活更感兴趣。他的医学理念是多方面的，强调以社区为基础的规划以及防治服务工作的结合。

To this end, he constantly focused the attention of students on conditions in their own country, choosing lecture material that was relevant for China. He always illustrated his points with local or regional examples and arranged for training outside the classroom to provide us with firsthand exposure to real-life situations. For many students, the face-to-face exposure to the suffering of clinical patients and their increasing awareness of the health problems of millions of Chinese men, women, and children in the countryside was a shocking experience. It was true, as Grant had noted, that poor health was in part responsible for China's weakness.

As we delved more and more deeply into public health studies, the critical relationship of public health to national renewal became increasingly clear. We saw public health promotion as an urgent issue, especially with respect to prevention. Private practice, however attractive, would not contribute much to society. In time several classmates and I decided to forego its rewards and devote ourselves instead to pioneering in the development of a health system to meet the needs of rural people.

On hearing Grant insist on the adaptation of practice to the realities of China, I reached a critical realization: rather than rely on a borrowed medical school model in our efforts to bring modern medicine to the people, China must create a new model, based on its own conditions and its own resources. Foreign models were fraught with risks and problems. That insight has remained with me throughout my life.

The issue then became how we could best introduce modern scientific medicine into a predominantly rural population and make it take root there for the benefit of the entire country. I have been concerned with this issue ever since I left medical school.

PRELIBERATION CHINA: 1912 to 1928

For most of the years I spent as a student in Beijing, the city was

为此，兰安生经常选择与中国有关的讲座材料，并引导学生关注本国国情。他总是用当地或地区的例子来论证自己的观点，并安排学生课外实践，让学生直接接触第一手的现实情境。对许多学生来说，直面患者的疾苦，并且越发意识到中国农村有数以百万计的男女老少存在健康问题，这是令人震惊的经历。正如兰安生所指出的，不良的卫生状况是造成中国衰弱的一部分原因。

随着公共卫生问题的深入研究，我们逐渐明确公共卫生与国家复兴有着密切关系。我们认为促进公共卫生是一个紧迫的问题，预防更是重中之重。尽管私人执业非常有吸引力，但对社会的贡献不大。后来，我和几个同学决定放弃高薪报酬，转而致力于开拓发展卫生体系，以满足广大农村人民的需要。

当听到兰安生坚持认为实践要适应中国的实际情况这一观点时，我深深意识到：中国必须根据自己的条件和资源，创建一个新的模式，而不是靠借用医学院的模式来提供现代医疗。外国的模式充满了风险和问题。这一认知一直伴随着我的一生。

问题在于我们如何能够最好地将现代科学医学引入以农村人口为主的地区，并使之在那里扎根，造福整个国家。自从我离开医学院后，我一直在关注这个问题。

解放前的中国：1912 年至 1928 年

我在北京的许多年是在协和医学院学习中度过的，那时北京

the internationally recognized capital of the Chinese Republic. China, however, was unable to achieve even nominal unity until 1928, and Beijing, meanwhile, was controlled by a succession of warlord regimes. The country itself was beset by civil strife and contending political-military forces in a prolonged crisis of power.[1]

The Health and Medical Setting

Comprehensive and reliable health data for the period 1912-1928 are unavailable because the warlords took no interest in public health, much less in the collection of vital statistics. A country the size of China could not be considered as one unit, and health conditions, of course, varied from place to place. Surveys of Beijing, Shanghai, and Harbin, in Manchuria, nevertheless confirmed the general impression of widespread medical problems.

It was safe to assume that the crude death rate probably exceeded 30 per 1,000; the infant mortality rate was probably about 200 per 1,000 live births; and life expectancy was probably about thirty-five years. Maternal mortality may have exceeded 20 per 1,000, especially in rural areas. Tetanus neonatorum was the number one cause of infant death. It was reported, for example, that in one of the twenty counties included in the municipality of Beijing, many children under one week of age died from tetanus, which at that time had been entirely eradicated from many Western countries. In fact, one village reported that, over the previous ten years, 60 percent of its live-born children had died. Infectious diseases, mostly preventable, accounted for one-third to one-half of all deaths. The birth rate was very high, and numbers of children suffered from various physical defects for which no treatment facilities existed. Intermittent famines caused considerable suffering.

In the mid-1920s there was, to all intents and purposes, no public health organization at the national, provincial, or municipal level. The health-related activities that did take place were conducted under the

是国际公认的中国最发达的城市。然而，1928 年以前，中国处在军阀割据的状态。在此期间，北京被一系列的军阀政权所控制。国家本身也饱受内乱和政治军事力量的争斗之困扰，陷入了长期的政权危机。

卫生和医疗机构

由于军阀对公共卫生不感兴趣，我们没有 1912 年到 1928 年期间全面而可靠的卫生资料，更不用说采集生命统计资料了。中国这样一个大国，各地区并不平衡，卫生条件当然也各不相同。对北京、上海和哈尔滨的调查证实了医疗问题普遍存在的这一总体印象。

按保守估计，当时中国粗略的死亡率可能超过 30‰；婴儿死亡率可能约为 200‰；而预期寿命可能约为 35 岁。特别是在农村地区，产妇死亡率可能超过 20‰。新生儿破伤风是婴儿死亡的首要原因。据报道，在北京所辖的 20 个县中，有一个县有许多不满一周岁的婴儿死于破伤风，而当时许多西方国家已经完全消除了破伤风。有一个村庄报道，在过去的 10 年中，60% 的新生儿夭折。1/3 ～ 1/2 的新生儿死于传染病，而大多数传染病是可预防的。当时出生率非常高，许多儿童患各种身体缺陷，但没有治疗设施，而断断续续的饥荒更加剧了群众的苦难。

在 19 世纪 20 年代中期，在国家、省或市一级都没有设立公共卫生组织机构。与卫生有关的活动是在内务部的支持下由警察

aegis of the Ministry of the Interior by police authorities. Such measures were few and far between, however, and as the chief of police was a returned student from Germany, German and Japanese models were emulated. They focused mainly on street cleaning, and even that was poorly done.

The single noteworthy government initiative in the health sphere during this period was the establishment in 1919 of a Central Epidemic Prevention Bureau. This move followed in the aftermath of an outbreak of plague in Manchuria that had taken 60,000 lives and an epidemic of pneumonic plague in Suiyuan in northwestern China in 1917. The agency produced some vaccine, mainly for smallpox. Regrettably, however, not long after its establishment, popular concern about disease abated, and most people lost interest in being immunized.

British-trained Wu Lien-teh, who directed the immunization activities in Manchuria, and a few other modern Chinese physicians, were convinced that prevention warranted more emphasis. As early as 1915, at the first meeting of the newly formed "returned student" group, the National Medical Association of China (NMAC), he and Yen Fu-ching had organized a public health committee. They also sponsored a motion making health education an NMAC goal. Wu and Yen also supported a subsequent NMAC recommendation for the formation of a national-level health administration agency and a call for government action against tuberculosis and venereal disease. Wu also attacked the opium problem. At his urging in 1917, the NMAC demanded prohibition of the importation of morphine. Later Wu himself went to Shanghai to destroy 1,200 boxes of imported opium.

Meanwhile, modern scientific medicine had established a strong position in urban China, dominated by medical missionaries whose activites focused on hospitals and clinical treatment. A1919 missionary report counted 900 Chinese physicians and 600 foreign physicians in China, nearly all in the cities. Medical missionaries were doing some

当局进行的。然而，这种措施很少，而且由于警察局长是从德国回来的留学生，所以照搬了德国和日本的模式。他们的工作主要集中在街道清洁上，即便如此也做得极差。

在此期间，政府在卫生领域唯一值得一提的，是在 1919 年成立了中央抗疫局。这一举措是因为 1917 年，东北地区爆发瘟疫，夺走了六万人的生命，并且西北部的绥远又爆发了肺鼠疫。该机构生产了一些疫苗，主要用于天花。然而，令人遗憾的是，在该机构成立后不久，人们对疾病的关注有所减弱，大多数人对免疫接种也就失去了兴趣。

曾在英国接受过培训的伍连德，在东北地区负责指导免疫活动，他和其他几位现代中国医生都认为应该更加重视预防。早在 1915 年，在新成立的"归国留学生"团体——中华医学会的第一次会议上，他和颜福庆就组织了一个公共卫生委员会。他们还倡议将健康教育作为中华医学会的目标。伍连德和颜福庆还支持后来的中华医学会关于成立全国卫生管理机构的建议，并呼吁政府采取行动防治结核病和性病。伍连德还抨击了鸦片问题。1917 年，在他的敦促下，中华医学会出面要求禁止进口吗啡。后来，伍连德亲自到上海销毁了 1200 箱进口鸦片。

与此同时，现代医学在中国的城市已经建立起了稳固的基础，由医学传教士主导，他们的活动集中在医院并进行临床治疗。一份 1919 年的传教士报告称，中国有 900 名中国医生和 600 名外国医生，几乎都在城市。医学传教士在湖南省农村和少数边远地

work in rural Hunan Province and a few other outlying areas, but this was an exception to the general urban orientation of missionary medicine.

Modern medical facilities included a few public hospitals and a proliferation of missionary hospitals, medical schools, and dispensaries and one or two private, secularly run institutions. One report estimated the number of missionary hospitals at that time to be well over 300.4 By far the most prestigious medical institutions, however, were the PUMC and its affiliated hospital. The Rockefeller Foundation had purchased the Union Medical College in Beijing from its missionary founders, and by the early 1920s had developed it into the leading institution in China for the training of physicians and nurses.

Standards in the PUMC hospital were impeccable, but those in many other hospitals were far from satisfactory. One medical missionary association report indicated that the great majority of hospitals lacked a potable water supply and that most had no means of sterilizing beds or mattresses. More than 30 percent lacked laboratory facilities of any kind. Despite these shortcomings, the missionary hospitals provided a large amount of service and in so doing contributed to building a more favorable popular attitude toward modern medicine among the urban population.

Political instability and lack of funds accounted in part for the poor conditions found in public hospitals; however, as important as these were, the low level of scientific awareness was probably still more important. A reporter for the Binying Weekly, a newspaper health supplement that several other PUMC students and I had established to raise health consciousness in the capital city, described a visit to a public hospital in Beijing in 1926:

The curtain at the room's entrance was very dirty; the air was putrid; and the basins at the bedside were filthy. No one seemed to look after the food for the patients, let alone give consideration to nutrition and cleanliness. As the drugs were kept by the patients themselves, there was no assurance they were taken care of properly. All this shows there

区做了一些工作，但这是教会医学普遍面向城市的一个例外。

现代医疗设施包括几家公立医院和大量的教会医院、医学院和药房以及一两家民间私营自主运行的医疗机构。据一份报告估计，当时的教会医院远超过 300 家。最负盛名的当属北京协和医学院及其附属医院。洛克菲勒基金会从传教士创始人手中购买了协和医学堂，并在 20 世纪 20 年代初将其发展成为中国培训医生和护士的最高学府。

协和医院的标准是无可挑剔的，但许多其他医院的标准却远不能令人满意。一份医疗传教士协会的报告指出，绝大多数医院缺乏饮用水供应，而且多数医院没有卧具和床垫的消毒措施。30% 以上的医院不具备任何类型的实验设施。尽管有诸多缺点，传教士医院还是提供了大量的服务，在城市居民中形成了对现代医学更有利的态度。

公立医院条件差，部分原因是政治的不稳定和资金的缺乏，但科学意识低下可能是更重要的原因。为提高北京居民的卫生意识，我和其他几名协和医学院的学生创办了一个报纸的健康副刊——《丙寅周刊》。该报的一名记者描述了他 1926 年参观北京一家公立医院的场景：

门帘很脏，空气腐臭，床边的盆子也很脏。似乎没有人照管病人的食物，更不用说营养和卫生问题了。由于药品是由病人自己保管的，所以不能保证他们会正确服药。所有这些都表明该院

existed no type of nursing.6

As long as the public remained ignorant of the consequences of such unhygienic conditions and unsound medical practices, little would be done to correct the situation.

Given the indifference of the urban population to health hazards, it was hardly surprising to find the situation incomparably worse in rural areas. Indeed, the difference in mentality between urban and rural communities was so great that any scientifically trained physician attempting to work in the countryside faced a formidable task. The relative impoverishment and lack of education of villages produced attitudes, values, and ways of thinking quite at variance with those of urban-born Chinese. The medical students that I knew came mainly from coastal cities and knew little or nothing about the concerns or circumstances of the villagers. In my own case, for instance, I still remember today how strange I found life in a village about ten miles from Chengdu, where I was taken for a visit as a boy of eight.

Two Medicines in Confrontation

Meanwhile, in urban China, intellectual currents emphasizing the application of scientific principles to transform society were being felt in the medical field, as elsewhere. Even traditional medicine was not entirely immune to the effect of these influences. For in- stance, one Qing dynasty scholar-physician, Wang Qing-ren, attempted to draw some biological inferences from an examination of the visceral organs of children who had died in a measles epidemic, eliciting some interest from a few of his colleagues.

After World War I, the fundamental question posed by Chinese intellectuals regarding Chinese and Western culture and their relative advantages and disadvantages provided the context for a rapidly escalating confrontation between traditional medicine and Western medicine.[7] A number of articles praising "Western medicine" appeared, along with occasional editorials demanding the outright abolition of traditional medicine.

缺乏任何形式的护理。

如果公众继续无视这种不卫生和不健全的医疗状况，政府就不可能会出台什么纠正措施加以改善。

鉴于城市居民对健康危害漠不关心，那么农村地区更加糟糕的卫生状况就不足为奇了。事实上，城市和农村社区之间的思想差异是如此之大，以至于任何受过科学训练的医生试图在农村工作都面临着一项艰巨的挑战。相对贫困和缺乏教育导致农民的态度、价值观和思维方式与出身城市的人截然不同。我所认识的医学生主要来自沿海城市，他们对村民的情况知之甚少或一无所知。以我自己为例，我 8 岁被带去一个离成都大约 10 公里外的村庄，我依然记得那里的生活是多么奇特。

两种医学的对峙

在中国的城市，医学界和其他领域一样，也涌现了将科学原理用于改造社会的知识潮流。即使是传统医学也未能完全避免这种潮流的影响。例如，清朝的一位儒医王清任试图通过检查死于麻疹的儿童的内脏器官，以得出一些生物学推论，这引起了他的一些同事的兴趣。

第一次世界大战后，中国知识分子提出了关于中西方文化以及孰优孰劣的基本问题，这一问题使得传统医学和现代医学的对抗迅速升级。一些赞扬"西方医学"的文章见诸报端，偶尔也有社论文章要求彻底废除传统医学。

Initially, scholar-physicians showed no great concern over this development, nor did it significantly diminish popular confidence in their modes of treatment. They outnumbered scientifically trained physicians, enjoyed high social status, and shared important political connections.

In 1922, however, the Ministry of the Interior, reacting to pressure from a group of returned students, promulgated a series of regulations governing traditional practice. In view of the freewheeling atmosphere that had prevailed under the Qing dynasty, this was a novel and decidedly unwelcome development for traditional physicians, and it aroused their concern and indignation. Not long afterward, controversy ensued regarding the right of traditional medicine to begin to organize its own formal schools of medicine on a par with modern medical colleges. In addition to this, in 1925 the Chinese Missionary Medical Association demanded that the government prohibit the teaching of modern medicine and that it enforce existing regulations requiring the licensing of traditional practitioners on the basis of a formal examination.

In the face of this onslaught, scholar-physicians organized for collective action, using their connections with the press and links to influential politicians to turn the situation around. Before the year was out, the provinces of Shanxi, Zhejiang, and Hubei had enacted resolutions specifically permitting the establishment and operation of institutions to provide formal instruction in traditional medicine. Further rounds in the struggle were to come.

FROM CHENGDU TO BEIJING: A STUDENT'S JOURNEY

As the struggle intensified, I was entering adolescence in Chengdu. My stepmother concluded her treatments at the French consulate and I continued to think about becoming a modern physician. My father, an old-style scholar, was sympathetic to this plan but had no more idea than

起初，儒医对这一事态发展并不太关心，而且当时这件事情也没有明显地影响民众对中医的信任。儒医的人数多于受过科学训练的医生，并且他们拥有很高的社会地位，还享有重要的政治利益。

然而，迫于一群归国留学生的压力，内务部于 1922 年颁布了一系列规范传统医学的条例。由于清朝时期盛行自由行医的氛围，这些条例明显不受传统医生的欢迎，引发了他们的关注和愤慨。不久之后，关于传统医学是否有权建立正规医学院并与现代医学院平起平坐的争论接踵而至。除此之外，1925 年，中华医学会要求政府明令禁止教授传统医学，同时请求政府强制执行既有法规，对传统医学执业者增设经正规医学考试方可取得执业许可的从业门槛。

面对这种冲击，儒医利用他们与新闻界和有影响力的政治家之间的联系组织了集体抗争，以期扭转局势。这年年底前，山西、浙江和湖北等省都颁布了决议，明确允许建立和运营提供传统医学正规教学的机构。这场斗争还将继续下去。

从成都到北京：一个学生的旅程

现代医学与传统医学的斗争日益加剧，而身在成都的我也步入了青少年时期。我的继母不再去法国领事馆求医治病了，而我继续考虑如何成为一名现代医生。我的父亲是一位老秀才，他很

I did how it might be accomplished.

In Chengdu proper, there was a missionary-run modern medical college, the West China Union University, but somehow I had never heard of it. Indirectly, however, I learned of another alternative. An article in the Shanghai press by Li Zhenpian, a male nurse at Hunan-Yale Medical College, attracted my attention. Its author argued the superiority of modern medicine over our own system so thoroughly and convincingly that I decided to contact him, asking him how I could become a student at Hunan-Yale. After a long delay, Li's response arrived. He wrote that an outstanding new- medical college had been organized in Beijing, and that it would be a better choice for me than his own school. That was how I first heard of the PUMC.

Gaining Admission to the PUMC

Studying modern medicine was a simple idea, but its realization was no easy matter. Years of preparation were required and thorny problems had to be overcome, not the least of which was cost. Our family's means were quite limited, certainly too restricted to finance my graduate education. Distance was another obstacle. Traveling to Beijing, a thousand miles to the northeast, would be uncommonly difficult, for Chengdu lay in a vast, remote part of southwest China, as yet unconnected by rail or highway to the northern or coastal cities. Most formidable problem of all, however, was the language barrier.

In the missionary medical colleges, instruction was typically offered in Chinese by teachers whose fluency in the language varied from fair to excellent. The PUMC, however, after what seems to have been considerable debate, chose to teach in English, admitting only students who qualified in terms of language capability.

While the PUMC decision was appropriate, it did require a great deal of effort by the candidate and posed enormous difficulty for almost any young Chinese who aspired to study medicine at that time. Some good

赞同我的想法，但对于如何实现这一计划也和我一样知之甚少。

当时成都有一所由传教士开办的现代医学院，即华西协合大学，但不知为何我从未听说过。然而，我间接地了解到另一种选择。上海出版社的一篇文章引起了我的注意，作者是湖南－耶鲁大学医学院的一名男护士李振翩。作者全面地论证了现代医学优于我们的传统医学，令人信服，于是我决定与他联系，问他我如何能成为湖南－耶鲁大学的学生。很久之后，李先生回复我说，北京新成立了一所优秀的医科大学，这个学校对我来说是更好的选择。这是我第一次听说北京协和医学院。

获得北京协和医学院的录取通知书

学习现代医学想起来容易，实现起来却不简单。多年的准备是必要的，还要克服很多棘手的问题，首当其冲的就是费用。我们家的财力相当有限，当然也就无法资助我的大学教育。距离是另一个障碍。成都位于中国广阔而偏远的西南地区，而北京位于远在 1600 公里以外东北部，那时还没有开通连接北方或沿海城市的铁路或公路。然而，最困难的还是语言障碍。

教会医学院通常是中文授课，老师们的语言水平都不错，有些是非常优秀的。北京协和医学院在经过了激烈论证后，最终选择用英语教学，只招收语言能力合格的学生。

虽然这个决定是无可厚非的，但考生必须为此付出巨大努力，对当时有志于学医的几乎所有中国年轻人来说，都是巨大的挑战。

students were excluded because of the language barrier, and others who circumvented the language requirement initially had to drop out later because their comprehension was inadequate.

In my own case, l began to realize the extent of the problem when a reply to my inquiry regarding admission, written in English arrived at our house in Chengdu. It suggested that, on the basis of the letter I had written, my English was insufficient to enable me to pass the entrance examination.

Not having realized just how inadequate my English was, I was naturally disappointed but became all the more determined to enroll. I found out about and joined a special English class given three times a week by my high-school language instructor, Song Chengzhi, at his church. Song later became an Anglican archdeacon. One of the texts we used was a collection of essays by Ralph Waldo Emerson. As I was doing fairly well, Song later introduced me to a British missionary who agreed to give me private instruction every Sunday. This instruction was concurrent with all my other high-school work.

Acquiring fluency in English was challenge enough in itself, but I soon discovered that to be admitted to the PUMC, I would have to pass English-language entrance examinations in various required subjects, including mathematics, physics, and chemistry. English-language textbooks for these subjects were not available in Chengdu. Few enough young persons studied these subjects in any language, and those who did undertook them in Chinese. After some exploratory correspondence, however, I found a supplier in Shanghai. My stepmother generously gave me funds to buy what was needed. The order took two months to fill, after which time I received a heavy parcel of books. A cousin of my stepmother who knew English and was familiar with scientific terminology offered assistance, and from then on we met every Sunday to work through these textbooks. Until my graduation in the summer of 1921, I studied day and night. Then it was time to try to get to Beijing and pass the admissions tests.

一些优秀的学生因为语言障碍而被淘汰，而另一些虽然起初勉强通过了语言要求的学生，后来也因为理解力不足而不得不退学。

就我本人来说，直到一封入学答复信寄到了我成都的家里后，我才开始意识到问题的严重性，因为信上说，鉴于我写的申请信水平，我的英语能力不足，不能通过入学考试。

我之前没有意识到我的英语有多差，自然感到失望，却更加坚定了入学的决心。我得知我的高中语言老师宋成之在他的教堂举办了一个特别英语学习班，每周三次，我就去参加了。宋成之老师后来成为英国圣公会的会督。我们使用的教材是拉尔夫·沃尔多·爱默生的散文集。由于我勤奋努力，宋老师后来把我介绍给一位英国传教士，他同意每周日给我提供个人补习。这项学习与我所有其他的高中作业同时进行。

掌握流利的英语本身就是一个挑战，但不久我就发现，要想进入北京协和医学院，我必须通过各种必修科目的英语入学考试，包括数学、物理和化学。这些科目的英文教科书在成都是买不到的。这些科目本来就没有多少学生学习，而那些要学习的人也是用中文学习。后来经打听询问，我发现上海有一家供应商。我的继母慷慨地资助我去购买书籍。我下订单两个月之后，收到了一包沉甸甸的书。我继母的表弟，懂英语且熟悉科学术语，他主动提供帮助，每周日我们一起学习这些教科书。我如饥似渴、不分昼夜地学习，直到 1921 年夏天毕业。接着我就要赶赴北京去参加入学考试。

Fortunately for me, a family relative, Mr. Wu, was moving to the capital at that time to work for the government. He had no objection to my accompanying him, and so with my family's approval, we set out, knowing that the trip would be rough and taxing. Sometimes we walked. Sometimes we were carried in a sedan chair. At night we stopped in small hostels, which were invariably dark and dirty. The rooms were illuminated only by small oil lamps similar to the one I had used in high school.

Our first destination was Chongqing, a city larger than Chengdu, lying southeast of it on the Yangtze River. There we boarded a sampan and sailed northeastward through the famous Yangtze River gorges. It was a dangerous voyage, but, as a youth of seventeen, I welcomed the challenge and excitement. Fortunately, we were able to reach Yichang in another ten days, where we changed to a small steamer, somewhat like a modern ferryboat. The boat was crowded, but we managed to find some sleeping space. After four days we reached Hankou in Hubei Province.

Because my traveling companion was exhausted, we rested in Hankou for several days before leaving for Beijing by train, a slow, northward journey of three days. Altogether it had taken us an entire month to cover the 1,000-mile distance between Chengdu and China's capital.

In Beijing, I stayed with the family of a former schoolmate, whose father had become a high official in the Ministry of Education. Eager to see the PUMC, I set off for there on foot at the earliest possible moment. The admissions secretary who had responded to my letter was astonished to see me and to find that I could understand what she said. She endorsed my decision to try entrance examinations.

They were scheduled to be held soon, and I began to prepare at once, moving into a small hotel. The room measured only about six or seven square meters, and a high wall directly opposite the window obstructed the daylight. Not being able to afford an electric reading lamp, I made do with an oil lamp, although this was hard on my eyes. I studied in that dim

幸运的是，当时家里的一个亲戚吴先生要到北京为政府工作。他同意我和他一起去，家人同意后我们就出发了。这次旅程十分艰辛费力。我们有时候步行，有时候坐轿子。晚上，我们借宿在那些又黑又脏的小旅馆里，房间里只有小油灯照明，和我在高中时用的那种油灯相似。

我们的第一个目的地是重庆。重庆比成都大，地处成都东南方向、长江上游地区。我们在重庆登上舢板，经过著名的长江三峡向东北方向航行。行程虽然危险，但是 17 岁的我面对挑战和冒险只觉得很兴奋。幸运的是，航行 10 天后，我们顺利到达了宜昌，并在那里换了一艘有点像现代化渡船的小轮船。船上拥挤不堪，但我们还是设法找到了睡觉的地方。航行 4 天后我们到达了湖北汉口。

我的同伴已经精疲力尽，于是我们在汉口休息了几天，才又乘坐火车北上，历时三天时间到达北京。我们花了整整一个月的时间，才完成从成都到北京之间 1600 公里的旅程。

在北京，我借住在一位老同学的家里，他的父亲已经是教育部高官。我迫不及待地想去看看北京协和医学院，便步行前往那里。给我回信的招生秘书看到我很惊讶，并发现我居然能听懂她说的话。她支持我参加入学考试的决定。

入学考试定于不久之后举行，我立即搬进一家小招待所开始准备考试。我的房间只有六七平方米，正对窗户的一堵高墙也挡住了光线。因为买不起电灯，我只好凑合着用油灯，尽管这样很费眼睛，我还是夜以继日地在灰暗的灯光下学习。

light, not only all day, but long into the night.

The decisive moment arrived, the first of two successive days of testing. The English-language examination took the entire first morning. We were given text to read from a book no one had ever seen before and were asked to explain its meaning. Dictation followed. The proctor looked for errors in what we had written down. In the afternoon, we were administered an intelligence test—a new concept to me. The time limit was rigid, and I felt a great deal of pressure.

Learning afterward that those who failed would have no further chance, I had difficulty sleeping. The next morning I awoke early and hurried to the school, where I was overjoyed to find my name among those who had passed. This meant that I was eligible to take the tests in Chinese, mathematics, physics, and chemistry, which were to be held that day. After finishing them, we were told to go home.

While awaiting these further results, I continued to study each day, living meanwhile free of charge at the home of a friend of my father, whose hospitality I greatly appreciated. Weeks later I received a notice of acceptance. I was elated, of course, and felt that all the effort of the preceding two years had been worthwhile. It was 1921. I would soon be eighteen years old. A new life was beginning.

Premedical School Experiences

The living conditions at the PUMC were much better than I had ever had before. An older student, Li Ting-an, who later became the first graduate to take public health as a career, showed me around Lockhart Hall, the old missionary building used as our classroom, and the dormitory behind it. He told me how to make use of all the facilities. I learned that I was the only student from Sichuan Province, in fact the only one from the entire southwestern part of the country. Most of the others were from the coastal cities, mainly Shanghai and Guangzhou.

为期两天的考试开始了，这也是决定性的时刻。第一天的整个上午都是英语考试。我们要阅读并翻译一篇文章，这篇文章出自一本大家都没有看过的英文书。接下来是听写，监考官会审阅我们所写的内容。下午，我们进行了智力测试——这对我来说是个全新的体验。考试有严格的时间限制，这也使我感到压力很大。

后来得知如英语考试不过关则再无机会，我彻夜难眠。第二天早上我很早就醒了，并急忙赶到学校，我欣喜地发现我的名字赫然在榜。这就意味着我有资格参加当天举行的语文、数学、物理和化学考试。完成考试之后，我们回家等通知。

我借住在我父亲的一位朋友家里，一边等待结果一边继续学习。我非常感谢我父亲朋友的热心招待，也不需要我花钱。几周后，我收到了录取通知书。我很高兴，觉得前两年的所有努力都是值得的。那是 1921 年，我马上就要 18 岁了。我的新生活即将开始。

医学预科阶段的经历

北京协和医学院的生活条件比我之前的学校要好得多。一名高年级的学生李廷安带我参观了娄公楼以及楼后面的宿舍，娄公楼原来是一栋旧教会大楼，现在用作教室。他还告诉我如何使用所有的设备。李廷安后来也成为第一位从事公共卫生事业的毕业生。我了解到自己是唯一一个来自四川省的学生，实际上是唯一一个来自西南地区的学生。其他学生大多来自沿海城市，主要是上海和广州。

The caliber of the faculty was high. The PUMC set itself apart from a number of other foreign educational institutions of the day not only in its insistence on English as the language of instruction but also in the distinction of its faculty. This was as true at the premedical school as at the medical school.

All the teachers at the premedical school were competent in their fields, and some went on to achieve academic prominence. Among the latter were physics instructor Dr. W. W. Stifler, later a full professor in physics at a leading university in the United States, and chemistry instructor Dr. S. D. Wilson, later dean of science at Yenching University in Beijing. Other teachers I remember particularly were Dr. Charles W. Packard and Helen R. Downes. Not all the best faculty were foreign, however. There were some particularly well qualified Chinese teaching assistants.

Curriculum requirements during this period compared with those of the best universities in the West. Among other subjects, we studied two foreign languages—English and German, as well as biology, physics, and chemistry. I worked particularly hard on English after the instructor, A. E. Zucker, to my embarrassment once copied out one of my letters on the blackboard so that he could use it to illustrate grammatical errors to the class.

As it was, students took their work very seriously, devoting their time to attending lectures, performing laboratory experiments, reading textbooks, and writing reports, and preparing for examinations, although there were always a few classmates who failed to make the grade. Apart from a glee club and a college publication, Unison, and an occasional physical education period, there was little to divert our attention from our main goal, acceptance into the medical school program.

After I passed that critical point in 1924 and was accepted for the medical school program, finances became a real problem. I had won a full-tuition Cochrane Fellowship at the end of the first year of premedical

协和与当时许多外国教育机构的区别不仅在于它坚持以英语作为教学语言，而且该学院的师资力量也非常雄厚。这点在医学预科和医学院都是如此。

医预科的所有教师在各自的领域具备很强的实力，有些后来在学术上也取得了卓越成就，包括物理学老师施福禄教授（后来在美国一所顶尖大学担任物理学教授）和化学老师威尔森教授（后来在北京燕京大学担任理学院院长）。其他教师我印象比较深刻的是查尔斯·帕卡德教授和海伦·唐斯教授。并非所有最好的教职员工都是外国人，也有一些非常优秀的中国助教。

这一阶段的课程要求是可以与那些西方顶尖大学相比的。其余的课程包括两门外语——英语和德语，以及生物、物理和化学。有一次，我的英语老师朱克把我的一封信抄在黑板上，作为反面教材向全班同学讲解语法错误。这让我很尴尬，之后我也特别刻苦学习英语。

事实上，学生们对待自己的学习和工作非常认真，他们把时间都投入到上课、做实验、看书、写报告和准备考试中，尽管总有一些学生没有达到要求。除了合唱团、大学期刊和偶尔的体育活动外，我们的主要目标就是被成功录取而进入到医学院，几乎没有什么可以令我们分心。

1924 年，我通过了关键考试并被医学院录取，但是学费成了问题。我在医预科第一学年结束时获得了全额奖学金，并通过担

school and had earned my room and board working as a college accountant and dormitory manager. To finance another five years of medical school, however, seemed out of the question. As an alternative, I briefly considered going into chemistry, but Professor Wilson argued that China was not in a condition to support people in careers in pure science at that time and recommended that I continue with medicine so as to assure myself of a reliable means of earning a livelihood. He arranged for the continuation of my Chochrane Fellowship for four more years. That meant that I had had to come up with only yuan 100 (¥100) for tuition during my entire academic career, the equivalent of about U.S. $50 at the time.

I have described these experiences in detail not because I am anyone special, but because they illustrate the enormity of the academic, financial, and linguistic obstacles faced by many young Chinese at that time in pursuing higher education. This was particularly true when one aspired to attain the best medical education available in China.

THE PUMC AS A FORCE FOR NATIONAL RENEWAL

A few words may be said about the characteristics of the PUMC from the standpoint of its early students. In the nation's capital, the PUMC stood as a proud symbol of the authority and legitimacy of science, the scientific method of studies and scientific medical knowledge. Contained within a walled compound were a faculty of high-ranking scientists trained in the West, residential and teaching facilities for a small, hand-picked group of Chinese students, and a teaching hospital furnished with the finest and most modern facilities and technological equipment available anywhere in the world.

The elitist character of the medical college and its technological and research emphasis reflected the specific pedagogical goal of its Rockefeller Foundation sponsors. That aim was to initiate the spread of scientific medicine in a revitalized China by preparing a small vanguard of superbly trained medical educators who would provide leadership for the long-term process.

任大学会计和宿舍管理员来赚取自己的食宿费用。但是，我很难再支付医学院五年的费用。作为权宜之计，我曾考虑进入化学部，但是威尔森教授认为按照当时中国的条件是不允许人们以从事纯科学研究工作来谋生的，他建议我继续学医以确保自己将来有可靠的谋生手段。他争取将我的奖学金延长了四年。这也意味着我只需要支付 100 元的学费，相当于当时的 50 美元。

我详细描述了我的经历，并不是因为我有什么过人之处，而是要借此说明当时许多中国年轻人追求高等教育时所面临的学术、经济和语言方面的巨大障碍。尤其是当一个人渴望获得中国一流的医学教育时，情况更是如此。

北京协和医学院在国家医学复兴的推动作用

北京协和医学院早期的学生可能会这样描述该学院的特点：北京协和医学院在科学研究和医学知识方面具有权威性，是一所令人自豪的学府。学院内有一支在西方接受过培训的高级科学家组成的教师队伍，住宿和教学设施供少数精选的中国学生使用，还拥有一个配备了世界上最先进的技术和设施的教学医院。

医学院的精英教育特点及其对技术和研究的重视反映了洛克菲勒基金会资助者特定的教学目标，其目标就是通过培养一批训练有素、具有领导能力的医学教育人才，在复兴的中国推动现代医学的长远发展。

To this end, no expense had been spared in constructing or operating the teaching institution, nor were academic standards any less rigorous than at the finest scientific institutions in the West. In a later era, the college would come to be regarded as something of a showplace because no developing country could duplicate such an institution. Still, it served an undeniably important role at that time, in that the quality of its diagnostic capabilities and treatment approaches provided a model that other medical schools attempted to emulate.

Emphasis on Scientific Excellence

In eight years of intensive study at the PUMC, students gained a solid appreciation of scientific methodology and were encouraged to engage in specialized research at advanced levels. The size of the graduating classes was small: three in 1924, five in 1925, three in 1926, ten in 1927, fourteen in 1928, sixteen in 1929, and eight in 1930. Later classes were larger, although rarely exceeding twenty-five.

Limiting enrollment was deemed necessary and appropriate, despite China's then critical shortage of modern physicians, given the institutional goal of producing an elite vanguard of medical educators and administrators. Quality, not quantity, was the object. Later developments may have vindicated this judgment, although in retrospect it seems likely that a somewhat larger number of graduates could have been turned out without lowering the standard—perhaps double the number who actually completed training.

Faculty and students performed research work of high caliber. The most widely publicized of these achievements was one that produced a major archeological breakthrough: the finding, outside Beijing, of skeletal remains of an extinct species, Peking man. In another example, the development of ephedrine from ma huang, a plant long familiar in Chinese pharmacology, facilitated treatment of respiratory diseases the world over.[8]

为此，北京协和医学院在教学机构的建设和运作方面不遗余力，学术标准的严格程度也不逊色于西方最优秀的科学机构。因为这样一个机构在任何一个发展中国家都无可复制，以至于后来这所学院可以被视作一个"名胜"。该学院在当时起到了不可否认的重要作用，因为其准确的诊断和高质量的治疗方法成为其他医学院的效仿对象。

强调科学上的卓越性

在北京协和医学院 8 年的紧张学习中，学生们对科学方法有了扎实的理解，也开展了高水平的专业研究。毕业班级的规模很小：1924 年 3 人、1925 年 5 人、1926 年 3 人、1927 年 10 人、1928 年 14 人、1929 年 16 人、1930 年 8 人。虽然后来班级人数有所增加，但也很少超过 25 人。

尽管中国当时严重缺乏现代医生，但考虑到学院的目标是培养一批医学教育和管理方面的优秀人才，因此有必要适当限制招生数量。学院注重的是质量而不是数量。后来的发展也证明了这一判断是正确的，尽管回想起来，在不降低标准的情况下，本来可以培养出两倍数量的毕业生。

协和师生完成了高水平的研究工作。最广为人知的一项成就是考古学的重大突破：在北京城外发现了北京人的骨骸。另一个例子是从麻黄中提取了麻黄素，麻黄是中国药典中早已记载的一种植物，麻黄素在全世界范围内应用于呼吸系统疾病的治疗。

Excellence was sought in the classroom as well as the laboratory. One of the best teachers I encountered, returned student and physiologist Dr. Robert S. K. Lim, earned the respect of students and colleagues alike for his facility in lecturing and laboratory experimentation. Another respected member of the faculty was Dr. Harther L. Keim, who interested me in dermatology so greatly that initially I chose this as my field of specialization.

For the development of the ideas and ideals that were to have a crucial impact on my subsequent life and accomplishments, however, it was John Grant to whom I was most in debt. He not only steered me into public health as a career but also recommended me for the position in rural health at Dingxian, where I was subsequently able to do pioneering experimentation in rural health care delivery under the aegis of the Mass Education Movement (MEM).

I regard that component of my life's work as particularly important, because it was the basis for the Dingxian model of community medicine, an innovative, new approach to the provision of rural health care marked by a fundamental reliance on village-based health practitioners. Postrevolutionary authorities were able to adapt ideas developed at Dingxian to great advantage in building a nationwide rural health care system after 1958, one that employed village-based "barefoot doctors" as its basic care providers.

The legacy of Dingxian suggests that, while the PUMC was undeniably elitist in conception, isolated within its own confines from the reality of China, some of its students nonetheless were thinking and acting along lines that went well beyond the conventional concepts of the college. A small but highly visible group of graduates, concerned about the welfare of the common people, showed no lack of imagination and initiative in using their education for the benefit of their own society.

协和师生在实验室也精益求精，追求卓越。归国留学生兼生理学家林可胜博士是我遇到的最好的老师之一，他以卓越的讲课和实验能力，赢得了学生和同事的尊重。另一位受人尊敬的是哈瑟·凯姆博士，他使我对皮肤病学产生了极大的兴趣，以至于最初我选择了这个领域作为我的专业。

兰安生对我后来的理想和信念以及人生发展有至关重要的影响。他不仅引导我从事公共卫生事业，还推荐我到定县从事农村卫生工作，使得我在平民教育运动的支持下进行了农村卫生保健的试验性工作。

我认为这是我职业生涯中相当重要的一部分，因为定县是社区医疗模式的基础，是一项创新的农村卫生保健手段，其特点是从根本上依靠以农村为单位的卫生从业人员。1958 年以后，政府采纳了定县医疗模式，由农村的"赤脚医生"来提供基本医疗服务，从而建立了全国性的农村卫生保健体系。

定县医疗模式的经验显示，尽管北京协和医学院采用的是精英主义教育理念，且脱离了中国的现实，但该学院的一些学生的思想和行动却远远超越了学院的传统理念。少数有远见的毕业生关注普通大众的幸福需求，充分发挥想象力并积极地运用他们学到的知识造福社会。

JOHN B. GRANT: FOCUSING ON THE REALITY

John B. Grant, whom I first met as a student in 1926, later became an internationally known public health leader. As a young man he already displayed the vision, originality of thought, and tough- minded pragmatism that marked his long career.

Assigned to explore the incidence of hookworm in China as a possible starting point for Rockefeller Foundation work in our country, he concluded that developing a program limited to curative measures alone would be relatively useless in the long term. What was needed was a two-pronged program combining curative and preventive measures. Grant believed, however, that it was impossible to undertake such a program without a functioning public health organization and sufficient numbers of trained personnel, of which China had neither.[9] The critical scarcity of modern physicians in our country as disclosed in the course of Grant's investigation was one of a combination of circumstances contributing to the decision to establish the PUMC, and it followed quite naturally that he was invited, in 1921, to establish its department of public health.

Realizing that local communities had to have their own permanent health agencies if health improvement was to be sustained, Grant applied himself particularly to developing pioneer public health leadership. He encouraged interest in public health careers in as many students as possible and never lost sight of those he considered the best and the brightest. Because he had the support of the Rockefeller Foundation and the PUMC, he was able to make opportunities for those in whom he took a special interest to pursue graduate studies abroad, and once they had finished their training, he often found key positions for them in the municipal health administrations being developed with his help.

A major component of his teaching philosophy was his insistence on experience outside the classroom. As an initial step, he established a course requirement that each student organize and conduct a complete

兰安生：关注现实

我第一次见到兰安生是在 1926 年的学生时代，后来兰安生成为一位国际知名的公共卫生领袖。他年轻时就已经具备远见卓识、创新思想和务实精神，这些品质贯穿他漫长的职业生涯。

兰安生受派研究钩虫病在中国的发病率，这是洛克菲勒基金会在我国开展工作的起点。他得出结论，从长远来看，开展一个仅限于治疗措施的计划是相对无用的。我们需要的是将治疗和预防措施结合起来。然而，兰安生认为如果没有一个正常运作的公共卫生组织和足够数量的训练有素的人员，就不可能开展这样的计划，而当时的中国两个条件均不具备。兰安生在调查过程中发现我国现代医生严重匮乏，这也是促成建立北京协和医学院的多种因素之一，而他也在 1921 年顺理成章地被邀请至北京协和医学院建立公共卫生系。

兰安生意识到，如果要不断改善人们的健康状况，当地社区必须建立一个稳定的卫生机构，因此他特别致力于培养公共卫生领域的先驱者。他鼓励尽可能多的学生投身公共卫生事业，并且从未忘掉那些他认为最优秀和最聪明的学生。由于得到了洛克菲勒基金会和北京协和医学院的支持，他能够为那些他关注的学生提供出国深造的机会。等他们学成归国，他也常会为他们在自己帮助建立的市政卫生管理部门找到重要的职位。

health survey in a locality of that student's own choosing. More importantly, after several years in China, Grant sought the cooperation of Beijing municipal police authorities and established an urban health station, where PUMC medical and nursing students were provided with an opportunity to practice what they learned in the classroom. The experimental Peking First Health Station served an urban precinct of about 50,000 persons. Internship at the health station gave valuable experience to many students who later served in staff positions in China's fledgling municipal, provincial, and national health administrations.

Throughout his years in China, Grant continued to hammer at the theme of integrating preventive and curative services, couching his ideas in such a way as to point toward the concept of state, that is, nationalized medicine. The progress of health care under missionary sponsorship dissatisfied him precisely because it failed to progress far beyond the provision of hospitals and clinics and the treatment of individual patients. He wanted to see instead the rapid institution of a health care approach encompassing both preventive and curative components, and one that was adaptable to China's particular needs.

He assembled these ideas more than fifty years ago into a set of principles and practice he termed "community health care," the forerunner of present-day community medicine. According to his definition, community health care entailed "the provision of preventive and curative services, using modern epidemiological techniques in assessing the health needs of population groups, the setting of priorities, and the assessment of results achieved." Such an undertaking necessitated careful experimentation with new methods of health care and the evaluation of results, as well as the provision of a realistic setting for instruction of medical, nursing, and health science students.

In 1934, after nearly fifteen years as head of the public health department, Grant left the PUMC to assume broader responsibilities for Rockefeller-funded programs in China. His influence continued well after

兰安生的教学理念中一个重要组成部分就是坚持课外实践。作为第一步，他规定了课程要求，即每个学生自己选择地方组织和开展一次完整的健康调查。更重要的是，在中国工作几年后，兰安生与北京市政领导合作建立了一个城市卫生站，为北京协和医学院医学和护理专业的学生提供实践机会。北平第一卫生事务所（简称"一所"）试点服务于一个约有五万人的市区。在一所的实习为许多学生提供了宝贵的经验，这些学生后来也在中国刚刚起步的市、省和国家卫生行政部门工作。

在中国的这些年里，兰安生一直坚持于防治结合的方针，想在中国推行国民医疗体系。他对教会医疗事业的发展感到不满意，因为这种做法没有超越医院诊所对病人治疗的范围。相反，他希望建立一个涵盖预防和治疗的卫生保健体系，以适应中国的特定需求。

他在这 50 余年将这些想法汇集成一套原则和行为准则，称之为"社区卫生保健"，是当今社区医学的前身。根据他的定义，社区卫生保健包括"提供预防和治疗服务，利用现代流行病学技术评估人群的卫生需求，确定工作重点，并对结果做出评价"。这项工作需要对新的卫生保健方法进行缜密的实验及效果评价，同时也为医学、护理和卫生科学的学生提供了实践环境。

1934 年，兰安生在担任公共卫生学院系主任近 15 年后离开了协和，并在洛克菲勒基金会担任更重要的职责。他虽然离开了，但影响一直持续。在 1924 年至 1942 年间，协和医学院至少有

his departure. Between 1924 and 1942, at least 17 percent of all medical and nursing students entered the field of public health.

Grant left a pervasive and enduring mark on public health in China, reflecting an intuitive understanding of the complexity of modern society and the fundamental responsibility of medicine in its well-being. He believed that no one was better suited to solve China's grievous problems than the Chinese themselves, and that the only appropriate solutions were those within the economic reach of the community involved, not those that required outside support.

If his judgment failed him at any point, it was perhaps in underemphasizing the value of clinical training. Most academics agreed on the paramount importance of such training, especially for a public health educator. It was difficult for anyone with inadequate clinical training to enlist public confidence or to command respect from his colleagues. Yet for reasons known only to him, Grant made arrangements for one medical student to graduate before he had served an internship of any length at all, and for another student to leave after an internship of only six months.

Looking back at my personal relationship with Grant, I see him as having been both teacher and lifelong friend. Our association not only spanned my student years at the PUMC but also several decades thereafter at a time when his professional responsibilities took him to other parts of the world.

Throughout that period, he intervened at many points to assist me in finding an appropriate position from which to experiment with new ideas about rural health development. Immediately after graduation, he drew my attention to a popular education program, where I went to work among the Chinese peasants for the first time. Later he made it possible for me to do graduate work in public health abroad. Then, after

17% 的医学和护理专业学生进入了公共卫生领域。

兰安生对中国的公共卫生领域影响广泛而深远，反映了他对现代社会复杂性的直观理解，以及医学在保障人民健康福祉的根本职责。他认为，没有人比中国人自己更适合解决中国的棘手问题，而且唯一合适的解决方法是依靠社区自己的经济能力，而不是外援资助。

如果说他的判断在哪一点上不足，那也许就是没有重视临床训练的意义。大多数学者都认为这种培训极其重要，尤其对公共卫生教育工作者而言更是如此。缺乏临床经验的人很难获得公众的信任或同事的尊重。兰安生让一名没有实习的医学生直接毕业，而另一名学生只实习了六个月就毕业了，个中原因只有兰安生本人知道。

回顾我与兰安生的私人关系，我将他视为我的良师，更是我一生的益友。我们的联系不仅限于我在北京协和医学院的学生时代，还持续了数十年之久，期间他因为事业的发展而去了世界其他地方。

他多次帮助我，使我获得了一个合适的职位，实践我的新想法，开展了农村卫生保健的试验。我刚毕业，他立即推荐我关注一个公众教育项目，于是我第一次深入中国农民中开展工作。随后，他想办法安排我去国外攻读公共卫生研究生。在我回国后，他向平民教育运动的主任晏阳初推荐我担任医学主任的职位。在

my return to China, he recommended to James Y. C. Yen, director of the Mass Education Movement, that I be offered the position of its medical director. In that post, I had the unique opportunity to do experimental work in rural health, leading to the unprecedented Dingxian health care delivery system. Many of the best years of my life were spent in close association with Grant's ideas and ideals.

STUDENTS AND THE NATIONAL AWAKENING

With their country in the midst of the National Awakening during the early 1920s, medical students in China were inevitably caught up in the ferment of the times. Along with intellectuals and workers, they provided the main impetus for protest against their own government and Japan in 1919, following the revelation that representatives at the Paris Peace Conference had accepted Japan's claim to former German holdings in Shandong Province. Stung by this concession—seen as an ultimate humiliation at foreign hands, urban leaders throughout the country commenced a critical assessment of Chinese life and culture. This culminated into pressure for the radical remaking of China along Western lines. In that call for renewal, students played a major role.

It would have been impossible, as a student in Beijing at that time, to have remained entirely oblivious to ongoing political and intellectual developments. Until the spring of 1925, nonetheless, many, if not most, PUMC students, including myself, were almost entirely absorbed in our studies. The killing of a number of street demonstrators by British police in Shanghai on May 30 of that year, however, shattered our concentration, and after joining the nationwide student protests that followed, a number of us became rapidly politicized and committed to working for change.

那个岗位上，我很难得地有机会在农村卫生方面做实验工作，促成了前所未有的定县卫生保健服务体系。我生命中许多最美好的岁月都与兰安生的思想和理想紧密联系在一起。

学生和国家的觉醒

20 世纪 20 年代初，随着整个国家民族觉醒浪潮的推进，中国的医学生也不可避免地卷入了时代热潮之中。1919 年，巴黎和会的代表同意将先前德国侵占的山东半岛主权转让给日本，唤醒了整个中华民族的爱国意识，学生与知识分子和工人民众同仇敌忾，成为共同抗议政府和日本的主要力量。这一割让协议被视为外国掌控势力带来的终极羞辱，妥协退让的协议刺痛了举国上下的城市领袖们，他们开始重新以批判性视角审视中国当下的生活和文化形态。至此，全国各地觉醒浪潮不断高涨，最终演变为要求国家沿西方路线彻底变革的呼声，学生成了号召变革的主导力量。

彼时，我正是一名身在北京的学生，虽身在学校，但对国家的政治和思想发展变化也不可能毫无知晓。尽管如此，直到 1925 年春天，包括我在内的许多北京协和医学院学生仍几乎完全埋头于茫茫学海之中。随后，也就是 5 月 30 日，英国警察在上海杀害了一些街头示威者，这一事件让我们的目光从学业转向了当下如火如荼的政治浪潮中，一些同学在加入随后的全国性学生抗议活动后，也迅速投身并致力于政治变革运动。

The May 30 incident in Shanghai seems to have been a turning point in my own life. Energies that had heretofore been applied to academic interests were now channeled into opposition activities. I volunteered as a teacher of politics in the middle schools and spent time in ideological debate and discussion with new friends. Then, as I began public health studies in the fall of 1926, heard Grant's lectures, worked in the Beijing First Health Station, and conducted the survey on health conditions in a rural areas, my thoughts began to crystallize. Unconsciously, I had been searching for a means for applying the knowledge I was acquiring in medical school to society, and the means was becoming increasingly apparent.

Political Activism at the PUMC

The deaths in Shanghai had fanned patriotic sentiment—already high—to a feverish pitch, spawning a wave of strikes, protests, and demonstrations that quickly spread to other cities. Very shortly the Beijing Student Union called for a general strike of university and college students to protest British imperialism and the ineptitude, corruption, and disunity of warlord rule.

Unlike students at Beijing, Qinghua, and other universities, PUMC undergraduates were generally quite apolitical, and until then had never engaged in any kind of collective political action whatsoever. Those who had attended missionary schools were, as a group, particularly unconcerned about politics, so much so that many seldom, if ever, read the Chinese newspapers. Nonetheless, in this instance, a significant portion of the student body, influenced by an experience in a government school, or by a teacher, parent, relative, or friend, favored participation, even at the sacrifice of their studies.

上海的五卅惨案似乎也成为我人生中的一个转折点。此前一心倾注于学业的精力开始转向了抗议活动。我自愿担任中学的政治教师，并常常与友人就意识形态领域的相关主题各抒己见、畅所欲言。然后，1926 年秋天，在我开始接触到公共卫生、倾听兰安生的讲座、就职于第一卫生事务所并在农村地区开展卫生状况调查时，我脑海里的想法开始逐步具体而明晰。潜意识里，我仿佛始终在探寻并摸索着一条未知的道路，这条道路有望让我在医学院的所学应用于社会，而此时，这条道路正在我眼前徐徐展开。

北京协和医学院的政治浪潮

上海的五卅运动将已经处于高涨的爱国情绪再次掀起了新的浪潮，同时催生了一波又一波的罢工、抗议和示威活动，并迅速蔓延至全国其他城市。紧随其后，北京学生联合会也呼吁高校学生举行示威活动，以抗议英帝国主义和军阀统治的无能、腐败和割据。

与北京大学、清华大学和其他大学的学生不同，北京协和医学院的本科生鲜少涉身政治活动，在此之前，他们从未参与过任何形式的集体政治行动。就读于传教士学校的学生群体对政治历来都抱持着淡然置之的态度，他们甚至几乎从不阅读中国报纸。然而，面对举国上下激烈的政治运动浪潮，加之公立学校、老师、父母、亲戚或朋友的影响，仍有相当一部分学生赞成参与抗议活动，甚至甘愿为此牺牲自己的学业。

This response caught PUMC authorities unprepared and placed them in a very difficult position. Some faculty members, while unsympathetic with the movement in any way, felt that the extent of government corruption justified the strike, and students should be allowed to participate. Certainly on balance, however, the administration would have preferred that they remain out of the fray, concentrating on academic pursuits. Dr. Heng Liu, medical administrator of the hospital and the first Chinese to hold a PUMC staff appointment, advised students not to participate.

In the end, however, the authorities capitulated, probably having no real option in the matter. They suspended classes for a few' weeks and postponed the scheduled examinations. Professor Robert S. K. Lim led the PUMC contingent in the demonstrations.

As it turned out, general interest at the PUMC was rather short lived, and political activism as a whole waned rather quickly. Only a few undergraduates, myself included, continued to involve themselves in the reform effort. Factionalism and dissension within the Beijing Student Union helped to damp my enthusiasm. My own sustained interest was attributable in part to the number of stimulating intellectuals I had come to know and who offered challenging opportunities for analysis and debate. They included Dr. Xu Shilian, a professor of sociology at Yanjing University, and Chen Yuren (Eugene Chen), editor of a prominent English-language newspaper, the People's Livelihood, and a close political ally of Sun Yat-sen.

Preoccupied with reform issues, I failed to concentrate on preparing for final examinations in 1926 and received a poor grade in physiology. Alarmed, I once again devoted my attention exclusively to scholastic work. Lim arranged for me to make up my poor grade by assisting on a special department project. This was an exhilarating prospect. Dr. Hou Xiangchuan was delegated to train me

面对学生们的反应，北京协和医学院领导层始料未及，这让他们陷入了甚为难堪的境地。一些教职员工虽然对这场政治变革浪潮未置可否，但他们仍然认为政府的极端腐败无能是导致这场抗议运动的导火索，应该允许学生参与。当然，行政部门仍更希望学生们能置身事外，将全部精力集中于学术研究。刘瑞恒博士是首位担任北京协和医学院院长的中国人，他劝导学生不要参加政治活动。

最终，学校管理层做出了让步，毕竟，这样的大环境之下，管理层并没有太多的选择余地。他们最终做出了停课几周的决定，并推迟了预定的考试。最后，由林可胜教授率领北京协和医学院的队伍参加了游行示威活动。

事实证明，北京协和医学院的学生对政治活动的兴趣极为短暂，政治示威活动的热情迅速降温。只有包括我自己在内的少数本科生继续活跃于革命运动中。北京学生联合会内部的派系之争和分歧浇灭了我的政治热情。我对政治活动的持续兴趣有部分来源于我结识的一些热血知识分子，他们提供了对形势的分析和辩论的机会。这些知识分子包括燕京大学社会学教授许仕廉博士，以及著名英文报纸《民生报》的编辑、孙中山的亲密政治盟友陈友仁先生。

由于那段时期我大部分的精力都投入了政治运动，所以未能集中精力准备 1926 年的期末考试，最终，我那学期的生理学学科成绩不尽人意。遭遇此次滑铁卢之后，我再次将注意力转向了学业。林可胜安排我参加一个特殊的研究项目，以弥补那次不尽人意的期末成绩。前行的路光明而令人向往。侯祥川博士成了我

in research, and later I had the thrill of having the work I had done under him appear in The Chinese Journal of Physiology, a prestigious professional publication.

By the time I completed my first year in medical school, I had already been exposed to two sides of student life, the academic and the political. As I began public health instruction under Grant in 1926, I had mixed feelings about their relative importance. On one hand, the student movement made me feel that one could not be purely technical; on the other hand, it was clear that one had always to give the lion's share of one's time and energy to academic subjects.

Relations between foreigners and Chinese were particularly fragile at that time, and students were very sensitive about the country's weakness and vulnerability. Grant taught his course in a very tactful way, however, using material he had collected in China to suggest that some of that vulnerability could be attenuated by improved socioeconomic well-being among the peasantry.

That idea was furthered by the several weeks I spent in the small village of Tongxian, a rural settlement about fifteen miles from Beijing that I had chosen to study in fulfillment of the public health requirement for a survey of rural conditions. My stay was brief. I was able to make only superficial observations of the needs of the local people and had no opportunity to experience rural life in any real sense. Still even in that brief time I saw many problems that could be improved through public health measures, while the lack of medical care and the very backward conditions in the villages left a deep impression. Other classmates had the same reaction. They began to feel that the misery of the peasants must be relieved, and that it was up to them to see that this was done.

的研究导师，后来，在他的指导下，我负责的研究成果有幸发表于《中国生理学杂志》这一著名的专业刊物上，让我内心为之一振。

就这样，当我结束医学院第一年的学习生涯时，我就已经接触到了学生生活的两个方面——学术和政治。1926 年，当我在兰安生的引导下开始从事公共卫生教学时，我感受到学术和政治都很重要。一方面，学生运动让我感觉到，我不可能心无旁骛一心扎身于学业中去；另一方面，我也清晰地意识到我始终必须将大部分的时间和精力投入到学业中去。

彼时，外国人和中国人之间的关系十分脆弱，学生们对政府的软弱无能和国家的动荡不安也处于高度敏感的状态。然而，兰安生以一种极富技巧性的方式讲授他的课程，他引用在中国收集的材料和数据表明，通过改善农民的社会、经济福利，有望部分改善当前国家面临的艰难境地。

我在距北京约 20 公里通县的小村里停留了数个星期，兰安生在课堂上所传授的理念在我的脑海中日渐深入，我选择将我所在的这个小村作为研究对象，以符合农村状况调查的公共卫生需求。然而，我在这个小村仅短暂停留，只能对当地人的需求进行甚为表浅的观察，并未真正意义上融入其中。在这颇为短暂的时光里，我注意到小村里存在着诸多可通过公共卫生措施予以改善的问题，同时，小村里医疗服务的匮乏和极为贫困落后的生活环境也让我久难忘怀。其他同学的感受也与我几近相同。大家开始意识到，让农民摆脱落后医疗状况一事迫在眉睫，而大家需为此竭尽所能。

Science and Social Conscience

Medical students in our country at that time were much attuned to the philosophical implications of the scientific knowledge they were acquiring. Sensitive students everywhere have reflected on the potential of science for the creation of a more equitable society and for the better management of human problems, and we were no exception. If anything, that special time in China's history made the question all the more important. Nevertheless, many students believed that because China's problems were so enormous, little could be done to them.

Consequently, the great majority of PUMC graduates planned their careers without much consideration of the immense medical needs of the country at that time. Some went into teaching and others into health administration. Most, however, like other recent modern medical graduates in China at that time, settled into urban medical careers in Beijing, Shanghai, or Nanjing. The prevailing attitude in the professional community concerning the enormous public health problems in rural China was one of apathy and inertia.

Choosing a public health career, as a minority decided to do, required a strong sense of social responsibility and considerable determination. For without a patriotic and idealistic motivation, opting for such a specialization made little or no sense. The work demanded sacrifice of the academic and financial rewards of research or private practice and had to be performed under very difficult conditions. One could not settle in the relative comfort of the city. The most urgent problems—isolation, poverty, ignorance, and disease—were found in rural areas.

科学与社会良知

彼时，我国的医学生对其所学知识的哲学意义甚为关注。思悟先人一步的学生都开始思考科学对于创造更公平社会和解决人类问题的潜力，我们也不例外。在置身于国家历史节点的这个特殊时期，与之有关的这个问题就显得更为重要了。然而，许多学生认为，彼时国家已经千疮百孔，可谓积重难返。

因此，绝大多数北京协和医学院的毕业生在规划其职业生涯时，并未过多考虑当时国家所面临的巨大医疗需求。一些毕业生进入了教学领域，另一些则进入了卫生管理领域。然而，与当时中国其他新近的医学毕业生一样，北京协和医学院毕业生大多都选择在北京、上海或南京定居，从事城市医学的相关工作。而对于中国农村所面临的巨大的公共卫生问题，医学界的普遍态度是置之不理，无动于衷。

正如少数毕业生所决定的那般，在做出从事公共卫生事业的选择时，需要一名医学生抱持强烈的社会责任感和笃定的决心，才得以不畏艰辛，知难而行。对于医学生而言，只有凭借一腔爱国主义和匡时济世的志向、热血，才可能做出这样的职业决定，因为选择这样的专业对个体而言几乎没有任何意义。公共卫生事业需要医学从业者牺牲学术研究的成就或私人行医的经济回报，且通常必须在极端艰辛的条件下开展工作。条件优越的城市不是公共卫生事业的理想之地。在农村地区，最紧迫的问题是隔绝、贫穷、愚昧和疾病。

Forming the Binying Society

The benefits of knowledge uncovered in the age of science in the West had barely touched China's rural areas, where 80 percent of the population lived under conditions little different from those of Europe several centuries earlier. Among the peasants, nutrition was inadequate and sanitation was ignored. Conditions among the urban poor were only marginally better, if that. The seeming fixity of suffering and disease and the magnitude of need in rural areas defied attempts at solution.

At the PUMC, however, a sentiment took shape among a nucleus of idealistic students that it was not only feasible, but imperative, to try to improve the living conditions of the general population. On the basis of the existing social and political situation, there seemed to be no time to waste. Thus a small group of first-year medical students, including myself, gathered together one evening in 1926 to consider what action we could take even before we had completed our medical studies.

We organized ourselves on a formal basis as the Binying Society, choosing that name because, in the sixty-year cycle of the Chinese calendar, 1926 was the Binying year, the year of the tiger. Zhu Changgeng was instrumental in our organizing effort. Other members included Yang Jishi, Jia Kui, and Zhu Futang, all of whom later became professors of medicine.

Defining Our Aims

Meanwhile, John Grant had introduced me to Yuan Dengli, a professor of physical education at the Normal University of Beijing. An instant rapport developed between this thoughtful older man and myself. We both knew that the backwardness of the government was an impediment to any effort to improve national health. Nonetheless, suggested Yuan, an inroad might be made through health education. If I were interested in

成立丙寅医学社

西方科学时代的知识财富并未惠及中国的农村地区，而这些地区 80% 人口的生活条件与几个世纪前的欧洲毫无二致。农民普遍面临营养不良及卫生条件落后的问题，城市贫民的状况较之前也只是略有改善。长期肆虐于农村地区的痛苦、疾病以及广泛的需求，其程度之甚，似乎已令医学界望而却步。

然而，在协和医学院，一群意气相投并抱持理想主义的学生们达成共识，他们认为，改善这一广大群体生活条件的行动不仅可行，更迫在眉睫。而在那个社会和政治形势风雨飘摇的年代，更是当务之急。因此，1926 年，包括我在内的几位一年级医学生在一个夜晚共聚一堂，思索在完成我们的医学学业前即设法为这一事业尽己所能。

随后，我们正式成立了丙寅医学社，其名称源于当时是农历丙寅年（虎年），即 1926 年。朱章赓在学社发挥了主导作用。其他成员包括严济慈、贾魁、诸福棠，他们后来也都成为了医学教授。

确定目标

当时，兰安生将我介绍给北京师范大学体育教育的袁敦礼教授。这位思虑深远的长者与我一拍即合。我们都甚为了解，对于改善国民健康的任何举措而言，政府的腐败落后都是难以逾越的障碍之一。然而，袁教授建议，健康教育可能是推进国民健康的可行途径之一。他表示，如果我的心思更偏重于社区医学，则应该精心钻研如何才能开展健康教育。他说："比如，就北京目前正大肆流行的斑疹伤

community medicine, he said, I should think more about how this could be done. "Take, for example, typhus fever, which is raging in Beijing," he remarked. "This disease can be completely prevented by personal hygiene, provided people are aware of the danger of louse bites. Take trachoma, for another example. If one could practice personal hygiene, if people knew how to protect their eyes from infection, then this disease would be controllable." Yuan believed that such things would not require much government support and thus were practical for China at that time.

Thinking along these lines, Binying Society members rather quickly agreed that our fundamental mission would be educational. Given the focus on technical excellence at the PUMC, we might easily have been blinded by technology and its immense, and seemingly immediate, potential for relieving our country's health and medical problems. Technological development had its place in any modern order, and because the West had assigned priority to the development of technical skills and the pursuit of advanced scientific research, we might readily have chosen to follow its example.

Conditions in China, however, were very different from those in the West. Far from being fundamentally healthy, our population was disease-ridden, and life expectancy was short. Far from being clean and sanitary, our environment was rife with health hazards, to whose dangers most people were wholly oblivious. The level of health consciousness was deplorable, and every year hundreds of thousands of persons died from preventable illness.

A few medical students alone could not change that situation. Before modern medicine could be introduced and successfully implemented in such a society, people had to be provided with a fundamental appreciation of science and a scientific point of view. The prospective benefits in health improvement inherent in scientific medicine had to be made clear. Only then would it be possible to impose public pressure on the government for improved conditions.

寒而言，只要民众知晓虱子叮咬的危险，则这种疾病其实完全可通过加强个人卫生来加以预防。再以沙眼为例，如果民众注重个人卫生，并知晓如何保护自己的双眼免于感染，则该病也是完全可控的。"袁教授认为，健康教育并不需要政府给予充分支持才可付诸实践。对当时的中国而言，健康教育确实是一条可行之道。

循此思路，丙寅医学社的成员迅速达成共识，我们的基本任务是教育。在此之前，由于我们所在的北京协和医学院对前沿医疗技术高度关注，故我们可能极易将目光仅仅投向一些似乎对改善国家健康和医疗问题具有巨大且直接潜力的技术，而忽略了更接地气的健康教育。技术发展在任何现代体系中均占有一席之地，鉴于西方国家始终将发展技术技能和追求先进的科学研究置于首位，故我们也极易仿之，认为技术高于一切。

然而，中国的社会环境与西方的社会环境存在天壤之别。我国仍远未达到基本的健康水平，民众饱受疾病之苦，且预期寿命极短。我们所处的环境也离清洁卫生相差甚远，环境中充斥着各类健康危害，且大多数人对其危险性完全视而不见。此外，民众的健康意识水平也极度低下，每年约有数十万人死于可预防的疾病。

仅仅依靠寥寥数名医学生，是无法改变这种状况的。在社会引入并成功施行现代医学之前，必须首先让民众懂得尊重并认识科学和科学理念，且必须充分阐明医学在改善健康方面的潜在作用。照此行之，才有可能向政府施以民众压力，要求其改善国民生活环境。

As it was, popular beliefs and practices about illness and disease had almost medieval overtones. In rural China, because the concept of infection was almost universally unknown, cleanliness and sanitation were assigned no importance, and the spread of disease through contagion was never considered. Traditional midwives often used mud to arrest umbilical-cord bleeding. People drank un-boiled water from wells just a few feet from unprotected latrines. Children with diphtheria and scarlet fever shared beds with the healthy children in the same family.

In urban China, the education and health consciousness levels were somewhat higher, but even there there was much ground to be covered. For example, missionaries, and now the government, were building and operating hospitals, but to most Chinese, including city dwellers, a hospital still was a very foreign and unfamiliar idea, and the ordinary person had no notion of how one should function, what standards should be maintained, or what was required in the way of equipment. The lack of health consciousness among the Chinese at that time may astound present-day readers, but that is, indeed, precisely what China was like at that time.

Under these circumstances, health education was clearly a critical priority. Through our public information efforts, we wanted to try to make people more knowledgeable concerning health and disease, increase their sense of personal responsibility in regard to their own health, and eliminate prevailing misconceptions about modern medicine and what it could or could not accomplish. As it was, to the extent that people thought about the difference between modern and traditional medicine at all, because most early medical missionaries had been surgeons, they tended to think that Western medicine was preferable for surgery, while traditional medicine was superior in its use of drugs.

We believed that if the public could be made aware of the fundamental differences between the two medicines and of the crucial

彼时，民众关于疾病的信念和和实践仍停留在中世纪。在中国农村，感染的概念几乎无人知晓，清洁和卫生历来未受关注，更无从理解传染病通过接触传播和扩散。传统的接生婆甚至常使用泥土来阻止脐带出血。民众喝生水，且水井距厕所很近，而厕所又未加防渗和防溢。患有白喉和猩红热的儿童与家庭中的健康儿童同床睡觉。

中国城市地区民众的教育和健康意识的水平较农村地区略好些，但即便如此，健康教育的任务仍然任重而道远。例如，教会及政府开办了一些医院，但对于包括城市民众在内的大多数中国人而言，医院仍然是一个极"外来"且陌生的概念，普通人群对于医院的功能、标准以及设备要求均一无所知。彼时的中国公民普遍缺乏健康意识，今天的读者们可能难以置信，但这确实是当时国家所面临的真实状态。

就当时的社会形势而言，健康教育显然应作为医学领域的重中之重。通过加大公共信息的传播，我们期望增进民众对健康和疾病的认识，提高其对自身健康的个人责任感，并消除其对现代医学的普遍误解，了解现代医学的优势与不足。事实上，就现代医学和传统医学之间的区别而言，由于大多数早期的医学传教士均为外科医生出身，故其通常认为西方医学在手术方面略胜一筹，而传统医学则在药物使用方面颇具优势。

我们相信，如果能让民众了解两种医学之间的根本区别，以及这些区别的关键含义，则能更快地建立民众对西方医学体系的普遍

importance of these differences, we could more quickly develop popular confidence in the new system imparted from the West. Essentially we hoped to convey the idea that scientific medicine was intrinsically set apart from our indigenous system in that it relied on the scientific method, and that scientific inquiry into the derivation of disease produced an inherent interest in prevention as a corollary to interest in treatment. Traditional medicine, by contrast, was largely indifferent to the issue of prevention.

As matters stood, aside from a few intellectuals, few Chinese at that time had any understanding of these crucial differences at all. Most people regarded modern medicine simply as something involving the prescription of medication or performance of surgery. Medical practitioners themselves contributed to this notion, perpetrating the idea that all one had to do was hang up a shingle and prescribe from a catalog of drugs or learn a few surgical techniques. If a patient recovered, the physician or the drugs that were prescribed were credited with the recovery. Seldom, if ever, did it occur to them that nursing care, rest, cleanliness, or diet might affect the outcome, much less that any patients get well by themselves without benefit of any medical input whatsoever.

Facing the Challenge

The Binying Society decided rather quickly on a plan to develop a publication to increase public awareness of health issues. We would try to persuade a leading newspaper publisher to agree to the insertion of a health supplement into copies of his newspaper on a weekly basis. It would be called The Binying Weekly, and I was elected its editor.

Both the missionaries and the Peking First Health Station were already undertaking some health education work. The station was training midwives and offering health education classes for schoolteachers. Its general thrust emphasized personal hygiene and maternal and child care

信心。究其本质而言，我们希望传达这样的理念：现代医学与我们的传统医学体系存在天壤之别，因为前者依赖于科学方法，通过对疾病起源的科学探究，如同对疾病治疗一样，也必定可以引发对疾病预防的固有兴趣。相比之下，传统医学对疾病预防则鲜有提及。

就当时的情况而言，除了少数知识分子外，了解中西医根本差异的民众寥寥无几。大多数民众认为现代医学仅是开处方和做手术等。开业医生本身也进一步加深了民众对此的误解，他们认为现代医学只不过是挂牌营业、开具药物和学习数项外科技术而已。如患者最终康复，则该功劳则归功于医生或其所开具的药物。他们几乎从未意识到护理、休息、清洁或饮食均可能是患者康复的因素，更未曾知晓患者可能在未行任何医疗干预的情况下即可自行康复。

直面挑战

丙寅医学社火速拟定了一项计划，即撰写刊物以增进民众的健康认识。我们计划请求一家主流报社同意每周在其报纸版面中插入一份健康副刊，该副刊则被命名为《丙寅周刊》，我也有幸被选为编辑。

教会和北平第一卫生事务所也开始着手开展一些健康教育工作。该所的助产士培训增加健康教育内容，也为学校教师提供健康教育课程。其倡导的主旨是强调个人卫生和母婴护理，同时也会论及一些当时当地的热点问题。一所采用的方法则是让学生直接参与至学习过程之中。我们对此予以支持，并相信该项目将有

and other topics of immediate and local interest. Its method was based on trying to involve the students directly in the learning process. We supported these ideas and believed in the program as far as it went. Our goal, however, was to try to reach a larger and more influential audience and to present some fundamental ideas about scientific medicine, rather than to teach specific techniques.

The missionaries had organized a Council on Health Education, whose plans included the education of teachers, the conducting of surveys on health conditions, and the organization of health propaganda campaigns in the streets. The hope was, whenever possible, to integrate these health education efforts with evangelistic programs. One of the best known missionary activists in health education was W. W. Peter.

Of the various missionary health education efforts, the most visible were their street campaigns, which were based on a strategy of arousing curiosity through audiovisual aides, mechanical devices, and occasionally, parades using floats and megaphones. This could be accomplished with some effect in cities and towns, but in outlying areas, there was no electricity with which to operate equipment. In any event when the campaigns were over, they were soon forgotten.

Accordingly, the idea of a newspaper supplement appealed to us on two counts. It would be a sustained, rather than sporadic effort, and it would appeal to a sizable and influential group of readers, rather than a disparate group of bystanders in the street.

In laying our plans, we were thinking specifically of trying to reach other medical students and graduate physicians. We were greatly disturbed by the prevailing inertia in the medical profession concerning our country's grave health problems, and we wanted to make our citizenry more aware that the national interest in health was their own. As it was, the concept of public responsibility was quite alien to those physicians who had not been exposed to the classical tradition. This was

望长足发展。然而，我们的目标是试图让健康教育惠及更多且更有影响力的人群，并阐述一些关于现代医学的基本观点，而非授之具体的技术。

教会组建了一个健康教育委员会，其计划涵盖教师教育、健康状况调查以及街头的健康宣传活动。希望在可能的情况下，这些健康教育工作能与宗教传播互为补充，相得益彰。在健康教育方面，最著名的教会活动家之一是彼得。

在各类教会的健康教育工作中，最引人注目的活动是其开展的街头宣传活动，该活动通过使用视听辅助设备、机械装置以及偶尔举办的游行活动（使用花车和扩音器）来吸引民众的关注。该做法在城市和城镇有望取得一定的效果，但在偏远地区，因为缺乏电力资源，故无法使用辅助设备。此外，这些宣传活动的影响极为短暂，随着活动的结束，其影响力即消失殆尽。

因此我们认为创建报纸副刊有两项要求，一是要能够产生持续的而非一时的影响，二是要能够吸引一个庞大读者群体，而非街头不同群体的旁观者。

制定计划时，我们特别希望将这些内容传播至其他医学生和毕业生。我们对医学界普遍不关心我国严重健康问题而感到甚为不安，因此我们力图通过健康教育增进民众的健康意识，使其认识到国家健康利益与个人健康利益密切相关。事实上，对于那些未曾接触过普通民众所处的境遇的医生而言，公共责任与他们所

particularly unfortunate in view of the backwardness of the common people, who were poor and needy and who could be taken advantage of rather easily.

Our planning for the publication was also premised on the recognition that a group of medical students alone could not possibly bring about significant improvement in health conditions. Our chief hope lay in being able to arouse influential intellectuals to take a stand on various health issues and bring pressure on the officials. We thus hoped to stimulate interest among readers whose views carried weight with the warlord regime as well as the general public.

Differences among members of the Binying Society had arisen initially as to what topics we should address. Some members favored very specific topical material, others a more generalized approach. Soon, however, we agreed that our first job was to help people understand what modern medicine was all about. We would be wasting our time talking about specifics, we concluded, before people understood some basic ideas. As it was, the Chinese public as a whole had not yet been introduced to such ideas as that that disease is transmittable; that infection occurs when microbes enter the body, gain a foothold, and multiply; and that wounds thus must be kept clean. Until we provided some basic groundwork in scientific principles, there was no use in teaching basic health practices, because anything that was not understood and appreciated would hardly be followed.

Moreover, if we taught people such things without first establishing the cause-and-effect relationships involved, they might not carry out our instructions properly, and in some cases the consequences could be dangerous. Once a basic education in scientific principles had been conveyed, we could teach the techniques rather rapidly.

The idea of a weekly newspaper supplement on health was quite innovative, but because it was without precedent, no newspaper publisher

关注的问题毫无联系。尤其不幸的是普通民众所处的落后状况，民众在穷困与迫切需求的苦海中挣扎时，易被不当利用。

我们计划出版前既已知晓，单单靠一群医学生无法使民众的健康状况得以彻底改善。我们的主要目的是唤起有影响力的知识分子，利用存在的各种健康问题向相关部门施压。因此，我们希望该刊能激发那些对军阀政权有影响力的读者以及普通民众的兴趣。

最初，在讨论刊物应纳入哪些健康主题时，丙寅医学社的成员出现了分歧。一些成员倾向于甚为具体的专题材料，另一些成员则更倾向于更具普适性的问题。然而，大家经简短讨论后迅速便达成共识，我们的首要任务是帮助民众了解现代医学的涵义。各成员意见一拍即合，一致认为民众在了解一些普遍概念之前即论及具体问题徒劳无益。彼时，整个中国的民众尚缺乏这样的理念：疾病是可传播的，当微生物进入人体，到达其相应的部位并繁殖时即可发生感染；必须保持伤口清洁。在为民众奠定一些科学原理的基本理念之前即授之以基本的健康实践毫无意义，因为民众通常不会遵从其尚未充分理解且赞成的做法。

此外，如果我们在尚未确定该实践所涉及的因果关系时即授之以具体做法，民众可能难以正确地掌握我们传授的健康技能，某些情况下甚至可导致严重后果，而将科学原理的基本教育传达到位之后，我们即可迅速授之以相应技能。

在报纸上开办健康周刊，在当时尚属创新之举，但由于此前尚

was easily convinced of its feasibility, much less its ultimate value. Obtaining publisher cooperation was difficult also because neither their editorial boards nor their readers regarded health topics as being of much importance. Worse still, there was a large market for patent medicine, prepared and sold by persons with little or no medical training, and newspaper editors were quite naturally more interested in the income derived from advertisements of these products than in subsidizing our efforts.

Much to our delight, though, we succeeded in time in getting the widely circulated and rather important Peking World Herald to agree to include our supplement. The paper already had several other supplements on different subjects. To obtain the publisher's agreement, we had to furnish all the material, for he had originally refused to consider our idea, saying that he had no one to write it. There was another problem, too. We had hoped to ask various prominent physicians and others to contribute articles. However, scientifically trained physicians proved to be unwilling, in many cases, to submit articles for editorial review by persons who themselves lacked any background in science. Even those who were willing, being unaccustomed to writing for a popular audience, often were unable to make themselves understood. So we ended up soliciting material from other medical students but by and large writing most of the articles ourselves. This required a sacrifice of time, energy, and other interests. It became very difficult to sustain our efforts while trying to keep up with our medical studies. The drain on our energies was tremendous, and we found ourselves working day and night to keep the publication going.

The Peking World Daily published the supplement until 1927, when political affairs preempted its news space, and the medical supplement was discontinued. New China, a scientific journal, picked up the idea, and we hoped to continue to collaborate with it on a permanent basis. Just two months after this arrangement began, however, its editors

无先例，故且不论其最终价值，就连其可行性都无任何报社对其抱之以充分信心。获得报社的合作过程也倍加艰难，因为报社编辑部和读者均未意识到谈论健康问题的重要意义。更为雪上加霜的是，彼时由几乎或完全由未接受过医学教育的人经营药品市场，报社编辑自然对这些产品可带来的广告收入更感兴趣，而无意资助我们。

然而，甚为欣慰的是，我们很快得到了《北京世界先驱日报》的同意，将我们的副刊纳入，该报发行量大且是当时主流的报刊之一。该刊此前已有其他几种不同主题的副刊。为了获得报社的同意，我们必须负责提供所有材料，他们最初拒绝了我们的请求，表示编辑部尚无人能完成编辑工作。此外，另一个棘手问题也令我们倍感困扰，我们曾计划邀请各位名医和其他专家提供文章。然而，事实证明，受过科学训练的医生大多不愿将文章提交给本身缺乏任何科学背景的编辑进行审查。即使是那些愿意撰写此类文章的医生，由于其在为大众读者写作方面经验匮乏，故也通常难以撰写通俗易懂的文章。因此，我们最终决定不从其他医生处征集材料，而是由我们自己负责完成大部分文章的撰写。这一过程需要我们付出大量的时间和精力。与之同时，我们还不能落下自己的学业，故要维持刊物的正常运营变得尤为困难。同时完成两项任务让我们精力消耗极大，我们日以继夜地工作才能维持刊物的正常发行。

《北京世界先驱日报》随后出版了此副刊，直至 1927 年因政治事务抢占其新闻版面，医学副刊才不得以停刊。此后，另有一份科学杂志《新中国》接受了副刊，我们希望能继续与其开展

decided to suspend publication of all supplements. We then moved to Da Gong Bao.

In time, the supplement gained recognition. It appeared regularly for five years, proferring hundreds of informative articles. A number of PUMC students contributed material, and some faculty members gave us encouragement. Of course, others thought that we were wasting our time. Even among students who wished us well, however, support was only nominal at best. A few students disapproved outright, regarding our activities as appropriate to a politician, but not to a scientist. Disappointment at this attitude was offset by success. When we began to receive letters from a number of intellectuals, we were convinced that our impact was growing. As the audience for the supplement increased, some articles prompted popular demands on the government for improvement in health services.

Content

Just a few excerpts from the supplement are presented here; readers who desire more may consult the files in the national library. Some of the views expressed are dated, and some of the problems that we raised have been resolved or become less important. Still, the material is of some importance; if for no other reason, it suggests what a small group of students at a leading medical college in China were thinking five decades ago and how many of the problems they wrote about are relevant in developing countries today.

One concern of the editors was to rid modern, scientific medicine of the disadvantage of being regarded as "foreign." At that time, it was common in our country, and still is today to some extent, to distinguish between so-called Western medicine and Chinese medicine. This tendency is unfortunate as it obscures the true, temporal basis for distinguishing between the two systems, one associated with ancient learning and the other with modern knowledge. While refraining from

长期合作。不巧，就在计划开始后的两个月，其编辑决定暂停出版所有副刊。随后，我们的阵地转移到了《大公报》。

短短一段时间，该副刊很快便获得了认可。副刊定期出版，共计 5 年，期间发表了数百篇内容丰富的文章。不少北京协和医学院学生为我们提供了文章，一些老师也给我们以勉励。当然，仍有不少人认为我们完全是在浪费时间。即使是那些对该刊抱以支持态度的学生，其给予的支持充其量也只是名义上的寥寥数语而已。有几个学生甚至直言反对我们的做法，认为我们开展的这项活动更像是政治家而非科学家应从事的事项。然而，随之而来的成功抚慰了我们因各种非议而萌生的失望情绪。随着副刊影响力的增加，我们不断收到一些知识分子的来信，这使得我们相信，副刊的影响力正持续增长。同时，随着副刊受众的增加，一些文章的影响逐步凸显，并促使民众要求政府改善卫生服务。

副刊内容

欲了解《丙寅周刊》更多内容的读者可查阅国家图书馆的档案。回顾起来，我们提出的观点有些已经过时了，有些已经得以解决或不再那么重要了。尽管如此，这些材料仍具意义；抛开加诸在其身上的众多光环，它起码再现了 50 年前中国一所顶尖医学院内一小群学生的所闻所想，且其所述及的诸多问题对于现今发展中国家仍颇具重要意义。

编辑们甚为关心的议题之一是使现代医学摆脱"外来"标签。当时，我国对所谓西医和中医的区分尤为显著，从某种程度而言，

judgments about which system was superior, we wanted the public to think, not in terms of Chinese as contrasted with Western medicine, but in terms of ancient as contrasted with modern medicine.

Medicine and medical knowledge belong to the whole world. Our people, deeply committed to traditional medicine, call the newly-introduced medicine from the West "western" medicine. This is natural, but actually in the West, there is only the difference between ancient and modern medicine.[11]

What was at issue, we tried to suggest, was not a value judgment between things Eastern and Western. That is, we were not arguing for "respecting medicine from abroad and despising our own." Rather, it was a case of wanting our population to benefit from the application of scientific medical knowledge, as japan had done. "Japan... has adopted modern medicine to the best advantage of its own people. This does not mean [however] that modern medicine has reached a stage of perfection." For that matter, we felt that there were shortcomings in either system. We believed it was foolish to assume that favorable outcomes resulted from modern medical treatment simply because there was some scientific justification for its application. We tried to emphasize to people that in modern or traditional medicine there is always an element in the outcome that is attributable to pure chance.

It is therefore important to tell the common people that chance sometimes plays an important role in determining their (confidence) in either one system or the other. We do not mean by that that traditional medicine cures disease by chance, and modern medicine all by scientific knowledge.[13]

We wanted to discourage blind faith in either one system or the other.

直至今日仍然如此。这种倾向对民众尤为不利，因为它掩盖了区分两个体系的年龄的差异与理论基础的差异，前者基于现代知识，而后者则基于古代学问。我们所应做的不是评判孰优孰劣，我们希望民众不是从中医与西医的角度来思考，而应从古代医学与现代医学的角度来加以分析。

医学和医学知识属于全世界。我国民众对传统医学感情深厚，其通常将从西方新引进的医学称之为"西医"。该做法无可非议，但实际上，在西方，医学流派存在着古代医学和现代医学的区别。

我们试图向民众阐明，问题的关键不在于东方和西方事物之间的价值判断。换言之，我们不是在争论"尊重国外医学，贬低我国医学"的问题。相反，我们的初衷是希望广大民众能够像日本那样从现代医学知识的应用中受益。"日本……应用了现代医学，为国民的健康广造福祉。当然，这并不意味着现代医学已经达到了完美的阶段"。就这一点而言，我们认为这两个体系均尚存不足之处。我们认为，仅仅因为现代医学的应用以一定的科学依据为基础，就认为其一定能带来有利结局的观念是愚蠢的。我们试图向民众强调，无论是现代医学还是传统医学，结局中始终有一部分因素可归因于纯粹的运气。

因此，必须让广大民众知晓，运气偶或在决定其对一个体系或另一个体系的（信心）方面时发挥着至关重要作用。当然，这并非表明传统医学的治疗仅仅凭借运气，而现代医学则完全基于科学知识。

我们的初衷是希望民众不要盲目地相信这个体系或者那个体系。

In the midst of the growing controversy between the two medicines, The Binying Weekly argued for equitable treatment. We editorialized that if regulations applied to one type of practice, they should apply to the other: "The Society is not sympathetic with the government in enforcing the kind of laws and regulations governing only the practice of traditional medicine."[14] We suggested that it was impractical to propose to deny traditional practioners the right to practice because "their number is quite large, and there are no available substitutes."[15] We asserted that there was value in both systems and proposed "the establishment of an institute of research on Chinese drugs, and also an academy of traditional medicine. "[16]

Opponents of traditional medicine at that time were charging that some of its practitioners were incompetent. As its editor, I pointed out that this could be said of modern medicine as well:

Now if we examine the status of so-called practitioners of modern medicine we may discover that they are quite varied in quality. One is composed of graduates of regular medical schools, of which only a few are well-equipped and staffed with well-trained people. Another group is composed of apprentices of missionary doctors; a third is composed of charlatans practicing so-called western medicine. As long as the last two groups are still practicing in the community, they bring disrepute to modern medicine. Medical control with uniform criteria for all practitioners is essential.

Our government should organize formal health education in normal, primary, and secondary schools, and also should promulgate laws governing not only medical practitioners, but also the use of drugs.

The government, in formulating laws, must proceed gradually, however. Without informed public opinion, laws are bound to meet with resistance. At the same time, we should also know that many schools of modern medicine must be strengthened. Our government should emphasize careful planning in education and law.[17]

在两类医学之间日渐火热的争议背景下，《丙寅周刊》主张公平看待两类医学。我们在社论中强调，如果法规适用于两者之一，则同样应该适用于其中另一类医学体系："丙寅医学社不认可政府实施只对传统医学实践进行管理的法律法规。"我们认为剥夺传统医师的执业权利是不切实际的做法，因为"传统医师人数众多，且无替代人员可执行其职责"。我们认为两个医疗体系均有其存在的价值，并提议"建立中国药物研究所和传统医学的学会"。

当时，传统医学的反对者指责一些传统医学的从业人员不能胜任工作。作为编辑之一，我指出现代医学中也存在同样的问题。

如对现代医学"所谓"从业者的状况加以分析，也可发现业者存在良莠不齐的情况。部分从业人员来自正规医学院的毕业生，但其中仅少数学校设备齐全且教职人员训练有素。另一部分为教会医生的学徒；还有一部分则是号称西医的"江湖骗子"。只要后两种人在社会上行医，则可为现代医学带来负面影响。因此，应该对所有从业人员采用统一的标准进行管理。

我们认为，政府应该在师范学校、小学和中学组织正规的健康教育，还应颁布相应法律对医生和药物使用进行规范管理。

然而，政府在制定法律时，必须逐以行之，才能日臻完善。缺乏知情的民众意见，则法律必然会遭遇阻力。同时，我们还应意识到，从事现代医学教育的许多所院校也仍待改进。我们的政府应着力加强在教育和法律方面的仔细规划。

Editorial attention focused on many other topics besides the encounter between two medicines. Because hospitals were regarded as nothing more than places where medications were dispensed or surgery performed, other matters that directly affected the patient such as diet, nursing care, and sanitary standards received little or no attention. The teaching hospital of the PUMC was excellent, of course, reputed to be the best equipped and best managed hospital in East Asia. Other hospitals were not so good, however. The editor described conditions a visitor to a Beijing hospital encountered in 1927:

When I raised the curtain of the entrance, I saw my friend, Mr. Shen, and a man—not a nurse—was handing him two bowls of rice. My friend looked pale and weak, and was breathing rapidly. In that room, there were two beds; one had a mosquito net and the other did not. There were a few packages of drugs on the table and a bottle of fluid without instructions. Each package had a label which read "one package three times daily. " While I talked to my friend, a few flies buzzed around in the room. I learned that the bedding was brought in by the patients without delousing. I used my hand to feel my friend's body and found that his chest and abdomen were covered with sweat, showing me he had never had a bath in the hospital.[18]

Since the government and the public at that time were aware of the need for hospitals, they were willing to fund them. Yet given the public tolerance for such conditions, the expenditures were almost self-defeating.

Another topic in which the editor was particularly interested was rural health care. A 1929 article pointed out that preventable illness was responsible in great part for the high mortality rates:

除两种医学交锋之外，编辑的注意力更多地集中于其他诸多议题上。鉴于民众普遍认为医院不过是配药或施行手术的场所，其他可直接影响患者的因素，如饮食、护理和卫生标准，鲜有或完全未得以任何关注。当然，北京协和医学院的教学医院是一所优质医院，其被誉为东亚地区管理及设备均最为优质的医院。然而，其他医院的情况则并非如此。编辑描述了 1927 年患者前往北京一家医院时所遭遇的情形。

当我掀开入口处的门帘时，我看到我的朋友沈先生和一位男士（不是护士）正向他递去两碗米饭。我的朋友看上去苍白无力且呼吸急促。房间内设有两张床，一张配有蚊帐，另一张则没有。只见桌上随意散放着几包药和一瓶无任何标签的液体。每个药包上均贴有"每日三次，每次一包"的标签。我与朋友交谈时，几只苍蝇一直在房间里嗡嗡作响。从朋友处我了解到，被褥均是由患者自己带入医院的，且未经灭虱处理。我用手摸了摸我朋友的身体，发现其胸腹部浸满汗液，说明他在医院住院期间从未洗过澡。

由于当时的政府和民众均已意识到医院需求的重要性，故纷纷愿意为医院提供资金。然而，让民众容忍这样的医疗条件，这些支出可谓几乎付之东流。

编辑尤为关注的另一项议题是农村卫生保健。1929 年的一篇文章指出，很大程度上，大多数导致高死亡率的疾病均为可预防的疾病。

If our health conditions could be improved to the degree comparable to those of many countries, we could probably cut the number of deaths by one half. The unnecessary loss of people is grievous to our economy and is a sign of a backward civilization.

Since 80 or more percent of those who die each year unnecessarily occur among the farming people, we naturally should pay close attention to [that group]. [At one time I] thought there were not many patients in the villages. After working in two rural communities, however I began to realize there were actually many sick persons in the countryside.

[When rural people became ill] they usually pray before gods, and if minor ailments get better, they say the gods cured the disease. Patients with serious ailments usually get worse due to delayed treatment. They first try herbs and patent medicine. They rarely use, and cannot afford to use, formal or so-called official medicine, which is drugs prescribed by scholar-doctors. Some patients we see at [modern medical] clinics mostly have tried witchcraft, conventional herbs, patent medicine, and traditional medicine without success.

The peasants generally believe that sickness is due to bad luck or lack of adaptation to water and soil [the ecological conditions]. They do not know that each disease has its own cause. Traditional medicine generally does not know the real cause of disease, and nothing can be said about prevention. . . . Smallpox, which had disappeared in some countries, is still prevalent in our villages. Diseases like smallpox and cholera are quite easily preventable; there is urgent need for a rural health service practicing scientific medicine.[19]

We noted, too, that the disinterest of modern physicians in rural practice contributed to the problem:

如果我们的卫生条件能够改善至与大多数国家相当的程度，则可能有望将死亡人数减少一半。非必要的疾病死亡不仅可导致经济上的重创，也同样是文明落后的标志。

由于每年发生在农业人口中的死亡病例，80% 以上是可以避免的，故我们自然应密切关注这一群体。我曾经认为农村地区的患者数量并不多。然而，在两个农村社区工作后，我开始意识到实际上农村地区的患者数量极高。

农村地区的民众患病时，他们通常会向神灵祈祷，如果小病自愈，则会认为神灵的庇佑治愈了其疾病。严重疾病的患者则通常会因延迟治疗而导致疾病进一步恶化，他们首先会尝试中草药和中成药，且鲜有使用、也无力承担正规的治疗药物或所谓的官方药物，即儒医开具的药物。我们在现代医学诊所所见的个别患者大多已尝试过巫术、常规草药、中成药和寻求传统医学帮助而无效者。

农民们普遍认为，生病是因霉运或水土(生态环境)不服所致。他们并不知晓每种疾病的发生均有其病因。传统医学通常无法了解疾病的真正原因，故自然也无从谈起疾病预防。一些国家已经消失的天花至今仍肆虐于我国农村地区。诸如天花和霍乱一类的疾病其实极易预防；我国农村卫生迫切需要实行现代医学照护。

我们还注意到，现代医生对服务农村的实践不感兴趣，这也是问题所在。

Graduates of modern medical schools do not go to poor villages to make a living. Government appointed doctors are unwilling to work in rural areas. Therefore, the peasant when sick, cannot get regular treatment. Patients travel two or three miles to see a doctor in a rural clinic. This shows the extreme shortage of doctors and medicine in our countryside.

Although we have thousands of doctors in the cities, in the villages of North China 40 percent of our people have no medical facilities of any kind. Western medicine has been in China for almost a century and only cities have slight contact with it. [20]

Another issue that interested the society was government responsibility for public health, and in that context we stressed the importance of effective health administration. We felt that even at that time health care should not be left entirely in the hands of private practitioners, and that it was time to introduce state- supported medicine.

An effective public health administration, of course, required appropriately trained professional personnel, of which there was a great scarcity. We might begin to remedy this glaring weakness, the editor felt, by using normal schools as a channel of health education for the general public.

An actual health officer, in The Binying Weekly, recommended that such a practitioner "should be a graduate of a good medical school; have special training in public health with understanding of local health conditions; have good character; and be capable, with leadership qualities."

The health officer further stated:

Lack of health knowledge is a [common problem] and a great obstacle to the operation of the Public Health Administration. The Beijing

现代医学院的毕业生不愿前往贫穷的农村谋生。政府委派的医生也不愿去农村工作。因此，当农民患病时无法获得正规治疗，且往往需要步行两三公里才能在农村诊所就诊。这些情况表明，我国农村严重缺医少药。

虽然城市里有数以千计的医生，但是在华北农村，40% 的农民无法获得任何形式的医疗设施。西医进入中国已近一个世纪之久，但仍然只是城市才有少许西医。

丙寅医学社感兴趣的另一个问题是政府在公共卫生领域肩负的责任问题，就这一领域而言，我们强调了有效卫生管理的重要性。我们认为，即使在那个时期，卫生保健也不应完全依靠私人开业医生，认为是时候由政府提供医疗了。

有效的公共卫生管理需由经过相应培训的专业人员承担，而当时严重缺乏此类人员。编辑认为我们可以利用师范学校对民众开展健康教育来弥补这个缺口。一位从事卫生的官员在《丙寅周刊》上建议：

此类从业者"应为好的医学院的毕业生；接受过公共卫生方面的专业训练；熟知当地卫生状况；具有良好的品格；同时兼具专业能力和领导品质"。

该官员进一步指出：

"缺乏健康知识是一个普遍的问题，也是推进公共卫生管理

Municipality has both high and ordinary normal schools, which are the best places for systematic health education. An important duty of the health officer is to train teachers and those preparing to be teachers. When young students have been trained by competent teachers with the proper teaching material, they will be educated from the standpoint of personal health and public health. Only then can the Public Health Administration advance satisfactorily.[21]

Editorial attention was also given to persuading readers that public health is a national asset:

Statistic[al] evidence shows clearly the relationship between health and productivity. People do not appreciate the economic value of health, but health can be shown as a great economic asset for a nation whose level of productivity is pitifully low.

It is easy to understand the economic value of a working individual in relation to his family, but it is hard to visualize the economic value of community health to the entire nation. ... In our country, the number of deaths due to preventable disease is estimated to be as high as 6 million per year. Cases of illness that could have been prevented accounted for almost 2 million. The economic loss calculated even at the present level of productivity must be enormous.

If infectious diseases such as typhoid fever, tuberculosis, diphtheria, and tetanus could be prevented, many lives would be saved, and socio-economic loss would be greatly reduced. ... So if our government and our people appreciate the objectives and techniques of preventive medicine, and practice them through organized community efforts, it would contribute to the prosperity of our country. The economic value of health is enormous, and requires much study to elucidate its significance.[22]

的巨大障碍。北京市云集了许多高等和中等的师范学校，而这些学校则是进行系统地开展健康教育的绝佳阵地。卫生官员的重要职责之一是培训教师和准备成为教师的人员。当年轻的学生经过有能力的教师采用适当教材进行培训之后，他们将有望从个人健康和公共卫生两方面获得教益。只有遵循此径，公共卫生管理才能得以稳步推进。"

编辑部还在周刊中不断告知读者，公共卫生是国家的宝贵财富。

统计学证据已清晰地表明了健康和生产力之间的关系。人们并不能理解健康的经济价值，但事实上，对于一个生产力水平极低的国家而言，健康可作为一种巨大的经济资源。

民众很容易理解一位劳动力对其家庭经济的价值，却难以充分理解民众健康对整个国家的经济价值。在我国，每年因可预防疾病而死亡的人数估计高达 600 万，其中，可预防疾病的患者高达近 200 万。即使按目前的生产力水平计算，其带来的经济损失也极为巨大。

如果伤寒、肺结核、白喉和破伤风等传染病能够得以预防，则大多数患者的生命将得以挽救，社会经济损失也将大为减少……如果我们的政府和人民了解预防医学的目的和技术，并通过组织社区的力量来进行实践，将促进我国的繁荣发展。健康带来的经济价值将无比巨大，需开展大量的研究来充分阐明其意义。

Finally, but perhaps most important of all, the Binying Weekly stressed the requirement for a spirit of social responsibility and of personal sacrifice among members of the medical profession. In one article the editor noted that he, too, like everyone else, had lacked the appropriate attitude when entering the field:

When I began to study medicine, I considered the duty of the medical profession to be "hanging up shingles" and prescribing drugs for patients.

(But) at 25, I have come to believe that medicine is not a profession over and above society. It is only a part of social enterprise. This seems to be a change of personal attitude on my part. For myself, without this change, I never would have decided to shift my direction of clinical medicine to social medicine and village life; and I would not discuss rural health with my readers.

For the last two years, I have believed that health without education cannot be practiced effectively and education without health is in vain.[23]

The Binying Society felt the need not only to popularize medical knowledge but also to help medical schools draw closer to society... through this weekly, the medical profession is expected to develop the real spirit of modern medicine, which includes correct diagnosis, treatment, and extension of preventive measures. It should also try to extend the use of various diagnostic techniques... Medical students should cultivate a spirit of sacrifice so as to protect the people's health. The government must take responsibility to support them especially since public health personnel should be employed in government institutions... We as students of medicine have to broaden our vision and do our best to advocate the justified claim of the people for protection of their health.[24]

最后，也许是最重要的，《丙寅周刊》强调了医疗从业人员的社会责任感和个人牺牲精神的要求。在一篇文章中，编辑指出，与其他医学生一样，他在初入医学之门时也缺乏相应的态度：

最初踏入医海之路时，我曾认为医学的职责就是挂牌开诊和为患者开药方。

然而，25 岁后，我开始逐渐意识到，医学并非一个凌驾于社会之上的职业，它只是社会事业的组成部分之一。这似乎是我个人态度的转变。就我个人而言，如果未曾经历这样的态度转变，我将永远不会立志将临床医学的学习转变为社会医学和农村生活；我也不会与我的读者讨论农村卫生问题。

在最近的两年里，我开始越来越笃定地相信，缺乏教育的卫生实践是无法发挥作用的，而缺乏卫生实践的教育也是徒劳无益的。

我们感到丙寅医学社的使命不仅仅是普及健康知识，还需要：帮助医学院校与社会紧密联系。通过该周刊，期望医学界树立现代医学的真正精神，包括正确诊断、治疗和扩展预防措施。该刊还将戮力扩大各种诊断技术的使用范围。应着力培养医学生具有献身的精神，以担负起保卫民众健康的责任。政府也必须承担其为医学生提供支持的职责，包括支持受雇于政府机构中的公共卫生人员。作为从事医学专业的学生，必须拓宽我们的视野，尽心竭力支持民众对保护自身健康的合理要求。

In another article, we noted:

In recent years, our country has suffered from internal and external troubles and people of all walks of life could not do their business peacefully. Our country is in danger. In the field of medicine, many returned students from Germany and America are in private practice. Some young doctors consider private practice as only a means to serve rich people and yet they still think they are not depending upon others to make a living. They are not trying to adapt what they have learned from abroad to our own conditions, showing that they do not truly appreciate the spirit of modern medicine. In particular they do not feel the responsibility for educating the younger generation in the proper way.[25]

From the standpoint of progressive thinking, the work of the society is of historic interest. Its record attests to what a few inspired young persons could accomplish at a time when the medical community as a whole was marked by inertia. That may be why, twenty five years later, Ho Chen, Vice-Minister of Health in the newly established People's Republic of China, commented to me in his office during the first national conference on health: "We know of your work in the past and look forward to your cooperation."

Nonetheless, a few decades later the Binying Society and its work seemed to have faded into oblivion. Personal collections of the supplement were largely destroyed during the Cultural Revolution. Only one complete set remained in the National Library at Beijing. Many of the original members were deceased, and few traces remained to alert scholars writing about the PUMC to the dedicated effort a few students had engaged in voluntarily, at considerable sacrifice of time and energy, to educate the public in health matters.

另一篇文章中，我们提到：

近年来，我国遭遇内忧外患，各行各业的民众都处于风雨飘摇之中。我们的国家正处于危难之中。就医学领域而言，许多从德国和美国回来的学生都开办了私人诊所。一些年轻医生认为私人诊所仅仅是权贵阶层服务的手段，但即使这样，他们仍然认为自己并非依靠别人来安身立命。他们并未将其国外所学与我国国情相结合，这也表明其并未真正领会现代医学的精神。最令人唏嘘不已的是，他们甚至未曾认识到自己有责任以适当的方式教育年轻一代。

从进步思想的角度来看，丙寅医学社所做出的贡献尤具历史意义。丙寅医学社的记录向后人表明，在整个医学界因缺乏活力而停滞不前之时，数位忧国忧民的年轻医学生曾齐心协力为改善民众健康奉献一己之力。源于此，时隔 25 年后，在第一届全国卫生工作会议期间，中华人民共和国卫生部副部长贺诚在其办公室对我说："我们知道您过去的工作，期望与您合作。"

尽管如此，几十年后，丙寅医学社及其所付出的贡献似乎已逐步湮灭在历史的洪流之中。副刊的个人收藏几乎损毁殆尽。目前仅存一套完整的资料保留在北京的国家图书馆。多位丙寅医学社的初创成员都已去世，仅留存寥寥痕迹，不断提醒撰写北京协和医学院相关历史的学者们关注那一道遥远的微光，彼时，数位忧国恤民的医学生齐聚一堂，敢为人先，自愿投入其自身大量时间和精力，为民众健康教育的促进奉献出自己的一份力量。

How much the Binying Society and its publications contributed to the reputation of the PUMC, therefore, is an open question. At a minimum, however, its existence may have helped later generations to see that the school was far more than a mere philanthropic institution populated by a community of scholars interested only in technical excellence. It offered evidence of concern with the broad concept of human welfare as well, requiring the support of the founders as well as the motivation of a few idealistic students to keep it going over quite a few years.

　　虽然丙寅医学社及其出版物对协和医学院的声誉究竟带来了多大贡献，仍需等待时间去回答。然而，丙寅医学社的存在至少让后辈们看到，学校的性质远不止是仅由秉持技术为先理念的学者群体所组成的慈善机构，丙寅医学社的存在也是医学界关注人类福祉这一广泛概念的证据，当然，这一倡议不仅需要初创者给予支持，还需心怀抱负的学生们持续推动，以使其在未来相当长的时间内恒久如常地发光发热。

译者：刘振谧，杨阳

Chapter 3

Pioneering in Rural Health Development

In the early 1930s, fresh from graduate study in the United States and Germany, I finally had an opportunity to experiment on a health system to reach the villagers. I was invited to become director of the Department of Rural Health of the Mass Education Movement (MEM), a privately sponsored experimental program aimed at improving rural life in China by nurturing self-reliance among the peasants through popular education and other reform measures.

The MEM operated in various parts of the country. Its headquarters, however, were in Dingxian, a rural district and town of the same name, less than 100 miles from Beijing. I worked at Dingxian from 1932 to 1938, developing the health program of the movement in close association with its founder, James Y. C. Yen.

With respect to medical relief and health protection, rural China presented a bleak picture. Communicable disease was widespread, death rates were high, and life expectancy was short. Hospital- and clinic-centered missionary medicine had had little impact. Traditional practitioners, relying mainly on herbs, provided essentially the only available form of medical relief. A sense of the importance of cleanliness and sanitation was conspicuously absent, even among the few rural inhabitants who had some sort of education.

第3章

农村卫生发展的先驱

20世纪30年代初，我刚从美国和德国的研究生院毕业，终于有机会在农村进行卫生系统试验。我应邀成为平民教育运动农村卫生处的主任，这是一个私人赞助的试验项目，旨在通过普及教育和其他改革措施培养农民的自力更生能力，从而改善中国农村的生活水平。

平民教育运动在全国各地开展活动。然而，它的总部位于离北京不到200公里的河北定县。定县是一个县镇同名的农村地区。1932年至1938年，我在定县工作，与平民教育运动的创始人晏阳初密切合作，开展平民教育运动健康项目。

在医疗救助和卫生防护方面，中国农村呈现出一片惨淡景象。当时的中国农村传染性疾病广泛流行，患者死亡率高，预期寿命短。以医院和诊所为中心的西方医学作用甚微。主要依靠中草药的传统医学基本上提供了唯一可用的医疗救助形式。即使在少数受过某种教育的农民中，也明显缺乏对清洁和环境卫生重要性的认识。

The MEM had begun simply as a popular education program, but it soon became evident that increasing literacy alone would do little to raise the standard of living. Accordingly, the program expanded as it matured, developing an integrated, multifaceted approach to rural reconstruction based on correlated programs for social change in related areas of village life. From education it moved quite naturally into agriculture and from there into health. As it undertook an increasing number of measures essentially in the public domain, the MEM tried to strengthen its relationship to central and district authorities so as to build up their cooperation and to develop a sense of government responsibility in these areas.

My particular task was to devise, through experimentation, a model system affording health protection and modern medical relief to rural Chinese, suitable for adoption in any one of the country's numerous and diverse rural districts. Nothing of the sort had been contemplated, much less tried, before. Not only was there no previous experience to guide us but also the paucity of resources in the rural areas, both economic and technical, taxed our inventiveness to the hilt.

Notwithstanding the difficulties, hard work and sacrifice were rewarded with success. By 1934, little over two years after beginning our work, we had developed a systematic rural health care organization so well regarded that the new central government in Nanjing had recommended its adoption throughout the entire country. By 1937, when hostilities with Japan forced us to cease operations, we had worked out further refinements in the system and had been operating a rural field training site for medical and nursing students for several years. More than a few international health leaders had come to Dingxian to observe our work.

In devising that first systematic rural health organization, we had been careful to avoid simply copying what the missionaries had done

平民教育运动开始时只是作为一个大众教育项目，但很快人们就发现，仅仅提高认知并不能提高生活水平。因此，随着项目的成熟，该项目不断扩大，发展出一种综合的、多层面的农村重建方法，该方法基于农村生活相关领域的社会变革相关项目。它很自然地从教育转向农业，再从农业转向卫生。由于它采取了越来越多的属于公共领域的措施，平民教育运动试图加强与中央和地方政府的联系，以建立与他们之间的合作，并促进了政府在这些领域发挥职能责任。

我的具体任务是通过实验，设计出一个为中国农村提供健康保障和现代医疗救治的模式系统，适合在全国众多的和多样化的农村地区中采用。以前没有人考虑过这种情况，更没有人尝试过。我不仅没有前人的经验可以借鉴，而且农村地区经济和技术都资源匮乏，给我们带来了极大的挑战。

尽管困难重重，但艰苦工作和牺牲得到了回报。到 1934 年，也就是我们开始工作两年多的时候，我们已经成功建立了一个系统性的农村卫生机构，得到了很好的评价，以至南京中央政府建议在全国推广。到 1937 年，在日本侵略战争迫使我们停止了工作之前，我们已对这个系统进行了进一步改进，并为医学和护理专业的学生开设了一个现场教学基地，这一基地存在数年之久。我们还接待了多位国际卫生领导人来定县视察我们的工作。

在设计第一个系统性的农村卫生机构时，我们小心翼翼地避免简单照搬传教士在中国城市的做法。我们确信如果这样做，将

in urban China. That, we were convinced, would have been a grave error. Missionary medicine, after all, had evolved under conditions very different from those in rural China. Its accent on private practice and hospital- and clinic-centered practice met the needs of a privileged urban elite that shared something in common with Western society but not those of the great mass of villagers.

Our system, a versatile one that could be adapted to varying social, economic, and regional conditions, differed from the missionary model in several crucial respects. It addressed the problems of an impoverished, ill-educated, and predominantly agricultural society. It focused on the concerns of not individual patients, but entire communities, making their economic limitations its first consideration. Our rural health system also provided the benefits of advanced medical knowledge not only to a tiny segment of society, but to a vast rural population, which it linked for the first time to key centers of scientific medicine in the cities.

PRELIBERATION CHINA: 1928 to 1937

While infighting among warlords had prevailed in North China, concurrently in South China, two groups had sought to unify and stabilize the country under their own authority: The Guomindang party, led until his death in 1925 by Sun Yat-sen, and the Chinese Communist party (CCP) founded in 1921 chiefly by leading scholars and activists of the May Fourth Movement. Befriended by the Soviet Union, the Guomindang and the CCP had formed a revolutionary alliance that from a base in Guangzhou for a time had imposed a modicum of unity in South China.

Like many other young people at that time, we medical students in Beijing were fed up with the constant struggle among the warlords and hoped for their defeat. We believed that China must be unified, and that Sun Yat-sen offered a leadership that would be concerned with the

是一个严重的错误。传教医学毕竟是在与中国农村大不相同的条件下发展起来的。它强调私人诊所以及以医院和诊所为中心，满足了与西方社会有共同之处的特权城市精英的需求，而不是专注于满足广大村民的需求。

我们的体系是多功能的，它可以适应不同的社会、经济和地区条件，在几个关键方面与传教士模式不同。它解决了贫穷、受教育程度低和以农业为主的社会问题。它关注的不是个体患者的问题，而是整个群体的问题，将他们的经济条件差作为首要考虑因素。我们的农村卫生体系不仅为社会上的少数人提供了先进的医学知识，也为广大的农村人口提供了医疗照护，它首次将农村人口与城市的重要现代医学中心联系起来。

解放前的中国：1928 年至 1937 年

在华北军阀混战时期，在华南，有两个党派试图在自己的势力下统一和稳定国家：国民党一直由孙中山领导，直到 1925 年孙中山逝世；共产党由五四运动的主要学者和活动家于 1921 年创立。在苏联的帮助下，国共两党结成了革命联盟，以广州为根据地，一度在华南地区实现了小范围的统一。

和当时其他许多年轻人一样，我们这些在北京的医学生对军阀之间的不断斗争感到厌烦，希望他们被打败。我们相信，中国必定统一，而孙中山提出建立一个关心人民福祉的领导层。基于

welfare of the people. Our high expectations were based on his political philosophy, which centered on 'Three Principles of the People": "people's rights," "democracy," and "people's livelihood."

Regarding the tie between the Guomindang and the CCP, we knew that the latter had been organized in 1921, and that it conducted activities in many cities, including Shanghai, Wuhan, and even Beijing. We were aware, too, that the Soviet Union was supporting the CCP rather than the alliance as such; however, we had little knowledge of ideological differences between the CCP and the Guomindang. All that we were conscious of was that the two groups seemd to be working effectively together in the interest of the country, and so we supported the alliance.

Sun Yat-sen died in 1925, however, and after his military commander, Chiang Kai-shek, launched a successful expedition into central China, our attitude toward the Guomindang began to change. For the success of the drive into central and then North China enabled Chiang Kai-shek to broaden his personal power base, whereupon he turned on his former Communist allies, and with all the forces at his command. After bitter fighting, the Communists eventually withdrew from their urban enclaves, regrouping along the border of Hunan and Jiangxi Provinces, where they struggled to maintain a territorial foothold in various "revolutionary bases" or "liberated regions." In 1928 Chiang Kai-shek proclaimed his authority over the entire country and established a new central government in Nanjing.

Whatever expectations early supporters of the Guomindang party might have had that a Nationalist government would govern in accordance with the Three Principles were quickly dashed. Leaders gave only lip service to the formula on which the party had been founded, and as far as the needs of rural China were concerned, authorities in Nanjing showed little concern. The only departure from this pattern appeared after 1932, in the aftermath of a series of defeats suffered by Guomindang troops in unsuccessful attempts to wipe out the remaining pockets of CCP strength in rural areas. This seems to have produced the conclusion at the apex of power that some concessions might have to be made for the sake of stability in rural areas.

他的政治思想，其核心是三民主义——民族、民权和民生，我们对此抱有高度期望。

关于国共两党之间的联系，我们知道，共产党在 1921 年已经成立，并在许多城市开展活动，包括上海、武汉，甚至是北京。我们也知道，苏联支持的是中国共产党；但是，我们对共产党和国民党之间信念上的差异知之甚少。我们所知道的是，这两个党派在为国家的利益而通力合作，我们支持联盟。

然而，孙中山于 1925 年逝世，在继任的军事统帅蒋介石成功远征华中后，我们对国民党的态度开始发生变化。进军华中和华北的成功使蒋介石扩大了他的个人权力基础，于是他调遣了所有力量对付他以前的盟友。经过艰苦的战斗，共产党最终撤出了城市领地，沿着湖南和江西的边界重新集结，在那里他们努力维持各种革命根据地或解放区。1928 年，蒋介石宣布在南京组建了一个新的中央政府。

国民党早期支持者对国民党政府按照"三民主义"治国抱有期望，但是很快就破灭了。就中国农村的需要而言，南京当局几乎没有表现出什么关心。唯一与这种模式不同的是在 1932 年之后，当时国民党军队试图围剿在农村地区的共产党，却遭遇了一系列失败。国民党最高权力层得出了一个结论：为了农村地区的稳定，可能不得不做出一些让步。

In one manifestation of this new strategy, the National Economic Council, under the direction of T. V. Soong, brought in several League of Nations experts to survey the situation in rural areas. One of them was Andrija Stampar, an internationally known public health leader, who visited us at Dingxian. Stampar apparently did apprise the group of the urgency of nutrition, sanitation, and health care needs in the villages, although what his specific recommendations might have been I do not know.

THE SHAPING OF HEALTH POLICY AND ADMINISTRATION

A new constitution called for the establishment of five yuan, or public bodies, including an executive yuan encompassing various ministries to carry out administrative functions. From the standpoint of the medical profession, the establishment of a Ministry of Health—the first central health administration the country had ever had—was marked progress.

It soon became clear, however, that this had been a more or less perfunctory step. The portfolio of the ministry was given to a warlord as a token of appreciation for his support of the party. Party leaders took little interest in the new agency and did not significantly participate in its activities.

In a sense, their indifference turned out to be a blessing in disguise, for the new minister looked to the PUMC and John Grant for help in formulating evolving health policy and in staffing his new agency. Grant was able to place several highly competent people in key positions. J. Heng Liu, for example, director of the PUMC hospital, was asked to serve as vice minister. Grant also guided the establishment of new municipal and province-level health administrations, placing many former students in these agencies as well.

这一新战略的一个表现是，国家经济委员会在宋子文的指导下，请来了几位国际联盟的专家调查农村地区的情况。其中一位是国际知名的公共卫生领导人安准加·斯坦帕尔，他访问了定县。显然，斯坦帕尔确实向该小组通报了各村在营养、卫生和保健方面的迫切需求，但我并不知道他的具体建议是什么。

卫生政策和管理的形成

国民政府的新宪法要求建立五院制或公共机构，包括一个行政院，可以执行行政职能的各个部门。从医学界的角度来看，建立卫生部——我国有史以来第一个中央卫生管理机构是一个显著的进步。

然而，很快就可以看出，这或多或少是一个敷衍了事的步骤。卫生部部长职位被移交给了一位军阀，以"感谢"他对国民党的支持。国民党领导人对新机构兴趣不大，也没有大量参与其活动。

从某种意义上说，他们的漠不关心变成了塞翁失马焉知非福，因为这位新部长指望北京协和医学院和兰安生帮助他制定和完善卫生政策，并为他的新机构配备人员。因此，兰安生得以把几个极有能力的人安排到关键岗位上。例如，北京协和医学院附属医院的刘瑞恒主任被任命为副部长。兰安生还指导建立了新的省级和市级卫生行政部门，将许多其以前的学生安排在这些机构。

Through Grant's activities and those of other current and former students and faculty members, the Rockefeller Foundation and the PUMC were able to exercise a substantial influence on evolving health policy and administration. Ties between the college and the world beyond the campus compound expanded considerably as compared with the era of the warlords.

During the decade from 1928 to 1937 there was a considerable amount of progress in the development of urban health care facilities and training institutions. Central, provincial, and municipal authorities opened hospitals and clinics. Missionary hospitals and other care agencies remained on the scene. Medical education facilities flourished as government and private groups opened new training centers. Much of this new urban aggregate developed randomly, however, without benefit of systematic planning in respect to real needs and conditions.

There was slight progress in rural areas. After 1934, for example, a few county hospitals were established. My own appointment to oversee health affairs for the Rural Normal School Movement in Xiaozhuang, too, resulted from the instigation of the central Ministry of Health. By and large, however, rural areas received little attention.

Graduate training in public health abroad was made available to a number of present and future health administrators through a program of government-sponsored fellowships and, at the instigation of John Grant, by the Rockefeller Foundation. Between 1929 and 1942, two dozen PUMC graduates were selected and sent to schools of public health in the United States. In 1930/31 I was able to complete a year's graduate work at the Harvard University School of Public Health and to pursue further work at Das Reichshaus für Hygienische Volksbelehrung in Dresden.

For a student like myself, coming from a country whose conditions were very unlike those in the United States, the Harvard experience had both positive and negative aspects. Various teachers—including Milton

140

通过兰安生的活动以及其他在校和以前师生的参与，洛克菲勒基金会和北京协和医学院能够对卫生政策制定和行政管理带来实质性的影响。与军阀时代相比，学院与校园外的联系大大加强。

在 1928 年至 1937 年的十年间，城市卫生保健设施和培训机构取得了相当大的发展壮大。中央、省和市当局开办了医院和诊所。传教士医院和其他护理机构仍然存在。随着政府和私人团体开设新的培训中心，医学教育蓬勃发展。然而，这些新的培训中心的发展大多是随机的，没有根据实际需要和条件进行有系统的规划。

同时，农村地区略有进展。例如，1934 年之后，建立了一些县级医院。我自己被任命监督晓庄的农村师范学校运动的卫生事务，这也是在国民党中央卫生部的推动下进行的。然而，总的来说，农村地区仍很少受到关注。

通过政府资助的奖学金计划以及在兰安生的倡导下，洛克菲勒基金会为一些现在和未来的卫生管理人员提供了国外公共卫生方面的研究生培训。1929 年至 1942 年期间，有二十几名北京协和医学院的毕业生被选送到美国的公共卫生学校。1930—1931 学年，我在哈佛大学公共卫生学院完成了一年的研究生课程，并在德累斯顿的国家卫生研究所继续深造。

对于像我这样一个来自条件与美国非常不同的国家的学生来说，哈佛的经历既有积极的一面，也有消极的一面。不同的老

J. Rosenau, Edwin D. Wilson, and at the Massachusetts Institute of Technology, Clair E. Turner—exposed me to analytical and theoretical material that exerted an important influence on my thinking as a public health specialist. The field training was disappointing, however. It consisted mainly of superficial observation, without much student participation, a decided contrast to the highly motivating, hands-on exposure to the health problems of ordinary people we had had at the Peking First Health Station.

In any event, to return to medical affairs in China under Nationalist rule, in 1928 Robert S. K. Lim was elected president of the Chinese Medical Association (CMA). By that time there was, to all intents and purposes, only this one association of modern physicians, rather than two competing groups, and from Lim's election forward, its leadership was dominated by Chinese nationals. Lim took over the CMA at a time when missionary influence in it was fading and, under his direction, its emphasis became scientific rather than chiefly social. Within a short time span, the CMA began to have a major impact on health policy and administration. By 1935, the CMA had 1,700 members.

Two types of individuals accounted for its expansive influence on public health in the 1928-1937 period: (1) medical scientists with a broad orientation, of the type represented by Lim, a British- educated physiologist; and (2) physicians specifically trained in public health, such as Dr P. Z. Jin. As noted, Lim was elected to the presidency in 1928. Japanese-trained Jin, who held a high-ranking post in the health ministry, was elected to the presidency in 1935. Both men played prominent roles in shaping health policy and administration through activities both within and outside the CMA. The country was fortunate to have had such public health- minded leadership at that time, for without them the influential CMA would have been much more concerned with pure technology, contributing very little to the more important topics of medical education and health protection.

师——包括米尔顿·罗森诺，埃德温·威尔森以及麻省理工学院的克莱尔·特纳让我接触到了相关理论知识，掌握了分析方法，对我作为一名公共卫生专家的思考产生了重要影响。然而，现场培训令人失望。它主要包括粗略的观察，没有太多的学生参与，这与我们在一所能接触到普通人（其具有健康问题的高度积极性和实践性）形成鲜明对比。

1928 年，林可胜被选为中华医学会会长。从那时起，中华医学会的目标和目的，表明其现代医生协会，而不是两个相互竞争的团体，而且从林可胜当选开始，其领导层就由中国人主导。林可胜接手中华医学会时，传教士的影响正在消退。在他的指导下，中华医学会的重点从社会转向了科学。在很短的时间内，中华医学会开始对卫生政策和管理产生重大影响。到 1935 年，中华医学会已有 1700 名成员。

1928 年到 1937 年，两类人对公共卫生产生了广泛的影响：一是具有广泛取向的医学科学家，以在英国接受教育的生理学家林可胜为代表；二是在公共卫生方面受过专门培训的医生，如金宝善博士。如前所述，林可胜在 1928 年当选为会长。曾在日本接受教育的金宝善曾在卫生部担任要职，并于 1935 年当选为会长。两人都通过中华医学会内、外的活动在塑造卫生政策和管理方面发挥了突出作用。国家很幸运当时有这样的公共卫生意识的领导，因为如果没有他们，有影响力的中华医学会将更多地关注纯技术，而对医学教育和健康保护这些更重要的话题贡献就会甚微。

As it was, they infused the association with their public health-oriented outlook. A public health committee became active in prevention of tuberculosis, venereal disease, and cholera and in promotion of maternal and child health. There was some interest in rural health and issues in medical education, in which I actively participated. There were actions to press the membership to support the central Ministry of Health in implementing various health measures. The committee also developed criteria for evaluation of the evolving municipal health administrations.

The shift within the organization to a more professional emphasis was further evidenced in the scholarly upgrading of the association's publication, The Chinese Medical Journal. In part the more scholarly content of the journal reflected the high quality of research by students at the PUMC, who contributed quite a few articles. The PUMC staff members also exercised an influence on medical affairs at that time through the CMA and the journal.

Nurses were also becoming influential health activists. The 1930 CMA meeting was held jointly with the Chinese Nursing Association. By this time 32 nurses had completed training at the PUMC, and 200 attended the joint meeting. By now nurses were so involved with public health activity that collaboration with them was seen as an important step forward, indicating growing recognition of the profession and a trend toward upgrading quality.

All told, during this period, the impact of the activities of physicians, nurses, and academicians associated with the CMA on public health and medical affairs was very strong. This circumstance was attributable in part to the new, businesslike and scientific orientation of the professional organization and also to generalized close collaboration with the government.

事实上，他们把以公共卫生为导向的观点注入了中华医学会。公共卫生委员会在预防结核病、性病和霍乱以及促进母婴健康方面发挥了积极作用。人们对农村卫生和医学教育方面的问题有一定的兴趣，我也积极参与其中。我们采取了一些行动，敦促成员支持中央卫生部执行各种卫生措施。委员会还制定了对促进城市卫生管理部门发展的评估标准。

协会内部向更注重专业的转变，体现在协会出版的《中华医学杂志》的学术升级上。该杂志在学术内容上反映了北京协和医学院学生的高质量研究，他们贡献了相当多的文章。北京协和医学院的工作人员也通过中华医学会和杂志对当时的医疗事务产生了影响。

护士也正在成为有影响力的卫生积极分子。1930 年的中华医学会会议是与中国护理协会联合举办的。此时，32 名护士已经完成了在北京协和医学院的培训，200 名护士参加了联合会议。护士们已经深入地参与到公共卫生活动中，与他们的合作被认为是向前迈出的重要一步，这表明人们对护士职业的认可度越来越高，并有提升质量的趋势。

总之，在这一时期，与中华医学会有关的医生、护士和院士的活动对公共卫生和医疗事务的影响非常大。这种情况部分归因于专业组织的创新、务实与科学，也归因于与政府的广泛密切合作。

Whatever doubts the CMA or other agencies working for social change at that time may have had regarding the ruling clique in the Guomindang, they were compelled to work closely with, as well as within, the bureaucracy. Otherwise they could not have accomplished much, for in that period a private organization without connections in the government counted for very little. Before 1928 such recommendations on public health as the CMA had made to government authorities had usually been ignored, whereas in the 1928- 1937 period, they were more usually accepted and implemented.

A positive step in the planning area in the 1928-1937 period was the formation by representatives of the Ministry of Health and the Ministry of Education of a Joint Commission for Medical Education. Its aim was to bring about some uniformity in the highly diverse medical training programs of various private and public medical colleges. The commission eventually recommended a standardized six-year medical curriculum, including a one-year internship in all medical colleges. This appeared to be quite adequate for the country at the time.

While the trends in health policy and administration that evolved in the Nanjing decade were generally favorable to long-term national well-being—although the rural population had as yet benefited little from the process—in one respect these trends were not favorable. The adverse relationship between some members of the modern medical community and traditional scholar-physicians escalated to new heights after World War I and erupted into open controversy during the 1920s and early 1930s.

The struggle between the two systems of medicine had become quite fierce even before the Guomindang had established itself in Nanjing. As noted, a minority of returned students and missionary medical supporters, convinced that traditional medicine was worthless, had organized a systematic campaign for its abolition. In the mid-1920S they had written scathing attacks in the press and had pressed through the CMA for measures to curtail its practice or teaching.

146

无论当时中华医学会或其他致力于社会变革的机构对国民党的统治集团有什么疑虑，他们都不得不与官僚机构密切合作，并在官僚机构内部开展工作。否则，他们不可能取得多大成就，因为在那个时期，没有政府人脉的私人组织是微不足道的。1928 年以前，中华医学会向政府当局提出的公共卫生建议通常被忽视，而在 1928 年到 1937 年，这些建议通常是更多地被接受和执行了。

1928 年到 1937 年，规划领域的一个积极举措是由卫生部和教育部的代表组成了一个医学教育联合委员会。其目的是在各种私立和公立医学院高度多样化的医学培训项目中实现某种统一。该委员会最终建议采用标准化的六年制医学课程，包括在所有医学院进行为期一年的实习。这对当时的国家来说，还是很恰当的。

虽然在南京十年间形成的卫生政策和管理的趋势总体上有利于国家的长期福祉——尽管农村人口还没有从这一进程中得到什么好处，但在一个方面这些趋势并不有利。第一次世界大战后，现代医学界的一些成员与中医之间的不利关系升级到新的高度，并在 20 世纪 20 年代和 30 年代初爆发了公开的争论。

甚至在国民党于南京成立政府之前，两种医学体系之间的斗争就已经相当激烈了。如前所述，少数归国留学生和传教士的医学支持者坚信中医毫无价值，他们组织了一场系统的运动，要求废除中医。在 20 世纪 20 年代中期，他们在媒体上发表了严厉的抨击文章，并敦促中华医学会采取措施限制中医行医或教学。

In 1928 they found some allies in the new Nationalist health bureacracy who shared their point of view, and were willing to further it through the promulgation of official rulings. For example, the ministries of health and of education issued a joint regulation decreeing that traditional practitioners must term their patient care facilities "clinics" rather than hospitals and their training institutions "courses" rather than schools of medicine. The regulations seemed to be aimed at diminishing the credibility of traditional medicine.

The regulations aroused strong resentment from scholar-physicians who, as a group, had important political connections of their own in the government and who, because of their high social standing and press connections, were in a favorable position to mold public opinion. They immediately organized a protest meeting in Shanghai that drew a large attendance from many provinces. The conferees agreed to send a petition of protest to the Guomindang leadership and to dispatch a delegation to meet with officials of the central executive yuan in Nanjing. One of their most powerful backers was Chen Guofu, friend and confidante of Chiang Kai-shek and a powerful figure in the Guomindang.

The long-term impact of the organization of scholar-physicians in their collective interest was substantial. The most significant outcome was the organization in 1930 of a Bureau of Traditional Medicine on a level with the Ministry of Health in the central government. Another important result was impetus given to the establishment of new institutions providing formal training in traditional medicine.

STEPS TOWARD RURAL HEALTH ORGANIZATION

The emergence of central, provincial, and municipal health administrations and facilities and the expansion of hospitals, clinics, and teaching institutions during this period was an essentially urban

1928 年，他们在新的国民党卫生部中找到了一些与他们观点相同的盟友，并试图通过颁布官方制度来推进自己的观点。例如，卫生部和教育部发布了一项联合条例，规定中医必须将其为患者提供护理的场所称为"诊所"而不是"医院"，以及将其培训机构称为"课程"而不是医学院。这些规定看来是为了削弱传统医学的可信度。

这些规定引起了中医的强烈不满，他们作为一个群体，在政府中拥有自己的重要政治关系，而且由于他们的社会地位高，与新闻界有联系，在塑造公众舆论方面处于有利的地位。他们立即在上海组织了抗议集会，吸引了许多省份的人参加。与会代表同意向国民党领导层递交抗议书，并派代表团到南京与中央行政院官员会面。他们最有力的支持者之一是陈果夫，陈果夫是蒋介石的挚友，也是国民党的一个重要人物。

中医组织对自己集体利益的长期影响是巨大的。最重要的成果是在 1930 年成立了与中央政府卫生部同级的中医药管理局。另一个重要成果是推动了提供中医正规培训的新机构的建立。

迈向农村卫生组织的步伐

这一时期，中央、省、市卫生行政部门和设施的出现以及医院、诊所和教学机构的扩大，基本上是一种城市内的现象。在我国的其他地方，实际上并没有公共卫生组织。事实上，城市卫生服务

phenomenon. In the rest of the country, to all intents and purposes, there was no public health organization. In fact, the expansion of health services in the cities only served to highlight the gap between urban and rural China, which was by far the most important of the many lines of social division prevailing in the country at that time.

Traditionally the rural population had been left more or less to fend for itself and for better or worse, it was county officialdom, rather than the provincial or central administration, that touched the lives of the millions of peasants. Above that level, the government had been too remote to concern itself with the people. Below it, it had been too weak. Even after the Republican Revolution of 1911, provincial governors continued to depend on district magistrates to maintain order and collect taxes.

The magistrates often ruled harshly, prizing obedience, and rarely showing interest in the improvement of the lives of their constituents. Peasants were left to educate themselves as best they could, and illiteracy was considered an individual problem. Peasants worked hard year after year but earned barely enough to support their families. Their fate lay in the hands of the district magistrate and the local landed gentry and as far as they were concerned, could be ameliorated only through prayers to various gods for intervention. In most of China, the lives of the peasants had a feudal quality, no less marked by poverty and disease at the time I went to work in Dingxian than in previous centuries.

There was no way of knowing what health conditions were like at that time in the few Communist-controlled areas. As far as the Communist fighting forces were concerned, the primary requirement was surgical care for the wounded. Also, it was critical to the fortunes of the CCP to prevent the outbreak of a devastating epidemic, which could bring a serious setback to the Revolution. In 1931, therefore, to assure an adequate number of medical personnel, the fighting forces organized their own medical school.

的扩大只会凸显中国城乡之间的差距，这是当时中国普遍存在的许多社会分界线中最重要的一条。

传统上，农村群众或多或少都是自谋生路，无论好坏，影响千百万农民生活的是县政府，而不是省级或中央政府。在县政府层面以上，政府一直过于遥远，无法做到真正关心农民。而县政府以下层面则太弱。即使在 1911 年的辛亥革命之后，各省省长仍继续依赖县级行政长官来维持秩序和税收。

县级行政长官的统治往往很严厉，崇尚服从，很少对改善百姓的生活表现出兴趣。农民只能尽其所能地接受教育，而文盲则被视为个人问题。农民年复一年地努力工作，但挣的钱仅够维持家庭生计。他们的命运掌握在地方长官和当地地主贵族的手中，而他们认为，只有向诸神祈祷才能得到改善。在中国大部分地区，农民的生活都带有封建性质，在我去定县工作时，他们的贫穷程度和疾病特征与前几个世纪相差无异。

我们无从得知当时在共产党领导的地区的卫生健康状况如何。就共产党的战斗部队而言，首要的要求是对伤员进行外科治疗。另外，防止毁灭性的流行病暴发至关重要，因为它可能给革命带来严重挫折。因此，1931 年，为了保证有足够数量的医务人员，共产党的战斗部队组建了自己的医学院。

Probably these medical personnel shared what resources could be spared with the local peoples. Most party members, including Mao Zedong himself, were of rural origin and understood the problems of the peasants on the basis of their own experience. Moreover, they valued good relations with the farmers, for the rural masses, rather than urban workers, were now seen as the future source of party strength.

It is only assumed that the CCP gave some medical assistance to the peasants in South China with whom they came in contact. It is well known, however, that in the area of North China to which the Communists repaired in 1936, they organized rural health care services in three provinces. By that time the Nanjing government had already recommended the Dingxian model as the prototype for systematic rural health organization around the country, but it is not known whether information about our innovative work was available in the party-controlled areas at that time.

Xiaozhuang and the Rural Normal Schools

The interlude between graduation from the PUMC in 1929 and the start of my work in Dingxian had included two professionally valuable experiences. One was the aforementioned academic year at Harvard for advanced public health studies in 1930/31. The other was an experience that preceded that, coming in 1929, immediately after graduation—my first full-time position in public health, when I served as Chief of the Xiaozhuang Rural Health Demonstration Program.

Like the MEM, the Rural Normal School Movement at Xiaozhuang was an ongoing popular education movement. Its founder, Tao Zhixing, was convinced, as was Jimmy Yen, of the need to educate the peasantry. Nothing, he thought, was more central to any attempt to improve their lives, and it was important, he believed, to integrate that education with the actual day-to-day realities of their lives. Whereas Yen focused on adult education, however, Tao believed in starting with children. Before

也许这些医务人员与当地农民分享了自己所能节省的资源。大多数共产党员，包括毛泽东主席本人，都是农民出身，他们可以根据自己的经验了解农民的问题。此外，他们重视与农民的良好关系，因为农村群众被视为共产党未来力量的源泉。

我们只能估计共产党给予他们有接触的华南地区的农民提供了一些医疗援助。1936 年，共产党人在华北地区的三个省组织了农村保健服务机构。当时，国民党南京政府已将定县模式作为全国系统农村卫生组织的样板，但我们不知道定县的创新工作是否也传到了共产党人领导的地区。

晓庄试验农村师范学校

从 1929 年北京协和医学院毕业到我开始在定县工作，其间有两段宝贵的职业经历。一个是前文提到的 1930—1931 学年，在哈佛参加高级公共卫生研究生培训。另一个是在这之前的经历。1929 年，我刚毕业不久在公共卫生领域获得的第一个全职职位，当时我担任了晓庄试验乡村师范学校项目的主任。

与平民教育运动一样，晓庄试验农村师范学校也是一场持续的民众教育运动。它的创始人陶知行和晏阳初一样，坚信有必要对农民进行教育。陶知行认为，没有什么比改善农民的生活更重要的了，而且他认为重要的是将教育与农民实际的日常现实生活相结合。晏阳初专注于成人教育，而陶知行则认为应从儿童开始。在此之前，必须对教师进行培训，因此陶知行开

this could be done, teachers had to be trained, so he began bv organizing a network of rural normal schools with affiliated primary schools where future teachers could practice their skills.

As a medical student interested in health education, I had found myself very interested in Tao's philosophy and activities, and as editor of The Binying Weekly I had written a number of articles calling attention to the Rural Normal School Movement. At the time, The Binying Weekly was being well received. We had drawn favorable response from many readers and no doubt had succeeded to some degree in making people more knowledgeable about medicine and disease. Nevertheless, I was beginning to think we needed to reach a larger audience and that, by whatever means we found of doing so, it should emphasize experimentation, demonstration, and popular participation. People should be able to actually see the benefits modern medicine could bring, rather than just reading about them.

In that context, the Rural Normal School Movement was of great interest as a potential vehicle for the education of a large, rural population in the basics of modern medical knowledge. A quotation from a 1929 editorial suggests its promise:

This... movement has attracted the attention of many people, as the education there is not limited to teaching children how to read, but teaching them how to live as well.

As Tao remarked to the editor:

Health is the starting point of life. Rural education should emphasize health protection. Primary schools and kindergartens should consider health as the most important part of education. If a child cannot live long and remain healthy, what is the use of education.

Educators like Dr. Tao Zhixing," I wrote, "know well how important health is for education. If teachers in the villages do not try hard to

始组织农村师范学校和附属小学网络，让未来的教师可以锤炼自己的技能。

作为一个对健康教育感兴趣的医学生，我发现自己对陶知行的哲学和活动非常感兴趣，作为《丙寅周刊》的编辑，我写了很多文章，呼吁大家关注晓庄试验农村师范学校运动。当时，《丙寅周刊》受到了广泛的欢迎。我们得到了许多读者的好评，无疑在一定程度上成功地让人们对医学和疾病有了更多的了解。然而，我开始认为我们需要接触到更多的受众，无论我们找到什么方法来做这件事，它都应该强调实验、示范和大众参与。人们应该能够真正看到现代医学带来的好处，而不仅仅是阅读。

在这方面，晓庄试验农村师范学校运动作为向广大农村人口提供现代医学基础知识教育的一种潜在工具，引起了人们极大的兴趣。1929 年的一篇社论这样描述它的前景：

这一运动吸引了许多人的注意，因为那里的教育不仅限于教孩子们如何阅读，而且还教他们如何生活。

正如陶知行对编辑所说的那样：

健康是生活的起点。农村教育应强调健康保护。小学和幼儿园应将健康视为教育的最重要部分。如果一个孩子不能活得长久并保持健康，那么教育又能起什么作用呢。

"像陶知行这样的教育家，"我写道，"深知健康对教育的重要性。如果农村教师不努力促进健康，农村健康的未来将没

promote health, the future of rural health would have no real foundation... Rural school teachers are persons directly responsible for rural health at a time when our government is unable to develop rural health in general.

Because of the respect I had for Tao, I welcomed the offer that I received after graduation in 1929 to develop a rural health demonstration program at Xiaozhuang. This was an early milestone in my career. The prevalence of conditions that could have been prevented or relieved by modern medical treatment among the children there impressed me very deeply.

Coming on the heels of my experience as a student taking the health survey in Tongxian, this rural health demonstration program reinforced my nascent sense of personal responsibility to the common people. I became increasingly concerned with the medical problems of the villagers, and I saw that I could do a great deal in the countryside with my valuable training. Possibly I could even accomplish more to improve the health of the people by remaining in a rural setting than by getting into urban health administration.

At Xiaozhuang, my approach to my work was premised on Tao's notion of integrating education with life reality and relied heavily on demonstration and participation. I provided the future teachers of primary schools with an introduction to the fundamentals of modern medicine, developing my own syllabus for the course. The emphasis was on prevention. They seemed to welcome this as an enrichment of their general educational background.

Far more engrossing to them, however, were the clinical sessions, where they observed me as I worked and often participated in what was taking place. We undertook a smallpox vaccination program that they heartily endorsed, knowing that the disease was often fatal or left survivors with ugly scars. They were amazed at my delivery of a dead fetus by means of decapitation. What may have impressed them most,

有真正的基础……在我国政府无法全面发展农村卫生事业的情况下，农村学校教师是农村卫生的直接责任人。"

出于对陶知行的尊重，我 1929 年毕业后欣然接受了在晓庄开办农村卫生示范项目的邀请。这是我职业生涯早期的一个里程碑。在农村，儿童中普遍存在着可以通过现代医疗预防或缓解的疾病，其流行情况和病情都给我留下了深刻的印象。

在我具有作为学生参加通县健康调查的经历之后，这个农村健康示范项目加强了我原已存在的对百姓的责任感。我越来越关心村民的医疗问题，我看到可以用我接受的宝贵培训在农村做很多事情。与进入城市卫生管理部门相比，我选择留在农村，我甚至可能在改善人民健康方面取得更大的成就。

在晓庄，我的工作方法是以陶知行的教育与生活现实相结合的思路为前提，并在很大程度上依赖于示范和参与。我为未来的小学教师介绍了现代医学基础知识，为课程制定了我自己的教学大纲，重点是预防疾病。我的课程很受欢迎，受训者认为这丰富了他们的教育背景。

然而，更让他们着迷的是临床治疗，他们除了在我工作时进行观察，还经常参与正在进行的工作。我们进行了一项天花疫苗接种计划，他们非常支持，因为他们知道这种疾病通常是致命的，或者会给幸存者留下丑陋的伤疤。他们对我用斩首的方式接生一个死胎感到惊讶。然而，给他们留下最深刻印象的是我设计的一

however, was a rather inventive method I devised to treat and prevent the recurrence of ringworm of the scalp, a commonplace problem among the primary-school children. The teachers were astonished at the results, and the students who suffered from it were very happy. They were rid of a condition that had produced an offensive odor, prejudicing the teachers and other students against them.

Besides the many conditions in Xiaozhuang that required the attention of a trained physician, however, I soon discovered that there were many other conditions against which action could be taken even in the absence of a trained physician. Teachers or others could be instructed in first aid. Habits of cleanliness could be impressed on the villagers. Vaccinations and disinfectants could be offered. Water supplies and sanitation could be improved. Observations on these matters at Xiaozhuang may have germinated the ideas I developed subsequently at Dingxian to train village health workers to take on some of these relatively simple tasks.

Dingxian and the Mass Education Movement

Before going to Xiaozhuang, and later to the United States for advanced public health training, l had become somewhat conversant with the history and objectives of the Mass Education Movement. John Grant had brought James Y. C. Yen to the PUMC to speak one evening, when I was still an undergraduate.

From my own reading, I knew that Yen, who had been educated at Yale University in the United States, had gone to France during World War I to serve as a YMCA aide among 160,000 or so Chinese contract workers recruited to augment the civilian labor force. The recruits were largely illiterate, but industrious, and eager to learn to read and write. So Yen devised a teaching method based on the use of 1,000 selected Chinese characters. Familiarity with these few basic characters, he believed, would enable the men to understand a simple newspaper article,

种相当有创意的方法，用于头皮癣的治疗和防止其复发，因为这是小学儿童中存在的一个普遍问题。老师们对这一结果颇感意外，而罹患该病的学生们则非常高兴。患儿摆脱了一种产生令人讨厌的气味、使老师和其他学生对他们产生偏见的疾病。

然而，除了晓庄的许多疾病需要训练有素的医生关注外，我很快发现，还有许多其他疾病，即使没有训练有素的医生，也可以对其采取措施。教师或其他人可以接受急救方面的指导。教师可以培养村民的清洁习惯，可以提供疫苗和消毒剂，可以敦促改善水供应和卫生设施。在晓庄对这些问题的观察，可能萌发了我后来在定县培养农村卫生工作者承担这些相对简单任务的想法。

定县与平民教育运动

在去晓庄之前以及后来去美国接受高级公共卫生培训之前，我对平民教育运动的历史和目标有了一定的了解。兰安生曾在一个晚上把晏阳初带到北京协和医学院演讲，当时我还在读大学。

通过读书，我了解到，曾在美国耶鲁大学接受教育的晏阳初在第一次世界大战期间前往法国，法国为增加平民劳动力而招募了 16 万左右的中国合同工，他担任基督教青年会助手。新劳工大多是文盲，但很勤奋，渴望学习阅读和写作。因此，晏阳初设计了一种基于使用 1000 个精选汉字的教学方法。他认为，熟悉这些基本的汉字，新劳工就能读懂报纸上一篇简单的文章，也能

to write letters home, and eventually to learn something through reading that could improve the quality of their lives. He called his text The One Thousand Characters.

On returning to China after the war, Yen was able to expand his literacy program, notwithstanding the fragmentation of the country under various regional military leaders whose cooperation he managed to obtain. By the early 1920s, the MEM had become a recognized national movement, with branches in all major cities. Given its essentially rural ethos, however, it was more appropriate for the movement to have a base in rural areas, so Yen moved to Dingxian, not far from Beijing. His organization collected support from sympathetic intellectuals, local officials, and the landed gentry. Also he secured partial funding from the Milbank Memorial Fund in the United States and numerous personal contacts at home and abroad.

Not long into his efforts in Dingxian, Yen began to question the impact of a program aimed at making the peasants literate, while ignoring their dire poverty, ill health, and other problems. "We can feed their minds, but not their stomachs," he lamented to a friend. Education, he soon concluded, must be tackled together with other facets of social work. He then started to plan for a broader social experiment, where an integrated program of reconstruction could be developed and tested under educated leadership. The MEM expanded into other realms—agriculture, transport, and the establishment of rural cooperatives.

With respect to health care, Yen sought the advice of the PUMC and John Grant, and to assure medical and nursing personnel for an intended health component, he spent time trying to motivate its students to work with the MEM after graduation. One evening in 1929, a small group of students gathered in the E ward of the hospital to hear Yen speak.

He opened by asserting that people are the foundation of a nation, and that national stability is dependent on their well-being. China's

写信回家，最终还能通过阅读学到一些东西，从而提高生活质量。他把他的文本称为《千字文》。

战后回到中国后，尽管在各个地区动荡不安，晏阳初还是扩大了他的扫盲项目。到 20 世纪 20 年代早期，平民教育运动已经成为公认的全国性运动，在所有主要城市都有分支机构。然而，考虑到其服务农村的本质，在农村地区建立根据地更为合适，因此晏阳初搬到了离北京不远的定县。他的组织得到了富有同情心的知识分子和地方达官贵族们的支持。此外，他还从美国的米尔班克纪念基金和国内外的众多个人联系人那里获得了部分资助。

在定县开展工作不久，晏阳初就开始质疑旨在让农民识字的计划的影响力，因为它忽视了农民贫困、疾病和其他问题。"我们可以丰富他们的头脑，但不能填饱他们的胃。"他对一位朋友这样感叹。他很快总结道，教育必须与社会工作中其他方面的问题一起解决。之后，他开始计划进行更广泛的社会实验，可以在受过教育的领导层下开发和测试完整的重建计划。平民教育运动计划扩展到其他领域——农业、运输和建立农村合作社。

在卫生保健方面，晏阳初征求了北京协和医学院和兰安生的意见，为了保证医疗和护理人员参与项目，他花时间试图激励学生在毕业后参与平民教育运动。1929 年的一个晚上，一小群协和医学院的学生聚集在医院的 E 病房听晏阳初演讲。

他开篇就说，国民是国家的基础，国家的稳定取决于国民的

stability, he asserted, was threatened by the condition of its peasantry, which suffered from four interrelated problems: ignorance, poverty, poor health, and lack of public spirit. At Dingxian, he went on to say, the MEM was using an experimental approach to try to remedy these problems, based on a four-pronged, integrated approach. This entailed the development of an educational system to combat ignorance, the introduction of modern agricultural methods to alleviate poverty, the diffusion of scientific knowledge in medicine and public health to deter illness and disease, and reform in the political system to foster a spirit of public service. The research results of this social laboratory, he suggested, would be of great value to China's overall task of rural reconstruction.

Yen was a strong believer in his own movement and a persuasive speaker, and over the years he recruited six PUMC graduates in medicine and four in nursing to form a nucleus of technical personnel for the MEM Department of Health. "Sacrifice," he said, "is often needed to start something uncommon," and for the work at Dingxian, he cautioned, "You need the mind of a scientist and the heart of a missionary." John Grant was instrumental in ensuring him technical persons of high caliber, selected in accordance with criteria Yen himself established: competence, creativity, commitment, and character.

Dr. Yao Xunyuan, a PUMC graduate of the class of 1925, was appointed as first Director of the Department of Rural Health of the MEM in 1928, apparently recommended by several friends of Yen and agreed to by Grant. Yao fit the post well in that he himself was a man of rural origin, an unusual background for a PUMC graduate. As a result of his premedical schooling under the missionaries and work as a staff associate in a missionary hospital at Baodang, however, he had unconsciously absorbed a conventional, hospital- centered approach to medicine. Naturally, therefore, his plan was to undertake some general clinical work in the town and build a small district hospital. Construction of the

福祉。他断言，中国的稳定受到其农民状况的威胁，他们遭受着四个相互关联的问题：无知、贫穷、健康状况不佳和缺乏公共精神。他接着说，在定县，平民教育运动基于四管齐下的综合方法，采用一种实验性的方法试图解决这些问题。这需要发展教育系统以消除无知，引进现代农业技术以减轻贫困，传播医学和公共卫生方面的科学知识以阻止疾病，并改革政治制度以培养公共服务精神。他认为，这个社会性的实验室的研究成果将对中国农村建设的整体任务具有重要价值。

晏阳初对自己的运动有着强烈的信念，他是一位有说服力的演说家。多年来，他共招募了六名北京协和医学院医学专业的毕业生和四名护理专业的毕业生，组成了平民教育运动卫生部的技术人员核心。他说："要想开创不寻常的事业，往往需要牺牲。"他提醒说，在定县的工作，"你需要有科学家的头脑和传教士的心。"兰安生帮助晏阳初确保了高素质的技术人员，这些人员是根据晏阳初自己制定的标准挑选的：能力、创造力、奉献精神和个性。

1925 年毕业于北京协和医学院的姚寻源博士于 1928 年被任命为平民教育运动农村卫生处的第一任主任，这显然是由晏阳初的几个朋友推荐并得到了兰安生的同意。姚寻源很适合这个职位，因为他本身就是农村出身，对于一个北京协和医学院毕业生来说，这是一个不寻常的背景。然而，由于他是在传教士手下接受的医学预科教育，并在保定的一家传教士医院担任过助理人员，因此他不自觉地吸收了传统的、以医院为中心的医学方法。因此，他

hospital was underwritten by the Milbank Memorial Fund, but within two years of his appointment, Yao received a fellowship for advanced public health study abroad and left the MEM.

Shortly after returning from my own graduate training in the United States and Europe, Yen and Grant offered his position to me and I accepted with alacrity. I thought that the health project in itself was quite insignificant. If the model could be used for training, however, I felt that its impact on rural inhabitants could be very great. I was convinced that this could be done, that Dingxian could be developed as a rural health training station, just as the Peking First Health Station had been developed as an urban site. As for Grant, although he wanted field training posts in both rural and urban settings, he was less sanguine than I about the prospects at Dingxian. Ultimately, however, he and Yen agreed to the attempt.

As it turned out, organization of the training programs proceeded rapidly, and over the nearly six years we were in operation, we were able to provide many types of training to many sorts of health worker. We began to train village health workers almost immediately. Shortly thereafter, we added special instruction for secondary medical school graduates employed in our subdistrict health stations.

In time, too, we developed an on-site rural health training facility, where we provided PUMC medical and nursing students an opportunity to practice what they learned in the classroom. To facilitate my leadership of this latter program, I was appointed to the faculty of the PUMC School of Public Health, serving concurrently in that capacity and as Director of the MEM Department of Public Health. By the time the Sino-Japanese War began in 1937, forcing us to close down, I had been teaching for some six years and held an appointment as an associate professor.

的计划自然是在镇上开展一些一般的临床工作，并建立一个小型的地区医院。医院的建设由米尔班克纪念基金资助，但在他被任命的两年后，姚寻源获得了出国进修公共卫生的奖学金，因此离开了平民教育运动。

我从美国和欧洲参加研究生培训回来后不久，晏阳初和兰安生向我提供了这一职位，我欣然接受了。我认为卫生项目本身不足为重。但是，如果这个模式可以用于培训，我觉得它对农村居民的影响是非常大的。我相信这是可以做到的，定县可以作为一个农村卫生培训站来发展，就像北京第一卫生站作为一个城市站点来发展一样。至于兰安生，尽管他希望在农村和城市都有实地训练岗位，但他对定县的前景没有我那么乐观。然而，最终，他和晏阳初都同意了这一尝试。

事实证明，培训项目的组织工作进展迅速，在近六年的运作中，我们能够为各个岗位的卫生工作者提供多样化类型的培训。我们几乎立即开始培训农村卫生工作者。此后不久，我们为受聘于我们分区卫生站的中等医学院毕业生增加了特别指导。

随着时间的推移，我们也建设了一个现场农村卫生培训基地，在那里我们为北京协和医学院的医学和护理学生提供了一个实践他们在课堂上所学知识的机会。为了促进我对后一个项目的领导，我被任命为北京协和医学院公共卫生学院的教员，同时担任平民教育运动公共卫生部门的主任。到 1937 年抗日战争爆发，学校被迫关闭时，我已经教了六年的书，并被聘为副教授。

THE DINGXIAN MODEL OF COMMUNITY MEDICINE

The interlude at Dingxian, spanning the period from January' 1932 to July 1937, was a milestone in my professional life, the opening phase of a career in public health work that has continued for well over fifty years. In practical terms, the experience marked the beginning of a lifelong quest for the best means of diffusing scientific medicine within China's rural population, which more than fifty years ago was so strikingly similar to that of many developing countries today.

The work put me in contact with a great diversity of people, ranging from peasant farmers to international health specialists, yielding new understanding and appreciation of their concerns. It exposed me to a great diversity of problems, old and new, and tested my ingenuity in trying to solve them. It also provided experience that enabled me to clarify and define many of the central points in my thinking about community medicine, public health, and medical education.

Our country has a history of many millennia. But the systematic health organization developed at Dingxian was the first that had ever existed in China, bringing the benefits of modern medical care to an agricultural majority that until then had had to rely solely on indigenous beliefs and practice for medical relief.

Dingxian was barren. Its people cultivated barely enough crops to live on: corn, millet, cabbage, and turnips. These items constituted the basis of their diet, which was supplemented by a little meat. The district (the equivalent of "county" in the postrevolutionary administrative system) had no modern manufacturing enterprises whatsoever, and the only marketable commodities locally produced were a number of eye medications.

 The district government supported one normal school, located in Dingxian itself, and a few primary schools. Heavy carts and donkeys,

社区医学的定县模式

1932 年 1 月至 1937 年 7 月间在定县的工作，是我职业生涯的一个里程碑，是我从事公共卫生工作长达 50 多年生涯的开端。从实际情况来看，这一经历标志着在中国农村百姓中寻求传播现代医学最佳途径的开始，50 多年前的中国农村百姓与 20 世纪 80 年代许多发展中国家的农村百姓是如此惊人地相似。

这项工作使我接触了从农民到国际卫生专家等各种各样的人，对他们所关心的问题产生了新的理解和认识。它让我接触到各种各样的问题，有旧的也有新的，并考验了我解决这些问题的独创性。它还丰富了我的经验，使我能够澄清我对社区医学、公共卫生和医学教育的许多核心观点并定义它们。

我国有几千年的历史。但在定县发展起来的系统卫生机构是中国第一个将现代医疗保健的益处带给了大多数农业人口的卫生机构，在此之前，农民只能依靠传统的信仰和实践来进行医疗救助。

定县很贫瘠。当地村民种植的作物仅够维持生计：玉米、小米、白菜和萝卜。这些食物构成了他们饮食的基础，并辅以少量肉类。该区没有任何现代制造企业，当地生产的唯一可销售商品是一些眼科药物。

区政府资助了定县的一所师范学校和几所小学。沉重的马车

the chief means of transportation, carved deep grooves and dents into the muddy roads. A few people owned bicycles, and a ricksha could be rented.

The houses were fashioned from mud. Each room usually had only one window, so that the interiors were dark. The peasants slept on mud beds (kang), warmed in winter by weeds burned beneath the surface. Coal was available only for cooking. Oil lamps supplied such artificial lighting as there was. Kerosene, which was imported, was far too costly. Electricity was available only within the city limits of Dingxian.

Personally and professionally, it was very difficult for medical and nursing personnel who came from a large metropolitan city to adapt to such conditions. By that time, I had been marrried for several years, and when my family joined me we shared a house with another family, occupying three rooms all told. There were six of us, including my wife's elderly mother, using these quarters. Our sources of pleasure lay chiefly in contemplating the results of our hard work and in receiving visitors from other places.

I still remember very clearly the day—January 16, 1932, when I actually set off from Beijing for Dingxian with a group of staff members of the MEM. We left from the West Railroad Station in Beijing. By the time we arrived, there were no seats left, but someone found me a place to sit on the floor of the train. We stopped at many places along the way, and it took almost twelve hours to cover fewer than 100 miles. On arriving, we rode by mulecart over the one narrow road leading into the town.

Arrangements called for me to stay temporarily with Dr. Qu Junan, who headed the Department of Education. This was a welcome interlude, for Dr. Qu was a brilliant young intellectual, with a Ph.D. in philosophy from Harvard University. Before joining the MEM, he had taught at Yenching University.

和驴子是主要的运输工具，在泥泞的道路上刻下了深深的沟槽和凹痕。少数人拥有自行车，也可以租到黄包车（人力车）。

当地的房屋是用泥巴建造的。每个房间通常只有一扇窗户，所以室内很暗。农民们睡在炕上，冬天燃烧杂草取暖，煤炭只用于做饭。油灯是照明工具。煤油是进口的，价格太高。只有在定县的县城范围内才有电力供应。

从个人和职业角度来看，来自大都市的医护人员很难适应这种条件。那时，我已经结婚几年，当我的家人和我住在一起时，我们和另一个家庭合住一幢房子，我总共占了三个房间。我们六个人住在那里，包括我年迈的岳母。我们的乐趣主要来自于思考我们辛勤工作的成果和接待来自其他地方的访客。

我还清楚地记得 1932 年 1 月 16 日，那天我和一群平民教育运动的工作人员从北京出发去定县。我们从北京西站出发，当我们上车时，车上已经没有座位了，但是有人在火车的地板上给我找了个地方坐下。我们沿途在许多地方停留，花了将近 12 个小时走了还不到 200 公里。到达后，我们乘坐马车穿过一条通往镇上的狭窄道路。

根据安排，我暂时住在教育部部长瞿菊农博士那里。这段插曲令人非常愉快，因为瞿博士是一位才华横溢的年轻知识分子，拥有哈佛大学的哲学博士学位。在加入平民教育运动之前，他曾在燕京大学任教。

The Beginning: Developing an Information Base

A research group affiliated with Jin Ling University had undertaken an ongoing socioeconomic survey project in Dingxian, begun eight years earlier, and the first task I set myself, after getting my bearings, was to seek out its director, Dr. Li Jinghan. I wanted to learn as much as possible about conditions in the district.

The survey reports provided useful information on population, income, and traditional medical practice. They indicated that there was a total of 400,000 inhabitants, distributed in the town of Dingxian, various outlying market towns, and a multiplicity of surrounding villages. Annual per capita income was yuan 30—at that time the exchange rate was about Yi = U.S.$.50. That income would provide only a bare subsistence diet for one person, mainly cereals.

The survey material also provided a certain amount of data on health and medical care, but we needed a great deal more. Yen and others of the MEM leadership were a bit skeptical about my intention to organize a local health survey, as the notion of making a field survey as the basis for formulating a health plan had no precedent.

In this particular survey we selected a sample population of about 45,000 persons. A priority interest was to establish the causes of illness and death in the district so as to determine roughly what proportion of such incidents might be prevented within the limits of medical knowledge at that time.

The results showed crude birth and death rates of 40.1 per 1,000 population and 32.1 per 1,000 population, respectively/ and an infant mortality rate of 199 per 1,000 live births. Communicable diseases were responsible for much, if not most, of the illness. Among children under six years of age, diarrhea and dysentery were major causes of death. Tetanus neonatorum, formerly known as "four-to-six-day fever,"

开端：建立信息库

一个隶属于金陵大学的研究小组在定县开展过一个持续的社会经济调查项目，该项目早在八年前就开始了，在确定方向后，我给自己定下的第一个任务是寻找该小组的主任李进汉博士。我想尽可能多地了解这个地区的情况。

调查报告提供了关于人口、收入和中医实践的有效信息。报告指出，定县共有 40 万居民，分布在定县镇、周边的各个集镇和众多的周边村庄。当时的人均年收入为 30 元，汇率约为 1 元兑换 0.5 美元。这一收入只能为一个人提供勉强维持生计的食物，主要是谷物。

调查材料虽然也提供了一定数量的健康和医疗方面的数据，但我们还需要更大量的数据。晏阳初和平民教育运动的其他领导对我组织地方健康调查的意图有些表示质疑，因为这种把实地调查作为制定健康计划基础的思路从无先例。

在这次调查中，我们选取了大约 4.5 万人作为样本。优先关注的问题是确定该地区疾病和死亡的原因，以便大致确定在当时的医学知识范围内可以预防多大比例的此类事件的发生。

结果显示，粗出生率和死亡率分别为每千人 40.1 和 32.1，婴儿死亡率在每千名活产儿为 199。传染病是造成大量（虽然不是绝大部分）疾病的原因。在六岁以下儿童中，腹泻和痢疾是其主要的死亡原因。以前被称为"四六风"的新生儿破伤风是婴儿

however, was the leading cause of death among infants, explained in large part by the local custom of dressing the umbilical cord with mud. Besides infant diarrhea and dysentery, scarlet fever, typhoid fever, tuberculosis, measles, and smallpox were also commonplace. Analysis revealed that out of 2,032 deaths reported, 37 percent may have been entirely preventable; 32 percent more arose from conditions that could be treated successfully if reached early. While these figures were in no sense absolutely reliable, because of the uncertainty of the diagnosis, they nevertheless made it very clear that our first responsibility was to prevent communicable and infectious disease.

Another survey that I designed, covering health conditions in the schools, showed that nearly 10 percent of the children were regularly absent from classes. The reason given most frequently was "working at home." Cited next most often was "illness." Conjunctivitis and trachoma, headaches, skin diseases (i.e., scabies and pyogenic infections), sore throat, and abdominal pain— usually caused by roundworms—were the most common complaints of the absent children. Most of these conditions could have been prevented.

However tentative, the statistics clearly revealed the consequences of the lack of modern medical care and lack of knowledge about infectious diseases and how they are spread. The Adult People's Schools were teaching some hygiene, but it was important for all the villagers to know a great deal more about the causes of illness and disease. Hence I saw that, in addition to the need to establish medical facilities, the health work of experimentation must be begun quickly and be closely integrated with the educational aspects of the MEM program.

The survey revealed that the medical care available to this community was nothing other than treatment dispensed by traditional practitioners. These practitioners on whom the villagers relied had little in common with the scholar-physicians I had known in the cities. With an occasional

死亡的主要原因，这在很大程度上是由当地用泥巴包扎脐带的习俗造成的。除婴儿腹泻和痢疾外，六岁以下儿童中，猩红热、伤寒、结核病、麻疹和天花也很常见。分析显示，在报道的 2032 例死亡数据中，37% 可能是完全可以预防的；还有 32% 是由那些如果早期发现可以成功治疗的疾病导致的。由于诊断的不确定性，这些数字在任何意义上都不是绝对可靠的，但它们非常清楚地表明，我们的首要责任是预防传染性疾病。

我设计的另一项关于学校健康状况的调查显示，近 10% 的孩子经常缺课。最常见的理由是"在家务工"，其次是"生病"。沙眼、头痛、皮肤病（即疥疮和化脓性感染）、咽喉痛和腹痛（通常由蛔虫引起）是缺课儿童最常见的主诉。这些情况中的大多数原本都是可以预防的。

尽管是试探性的，但这些统计数字清楚地揭示了缺乏现代医疗保健和对传染病及其传播方式缺乏了解所带来的后果。虽然成人学校也教授一些卫生知识，但对所有村民来说，更多地了解疾病的病因是很重要的。因此，我认为，除了建立医疗设施之外，试验性的医疗卫生工作必须迅速开始，并与平民教育运动计划的教育方面紧密结合。

调查显示，定县当地所能得到的医疗保健只有由中医提供的治疗。村民所依赖的这些医生与我在城市里认识的学者型医生几乎没有共同之处。他们只是以卖草药为副业的普通农民，只是偶

exception, they were simply ordinary farmers who sold herbs as a sideline. They had had no special medical training and could not even read a pulse. Many were illiterate.

Even these village practitioners were not uniformly available. In fact, one-third of the district's 446 practitioners and 256 herb stores were located in a single subdistrict, whereas nearly half of the subdistricts had neither. The remaining subdistricts had anywhere from 30 to 85 practitioners and 25 to 70 herb stores.

In thinking about the quantitative and qualitative aspects of available medical care and how they could be improved, I knew that the establishment of a modem hospital, or even a series of clinics, in itself, would not remedy this situation. The only system that would have any real value was one that would extend down into the villages and improve the level of health consciousness among their inhabitants.

It was clear that in considering any solution, economic constraints would have to be constantly borne in mind. Few of the practitioners charged fees, although they did expect a compensatory gift of some sort from the patient. In actual cash outlay, villagers were spending an average of ¥0.30 per capita annually on medical relief, mostly for drugs. What could possibly be accomplished on such a small amount? Expended on an individual basis, it amounted to practically nothing; however, if it were used collectively, perhaps something could be done with it.

Even with its resources pooled, no village could support a modern physician. It could not even support a nurse. Assuming an average of 100 families per village, averaging five persons each, the combined sum of available resources was only ¥150. Nurses at that time were earning double that amount. An inventive solution had to be found.

有例外。他们没有受过专门的医疗训练，甚至都不会数脉搏，很多都是文盲。

即便如此，并非所有村民都能得到这些农村医生的服务。事实上，该区的 446 名执业医师和 256 家草药铺有 1/3 位于一个分区，而近一半的分区两者都没有。其余的分区有 30 至 85 名从业人员和 25 至 70 家草药铺。

在思考现有医疗服务的数量和质量问题以及如何改善这些问题时，我意识到建立一家现代化的医院、甚至是一系列的诊所并不能补救这种状况。唯一真正有价值的系统是能够延伸到村庄并提高居民的健康意识水平的系统。

显然，在考虑任何解决办法时，都必须不断考虑到经济方面的限制。很少有医生收取费用，尽管他们确实希望从患者那里得到某种补偿性的礼物。在实际的现金支出中，村民每年在医疗救助方面的人均支出为 0.3 元，主要用于购买药物。这么少的钱能做成什么事呢？就个人而言，这些钱几乎没有什么用处；但是，如果集体使用，也许就能有所作为了。

即使集中了资源，也没有哪个村庄能养活一个现代医生，甚至都不能养活一名护士。假设每个村子平均有 100 个家庭，每个家庭平均有五个人，可用资源的总和只有 150 元。而当时护士的收入是这个数字的两倍。因此，我们必须找到一个创新性的解决方案。

DEVELOPING THE METHODOLOGY

Our survey had provided us with data on health problems and socioeconomic conditions in the district. The next step was to plan a system of health care services for the inhabitants. This required considerable thought and creativity, since there was no forerunner of any kind on which we might model ourselves. I had no idea what might or might not be practical; thus, our ideas evolved as we went along.

Thinking through the development of a health program, however, I concluded that there were at least four premises on which our system should be based: it must be grounded in the village— the basic administrative unit of the district, its cost must be in accordance with the economic resources of the village, its basic personnel must come from the village, and its proper functioning must be the responsibility of the village leadership.

An Integrated Village-Based System

For purposes of administration, rural districts at that time were divided into subdistricts, and these, in turn, into villages. The subdistricts were made up of 40 to 100 villages. Only a minority of the inhabitants of any district were found in the district center or in one of its other market towns. The majority lived in rural villages. These links to each other and to the district center were slight, for travel was difficult and roads were few. Under such circumstances, a hospital- or clinic-centered approach to health care such as that used in urban China had little to recommend it. Our system had to reach everyone, not just the fortunate few in the towns. Nor were mobile clinics a practical solution for several reasons, including the inaccessibility of many villages to road traffic.

The solution I reached in time was a rural health organization that provided three levels of service built on the resources of the three administrative units: district, subdistrict, and village. The accent on

制定方法学

我们的调查为我们提供了有关定县健康问题和社会经济状况的数据。下一步是为村民规划一个保健服务系统。这需要相当多的思考和创造力，因为没有任何一种先例可以作为我们的榜样。我不知道什么是实际的，什么是不实际的；因此，我们的想法随着我们的前进而发展。

然而，通过思考卫生项目的发展，我得出结论，我们的系统至少应基于四个前提：它必须立足于村（地区的基本行政单位），其成本必须与村的经济资源相一致，其基本人员必须来自于村，其适当运作必须由村领导负责。

以村为基础的综合系统

为了便于管理，当时的农村地区被划分为分区，而这些分区又被划分为村。这些分区由 40 ~ 100 个村组成。在任何一个地区，只有少数居民居住在该地区的中心或其他集镇，而大多数人都住在农村。由于交通困难，道路稀少，他们相互之间的联系以及与地区中心的联系都很薄弱。在这种情况下，中国城市采用的那种以医院或诊所为中心的医疗保健方法没有什么可取之处。我们的系统必须覆盖到每个人，而不仅仅是城镇中少数的幸运儿。由于一些原因，包括许多村未通公路，流动诊所也不是一个实用的解决方案。

我及时找到的解决方案是建立一个农村卫生组织，该组织基于三个行政单位的资源提供三个级别的服务：区、乡和村。应特

integration in this structure cannot be overstressed. Units at each level in the system were supervised and supported by those at the one above, and effective interrelationships among the various parts were crucial to the effective functioning of the whole. The village nevertheless was the basic unit.

Economic Feasibility

Another premise on which the Dingxian model was based lay in the realm of economics. As already mentioned, I felt it was crucial that the village be able to financially support whatever services were to be provided at that level. Poor as the villagers were, there was no use in developing a system of health service that was inconsistent with their own resources. Commendable as such a system might be in other terms, its economic foundations were impossibly fragile. When outside aid was withdrawn, it would collapse.

The Use of Village Health Workers

My idea of using ordinary, lay people as the basic personnel of the system of rural health service seemed appropriate for essentially three reasons. First, assuming that a few villagers could be trained to undertake some preventive measures and to motivate the entire community to seek and maintain a cleaner, more sanitary environment, sources of infection could be reduced. With a lessening of illness, such skilled and technically trained personnel as were available to the system could be used to better advantage.

Second, if a few villagers could be trained to offer leadership in prevention, they could also be taught to provide initial care in emergencies or relief in simple cases, and their skill at this level could be trusted.

别强化对这种结构的整合性。系统中每一级的单位都受到上一级单位的监督和支持，各部分之间有效的相互关系对整个系统的有效运作至关重要。然而，村是基本单位。

经济上的可行性

定县模式能否成功的另一个前提取决于经济方面。如前所述，我觉得至关重要的是，无论在那个层面上提供什么样的服务，村里都要能够在财政上支付得起。村民很穷，要建立一个与他们自己资源不匹配的卫生服务系统是不行的。换句话说，这样一个体系或许值得称赞，但它的经济基础却极其脆弱。当外部援助撤走时，它就会崩溃。

使用农村卫生工作者

我的想法是使用普通的非专业人员作为农村卫生服务系统的基本人员，这基本上有三个原因。首先，估计可以培训少数村民来进行一些预防措施，进一步动员整个社区寻求和保持更清洁、更卫生的环境，那么传染来源就可以减少了。随着疾病的减少，系统中可利用的熟练和受过技术培训的人员就可以在其他领域中得到更好的利用。

其次，如果可以培训少数村民在预防方面发挥领导作用，就也可以教他们在紧急情况下如何提供初步护理或在简单情况下提供救助，他们在这一级别的技能是值得信任的。

The post-1958 expansion of rural services in China vaulted the term "barefoot doctor" into the global lexicon, leaving many outsiders with the impression that village practitioners represented something entirely new in rural health care delivery. Actually, however, the idea of village-based lay health workers originated neither at Dingxian nor in the postliberation period. Since time immemorial, Chinese villagers had been seeking medical counsel and obtaining their medication from other villagers whose knowledge of medicine was only slightly greater than their own.

Third, it seemed theoretically plausible to use villagers—who lacked advanced technical knowledge—as the primary health workers: they were already there, and they were apt to remain there. Whereas an outsider accustomed to more amenities and less isolation might well be reluctant to suffer the hardship of village life for very long, the inhabitants were accustomed to the local conditions and were bound to their communities by kinship and other ties. Villagers who were trusted by their fellow villagers, moreover, would have an advantage over outsiders, who would have to spend precious time demonstrating their reliability.

Community Responsibility

Finally, it was our intention that, in our system, medical knowledge would filter downward, through various training programs, while medical cases would be referred upward, according to increasing complexity of condition. Success depended on the personnel at each level performing their assigned functions and performing only those functions assigned to them, or certainly in any case, nothing for which they were not trained. So those at the base level could make or break the entire system.

We knew of other rural health systems using village health personnel that had failed because insufficient attention had been given to selection, training, and supervision of such workers. Inadequate supervision could lead to any one of several unwanted outcomes. Crucial measures of prevention could be neglected. Individual patients could suffer when

1958 年后，中国农村医疗服务的扩大使"赤脚医生"一词进入了全球词典，给许多外来者留下了这样的印象：农村医生代表了农村医疗服务的一种全新形式。然而，实际上，以村为单位的非专业卫生工作者的想法既不是起源于定县，也不是起源于解放后。自古以来，中国的村民就一直向知识只比自己强一点点的其他村民寻求医疗咨询和用药。

第三，使用缺乏先进技术知识的村民作为初级卫生工作者在理论上讲是合理的：他们已经在那里，而且倾向于留在那里。一个习惯了更多便利设施和孤立的外来者很可能不愿意长期忍受农村生活的艰苦，而居民们习惯了当地的条件，并通过亲属关系和其他纽带与他们的社区联系在一起。此外，得到同乡信任的村民比外人更有优势，因为外人需要花宝贵的时间来证明他们的可靠性。

社区责任

最后，我们的意图是，在我们的系统中，医疗知识将通过各种培训项目向下渗透，而医疗案例将根据病情的复杂性向上转介。成功取决于每个级别的人员履行其指定的职能，并且只履行分配给他们的职能，当然，在任何情况下，都不能履行他们没有接受过培训的职能。因此，这些在基层的人可能会对整个系统起造就或摧毁的作用。

我们知道，其他使用农村卫生人员的农村卫生系统之所以失败，是因为对这些工作人员的选择、培训和监督没有给予足够的

health workers without special expertise tried to minister beyond their capacities, or individual practitioners might begin trying to charge fees. We certainly did not want our village health workers to try to practice medicine on their own, nor did we want them to extract fees from the patients.

Such an approach would have destroyed our whole intention to make medical relief available to the entire community on a shared- cost basis. We were trying to move toward state medicine, and in the meantime we were trying to develop cooperation between the village authorities and higher officials to launch a public-supported system of medical relief that would eliminate the great economic wastage of unnecessary illness and death. I had been interested in state medicine since my student days and had written several articles on the subject for The Binying Weekly.

China at that time was not ready for socialized medicine, however. So in Dingxian, for the time being, we were trying to implant habits of cooperation for community welfare and to recruit volunteer labor to take preventive measures and give first aid relief. At the subdistrict health stations, where a physician was in attendance, we charged a fee that amounted to the equivalent of U.S. $0.01 or less.

The use of unpaid and only briefly trained village farmers as our basic personnel made the matter of their supervision all the more important. To maintain the confidence of the people, the health worker needed constant technical assistance and supervision. So we arranged for regular weekly exchanges between the health workers and the subdistrict physician. The health workers were in no way to be independent functionaries, acting on their own judgment and authority. Precisely the opposite; they were to be closely supervised and supported all the time. To ensure that these workers lived up to the responsibilities of the position, we made them accountable to the most powerful community organization in the village, the Alumni Associations of the Adult People's Schools. If a worker

重视。监管不力可能导致以下任何一种不想要的结果；关键的预防措施可能被忽视；当没有特殊专长的卫生工作者试图提供超出其能力范围的服务时，有些患者可能会受累；或者个别医生可能开始试图收费等等。我们当然不希望我们的农村卫生工作者试图独自行医，也不希望他们从患者身上榨取费用。

这样的做法会破坏我们在分担费用的基础上向整个社区提供医疗救助的整体意图。我们试图向国家医疗的方向发展，同时，我们也试着发展村官和高级官员之间的合作，以启动一个由公共支持的医疗救助系统，消除因不必要的疾病和死亡所造成的巨大经济损失。从学生时代起，我就对国家医疗感兴趣，并为《丙寅周刊》写了几篇有关国家医疗的文章。

然而，当时的中国还没有为社会化的医疗做好准备。因此，在定县，我们当下只是试图为社区福利植入协作模式，并招募志愿劳工来从事各种预防措施和提供急救救治。在有医生在场的分区卫生站，我们收取的费用相当于 1 美分或更少。

把没有报酬且只接受过短暂培训的农民作为我们的基本人员，因此对他们的监督就日益重要。为了保持人们的信心，卫生工作者需要不断的技术援助和监督。因此，我们安排卫生工作者和分区医生之间每周定期交流。这样卫生工作者就不可能成为独立的职能部门，而仅根据自己的判断和权威行事。恰恰相反，他们要一直受到密切的监督和支持。为了确保这些农村卫生工作者履行其岗位职责，我们让他们对村里最有影响力的社区组织 – 成

needed to be replaced for one reason or another, the Alumni Association had the authority to do so. These arrangements were of absolutely critical importance to the proper functioning of the system.

The worker needed not only supervision but also support and appreciation, which we hoped would be forthcoming from the collective membership of the Alumni Association as well as the community. Without appropriate recognition and appreciation, the morale of the village health workers, who were, after all, contributing their services free of charge, would be apt to slip. This was a great risk, because unless prevention was maintained on a continuing basis, our whole rural health effort would have very little long-term impact.

Persons examining the model of community medicine developed at Dingxian should consider it from the standpoint that it was, in fact, a community-based system, rather than that it used lay personnel (village health workers) as assistants within that system. The important points were not that the community-based system used voluntary village health workers for certain tasks but rather that village health workers constituted the lowest tier of a health maintenance system whose effective functioning began with them, and that their performance was monitored by a strong community organization responsible to ensure that quality was maintained.

It was economically unfeasible, and would remain so for many decades, for the average village to support a qualified physician or nurse, even if sufficient numbers of such personnel were available, which they were not. Yet if we were unable to reach the villages, we would have made little progress in the application of scientific medicine to improve rural health. Our solution, therefore, was to make the villagers themselves aware of the problems and arouse their sense of community responsibility and their motivation to work on the problem. That was the philosophy underlying the Dingxian model of community medicine.

人学校校友会负责。如果一名农村卫生工作者因为某种原因需要被替换，校友会有权这样做。这些安排对该系统的正常运作具有绝对的重要性。

对农村卫生工作者不仅需要监督，还需要支持和赞赏，我们希望校友会的集体成员以及社区都能提供支持和赞赏。如果没有适当的认可和赞赏，农村卫生工作者的士气就会减退，因为毕竟他们是在免费地提供服务。这是一个巨大的风险，因为除非预防工作持续进行，否则我们整个农村卫生工作的长期影响将非常小。

研究定县发展的社区医学模式的人应该从这样的观点来考虑：它实际上是一个以社区为基础的系统，而不是在该系统中使用非专业人员（农村卫生工作者）作为助手。重要的一点不是以社区为基础的系统利用自愿的农村卫生工作者来完成某些任务，而是农村卫生工作者构成了健康维护系统的最低层，其有效运作始于他们，而且他们的表现由一个强大的社区组织负责监督，以确保质量得到维持。

要让一个普通的村庄养活一个合格的医生或护士，在经济成本上是不可行的，并且在几十年的时间里都是不可行的，即使有足够数量的此类人员（实际上也没有）也不可行。然而，如果我们无法到达村，我们在应用现代医学改善农村健康方面就不会有什么进展。因此，我们的解决方案是让村民自己意识到这些问题，并唤起他们的社区责任感和调动他们对解决问题的动力。这就是定县社区医疗模式的基本理念。

The model, we fully realized, was based on the assumption of effective cooperation and collaboration of technical and nontechnical personnel. These would eventually include village health workers, to whom we gave brief training; mid wives and nurses with more extensive degrees of local training; young graduates of provincial medical schools, who had completed a regular six-year medical curriculum; and physicians, graduate nurses, and students from the PUMC, who had received training on a par with that of the most advanced universities in the West. At the outset no one who was responsible for the entire area, including myself, could be absolutely certain how well the system would work.

Organizational Basis

Two steps in building the unprecedented system of organized health services in Dingxian had now been completed. We had collected the necessary epidemiological data and had decided on the key elements of our plan. We were now ready for the next step, development of the various levels of the three-tiered structure and of the linkages between the levels.

We went about this in short order, developing an organization at the apex of which was a district health center, encompassing administrative offices, a fifty-bed hospital, a laboratory, and classrooms for training. Below the district center were the various subdistrict health stations and below that, the village health workers. (A flowchart of this system is shown in fig. i.) The system expanded quite rapidly. We began in 1932 with a district health center and two subdistrict health stations serving thirteen villages. By 1934, there were, besides the district health center, seven subdistrict health stations, serving more than seventy-five villages.

我们充分认识到，该模式是基于技术人员和非技术人员有效合作和协作的假设。这些人员最终将包括下述人员：农村卫生工作者，我们对他们进行了简单的培训；在当地受过更广泛培训程度的助产士和护士；已经完成常规六年医学课程的省级医学院的年轻毕业生；以及医生、护士和北京协和医学院的学生，他们接受的培训与西方最先进的大学一样。在一开始，包括我自己在内，负责整个地区的人都不能绝对肯定这个系统会运作得如何。

组织基础

在定县建立这个前所未有的有组织的卫生服务体系的两个步骤现已完成。我们已经收集了必要的流行病学数据并确定了我们计划的关键要素，并且现在已经为下一步做好了准备，即：搭建三级卫生保健体系中每个层级，并建立不同层级之间的联系。

我们很快就完成了这项工作，其最高一级建立的组织是区卫生中心，包括行政管理办公室，一个拥有 50 张病床的医院，1 个实验室以及若干用于培训的教室。区卫生中心之下的层级是各个乡卫生站，乡卫生站之下的层级是村卫生员（见图 1）。这个体系扩展得很快。1932 年开始时，我们只有 1 个区卫生中心和 2 个乡卫生站，为 13 个村庄提供服务。到了 1934 年，除区卫生中心外，已经有 7 个乡卫生站，服务超过 75 个村。

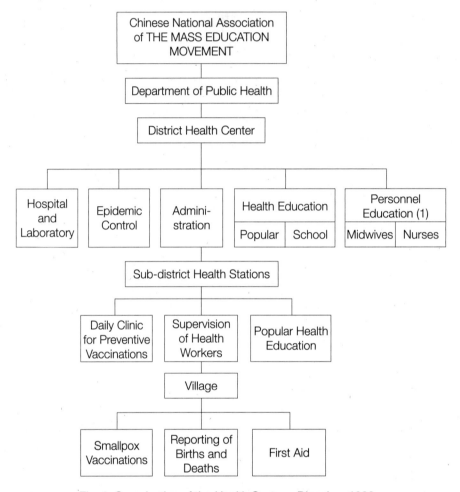

Fig. 1. Organization of the Health System, Dingxian, 1933.

We put a great deal of thought into the selection, training, and supervision of the lay personnel who constituted the foundation of our system. We knew that the village worker concept had been tried in India, but had failed to take root there, perhaps because the village health workers had been selected by the physicians in charge of the program rather than by a peer group within the village.

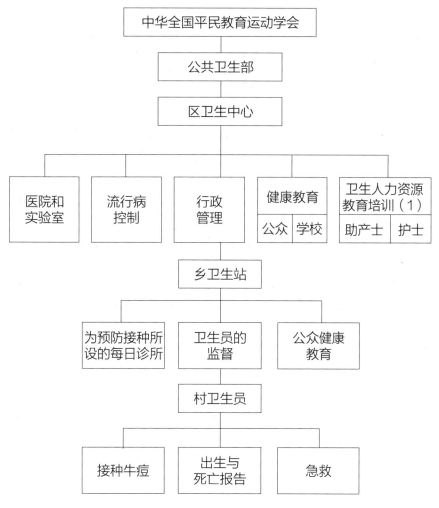

图 1 定县卫生系统的组织架构图（1933 年）

　　我们在对该体系工作的基层非专业人员的选择、培训和督导方面进行了诸多考量。我们知道村卫生员的概念曾在印度尝试过，但并未能在那里扎根，或许是因为村卫生员是由负责该项目的医生而不是由村里同等地位的村民小组选拔的。

In this context, I turned to the Alumni Associations of the Adult People's Schools of the MEM. The People's Schools not only gave their students basic competency in reading and writing but also tried to change their fundamental attitudes and values by imbuing in them self-reliance and community solidarity. The impetus for social change through self-effort was carried on through the Alumni Associations, whose members were spearheading the organization of agricultural cooperatives and other means of socioeconomic improvement. The basic philosophy of the MEM emphasized a correlated program of reconstruction. By training and this perspective, therefore, the members of the Alumni Association were eminently qualified to undertake a constructive project in health.

As far as the selection of village health workers for our program was concerned, my idea was to rely on the judgment of the Alumni Associations, assuming that they would choose whomever they regarded as most trustworthy and reliable. So our village health workers were elected to their positions by fellow members of these associations. With a few exceptions in villages where the organization itself was weak, the results were excellent. Our workers were generally hardworking, honest, and public-spirited.

As to the scope of their responsibilities, after careful consideration, we concluded that these should be limited to the prevention of disease and the provision of simple medical relief measures. Training, however limited, could prepare the health workers for these tasks. Emphatically, however, it could not prepare them to make accurate diagnoses of other than the simplest complaints.

It was a cardinal principle in our system that the health worker should never act, or be called on to act, as a physician. The worker's three tasks, as we envisioned them, were to record births and deaths in the village, to vaccinate the community against smallpox, and to render simple treatments from the contents of a first aid box that contained a few essential and nonhazardous items. Those contents included, for example,

在这种情况下，我求助于平民教育运动的成人学校校友会。成人学校不仅培养学生基本的阅读和写作能力，而且还试图通过灌输自力更生和社区团结来转变他们的基本态度和价值观。校友会通过自身的努力推动社会变革，其成员带头组织农业合作社和其他社会经济改善手段。平民教育运动的基本理念强调了一个与重建相关的计划并借助这种观点，校友会的成员在经过培训后都可以合格地开展健康方面的建设性项目。

在为我们的计划选择村卫生员方面，我的想法是依靠校友会的判断，认为校友会将选择他们认为最值得信赖和最可靠的人。因此，村卫生员都是由校友会的成员选举产生的。除少数村庄由于自身组织比较薄弱外，大多数村卫生员开展相关工作结果都非常好，他们普遍勤奋、诚实、热心公益。

至于村卫生员的职责范围，深思熟虑后，我们认为他们的职责应该仅限于预防疾病和提供简单的医疗救助措施。对卫生院的培训虽然简单，但可以使他们具备从事这些工作的能力。但需要强调的是，这些培训职能只让他们处理最简单疾病，并不足以让他们对疾病做出准确的诊断。

在这个卫生体系中，卫生员永远不会承担医生的职责，我们也不会要求他们承担医生的职责，这是一项基本原则。正如我们所设想的那样，卫生员的三大任务是记录村子里的出生与死亡，为社区接种天花疫苗，用急救药箱中的基本、无害的少量物品。

aspirin, soda mint, ointment for the treatment of trachoma, a disinfectant, and bandages. With these few simple items the health worker could not commit serious errors and might be able to alleviate much unnecessary physical discomfort.

Prevention was in our minds as well. Properly trained, the worker could prevent serious conditions from developing and could refer patients upward in the system to, and through, the physician at the subdistrict health station. With physicians and students from the PUMC serving in the district health center, this put the simplest villager in a direct line of access to the best scientific medical knowledge in the country.

Health workers would perform their duties on a voluntary, nonre-munerative basis. We had no intention of building a new profession, nor, more importantly, of creating competitive pressure on traditional practitioners. The health workers would continue to derive their income from farming and would receive no direct remuneration for their efforts. For now, their reward would have to be essentially spiritual, although perhaps in time some recompensation might be arranged for their leadership in prevention.

Village workers were in regular contact with the provincial medical school graduates who served as physicians and administrative heads of the subdistrict health stations. In fact, although the station physician provided treatment to certain types of patient, the training of the village health workers was the physician's first duty. This required that the physician visit the villages at regular intervals, and that the workers attend training sessions at the health station once a week.

Worker attitudes tended to reflect the varying attitudes and abilities of the health station physicians. Those physicians who were enthusiastic, took an obvious interest in what the workers were doing, and exhibited a reasonable level of competence in diagnosis and treatment earned the confidence and respect of the village health workers, who saw them as teachers, able to deal with problems they themselves could not handle.

如阿司匹林、苏打薄荷、治疗沙眼的软膏、消毒剂和绷带等，简单地处理小伤病，这样做，既可以让卫生员免于医疗事故，还能减轻患者许多身体不适。

卫生员还会开展预防工作。卫生员经过适当培训，可以预防严重疾病恶化，并且能够将患者转诊到上一级的乡卫生站医生处，或通过乡卫生站医生再往上一级区卫生中心转诊。北京协和医学院的医生和学生们在区卫生中心提供服务，这使得那些纯朴的村民能从这个国家最好的医学科学资源中受惠。

卫生员开展这些工作都是志愿、无报酬的。我们无意开辟一个新的职业，更重要的是，我们无意给传统医务工作者制造竞争压力。与从前一样，卫生员从农业劳动中获得收入，他们的付出并不能得到直接回报。虽然迟早可能会对他们在预防工作中的作用给予一些补偿，就目前而言，只能在精神上给予他们鼓励。

村卫生员保持常规沟通与毕业于省级医学院的乡卫生站的医生和行政负责人联系。事实上，虽然卫生站医生能为患有某些病的患者提供治疗，但对村卫生员进行培训才是他们的首要工作。这就要求医生定期访问各村，卫生员每周参加一次卫生站的培训课程。

卫生员的态度往往反映了卫生站医生的不同态度和能力。热心、对卫生员的工作表现出明显兴趣、具备良好诊疗水平的医生赢得了村卫生员的信任和尊重，村卫生员将他们视为能处理自己不能应付的问题的师长。

The provincial medical school graduates were unprepared for many of the situations they encountered in both practice and teaching. Therefore, we had to supplement their education with formal instruction in vital statistics, epidemiology, and other subjects. Nevertheless, with proper supervision and help from the district health center, in spite of their inadequate foundation, most proved to be quite effective, and certainly they were able to do far more than could have been expected of a physician working entirely alone. They offered medical care at a far more skilled level than village health workers were able to provide, especially after completing the continuing education courses that were offered at the district center. Fortunately, only a few exhibited indifference to their villager patients and clearly expressed their preference for working in an urban area.

As mentioned previously, we began in 1932 with two subdistrict health stations, each staffed by a physician and a trained lay worker. Both the physician and the aide received a small salary. Later on we added a nurse to the staff of those stations that undertook school health activities. Equipment was simple, but asepsis and general cleanliness were always emphasized. The minimum setup in these stations provided the crucial link between the basic services of the village and the relatively specialized service of the district health center.

Each station was situated in a market town, which had its own subdistrict administration and one or more higher primary schools. We chose the station sites in accordance with one or the other of the two patterns of population distribution prevailing in North China at that time. One served a fairly broad area containing a few large villages separated by considerable distances. The other served a relatively small area with many small villages, separated by only short distances. Areas typified by this latter distribution pattern were usually poorer than those with a few large villages. Within a short time, the number had increased to four, including, besides the two MEM-supported units, two others financed by the local authorities.

省医学院的毕业生并不一定能应对医疗实践及教学中的诸多问题。因此，我们必须通过正规教育，教授他们生命统计、流行病学和其他课程，以完善他们的知识体系。尽管他们的基础不够，在区卫生中心的监督与帮助下，他们大多工作都被证明是相当有效的，而且肯定远比一个单独工作的卫生员预期能够完成的更多。他们提供的医疗照护水平远远超过村卫生员，特别是在完成区卫生中心的继续教育课程之后。幸运的是，仅有少数人对村民患者表现出漠不关心的态度，并明确表示他们更喜欢在城市里工作。

如前所述，1932 年起步阶段，我们只有两个乡卫生站，每个卫生站内配备一名医生和一位训练有素的非专业卫生员。医生及其助手仅可领到一点微薄的工资。后来，我们为那些开展学校卫生健康工作的卫生站增添了一名护士。尽管设备简陋，但始终强调无菌和清洁。这些卫生站的最基本配置有效地衔接了村级基本照护和区卫生中心比较专业化的照护。

每个卫生站都设在一个集镇上，集镇设有乡行政机关和一所或多所高级的小学。我们根据当时华北地区普遍存在的两种人口分布模式之一来选择乡卫生站的地址。其中一个卫生站服务于几个相隔很远的大村庄，覆盖区域相当辽阔。另一个则服务于相对较小的地区，包括间距很近的众多且更穷的小村庄。不久后，卫生站数量就增加到了四个，两个由平民教育运动支持建立，另外两个由地方当局资助。

Responsibility at the top of the system rested with the district health center, which was expected to coordinate and supplement all the activities of the subordinate agencies. The center trained the provincial medical school graduates and other local health personnel, conducted studies of special health problems, and prepared and distributed educational materials.

Additionally, the district health center operated a 50-bed hospital, whose standards were maintained at the highest possible level, while the cost of equipment and supplies was intentionally kept as low as possible. For example, patient beds were simple frame structures covered with locally produced sheets. The operating tables, also locally made, were constructed at one-sixth the price of imported tables used elsewhere. A laboratory attached to the hospital was equipped to perform routine work related to district health programs, and its staff occasionally conducted outside investigations.

From time to time, the center engaged in special projects, such as devising control measures during a cholera epidemic in 1932. Dingxian civic leaders, at the recommendation of the center, established a control committee that included, besides the magistrate, the heads of the Bureaus of Police, Education, Finance, and Public Works, several prominent tradespeople and some MEM staff members. The committee distributed wall posters, telling people how to avoid infection and urging them to be inoculated. Special police were employed to comb the countryside, looking for victims, whom they urged to seek hospitalization in the district center institution, which at that time had been in operation for less than a month. Not a single death occurred among the forty-five persons who were hospitalized with cholera. The special police supervised the disinfection of wells—which, we were told by authorities later, it was almost impossible to do in many other parts of the country because the people refused to allow it. Our villagers, by contrast, had already had some health education and understood the need. Eventually, people from neighboring areas came to us, begging for help with disinfection of their wells.

196

这个体系最顶端是区卫生中心，下级机构的全部活动都应由该中心来协调与补充。该卫生中心负责对省医学院校毕业生及其他当地卫生人员进行培训、开展特殊健康问题研究并编写和分发教材。

另外，区卫生中心还运营一所拥有 50 张病床的医院。该医院尽可能按照高水准建设同时还要控制设备和用品的成本。如病床是简单的支架结构，铺着当地生产的床单。手术台也是当地制造的，其制造费用仅为其他地方使用的进口手术台的六分之一。医院附属实验室配备了与开展区卫生项目有关的日常工作所需的设备，工作人员有时也会外出进行调查。

区卫生中心不时参与特殊项目，例如在 1932 年霍乱流行期间制定防治措施。在中心的建议下，定县市领导成立了一个防治委员会，除地方行政长官外，委员会成员还包括警察局长、教育局长、财政局长和民政局长，还有几位知名商人和平民教育运动的工作人员。这个委员会发张贴墙报，告诉人们如何避免感染，并督促人们接种疫苗。当时区中心医院开办还不到一个月，就雇用了专职警察来搜寻各村落以寻找霍乱患者并督促他们去区中心医院住院治疗，住院的 45 例霍乱患者无一例死亡。专职警察还监督水井消毒，事后当局告诉我们，此举措在我国其他地区由于群众反对只能束手无策。相比之下，我们的村民已经接受了一些健康教育知识并理解这样做的必要性。最终，邻近地区的人们来到我们这里，请求帮助他们对水井进行消毒。

Only highly trained personnel could capably carry out the functions of the district center, so the best-educated nurses, technicians, and midwives available to us were assigned there. The project was fortunate in that these individuals were able to provide exactly the right type of leadership, without which no organized practice could succeed. Their energy, confidence, and personalities influenced the outlook of those at other levels, determining to a great extent the quality of the overall effort.

Effective communication among the three levels, in fact, was vital to proper functioning. District-level physicians met regularly with those at the subdistrict level, who, in turn, met regularly with the village workers. Through this and other integrative features, the three components of the system operated a mutually supportive network, and their joint effort represented the best form of practice that could be arranged under extremely difficult conditions.

Mapping out all the foregoing matters had been a complex and difficult task. Our reward came when the Dingxian model proved its effectiveness and we were able to gradually expand its activities, and when the central government selected it as the prototype for other district governments to follow in developing their health systems.

Field Activities

Once we had implemented and staffed our organization, we launched a wide variety of field activities. From 1932 to 1935 we emphasized experimentation in refining these various activities to ensure that the principles and methods of our work would be suitable for adaptation elsewhere. Then in 1935 we were ready to move from the experimental and demonstration phase of our work to that of training.

只有训练有素的人员才能执行区卫生中心的职能作用，所以我们将受过良好教育的护士、技术人员和助产士都分配在这里。这个项目很幸运，因为这些人员能够发挥完全正确的领导职能；如果没有正确的领导，任何有组织的实践活动都无法取得成功。他们的能力、信心与人格影响了其他层次相关人员，在很大程度上决定了项目的质量。

事实上，三级体系中不同层级之间有效沟通对于正常运作至关重要。区级医生定期与乡级医生会面，而乡级医生定期与村卫生员会面。通过这种方式和其他整合性措施，该体系的三个组成部分形成一个相互支持的网络，他们的共同努力代表了在极端困难条件下可安排的最佳实践形式。

对以上所有事项的勾勒、安排是一件复杂而艰巨的任务。当定县模式证明是有效的，我们能逐渐将其拓展，以及中央政府选择定县作为其他区政府建立卫生系统的样板，我们才真正得到了回报。

现场活动

在我们的组织建立并配备了人员后，我们就开展了广泛的各种各样的现场活动。从 1932 年到 1935 年，我们开展了改进这些不同活动的试验，以确保我们工作的原则和方法能适用于其他地方。随后在 1935 年，我们准备将我们工作从试验示范阶段转向培训阶段。

Collection of Vital Statistics

In the experimental areas where we had already established the three-tiered infrastructure, with village health workers trained and working, we were able to keep a reliable register of vital statistics. By 1934, the number of village health workers had increased to eighty, and the number of villages in the register had tripled from our starting point. The total population in the registration area was 103,087, almost one-fourth of the district's population. Births and deaths went unreported still in other parts of the district, but in this closely controlled area, supervised by an inspector, the registration was relatively complete. The system of registering births and deaths had no counterpart elsewhere in China at that time.

Our 1934 figures for the controlled area, where we were fairly certain of the data, give an indication of important health problems. The reported rate of infant mortality was 185.2 per 1,000 live births; deaths among persons under five years of age, as a percent of all deaths, amounted to 44.5 percent, in part because of epidemics in that year from both dysentery and scarlet fever. The death rate due to dysentery was 2.3 per 1,000. Other leading causes of death included scarlet fever, pulmonary tuberculosis, tetanus neonatorum, and kala azar—a tropical fever transmitted by sandflies. Specific death rates from these causes were respectively 653, 178, 73, and 42 per 100,000 population. The death rate among children under two years of age from diarrhea and enteritis was 200 per 100,000. While these figures reflected a lamentably low health level, we were making progress. The rates of puerperal sepsis, tetanus neonatorum, and problems related to childbirth and early infancy in general were declining.

Provision of Medical Relief

By 1935, three years after the Dingxian experiment had begun, its various agencies were providing an impressive volume of medical relief.

生命统计数据的收集

在我们已经建立基本的三级卫生保健网的试验区，依靠经过培训和正在工作的村卫生员，我们有能力开展可靠的生命统计登记了。到 1934 年时，村卫生员人数增加到 80 人，开展生命统计登记的农村数量也已经增加到最初的三倍。登记地区的总人口为 103 087 人，几乎占全区人口的 1/4。在该地区其他地方仍然存在出生和死亡漏报，但在这个严格管理的地区，在检查员的监督下，登记相对完整。当时，在中国其他地方都还没有类似的出生登记和死亡登记制度。

我们对管辖区 1934 年收集的数据准确性非常有把握，这些数据反映出一些重要的卫生问题。报告的婴儿死亡率为 185.2‰人；五岁以下死亡人数占全部死亡人数的 44.5%，部分原因是当年痢疾与猩红热疫情。痢疾的死亡率为 2.3‰，其他主要死因包括猩红热、肺结核、新生婴儿破伤风与黑热病（一种由白蛉传播的热带发热疾病），具体死亡率分别为 653/10 万，178/10 万，73/40 万和 42/10 万。两岁以下儿童腹泻与肠炎死亡率为 200/10 万。尽管这些数字反映出健康水平低下，让人悲观，但我们还是取得了一些进步：产褥期脓毒血症、新生儿破伤风以及与分娩和婴儿早期相关的问题的造成的死亡率总体呈下降趋势。

提供医学救助

到 1935 年，即定县试验开始三年后，各个机构提供了数量

In that year, the hospital admitted 600 patients, providing a total of over 10,000 days of hospital care. Staff physicians performed more than 260 operations without losing a patient, and they made nearly 200 outside calls. Subdistrict stations treated more than 65,000 persons, of whom 15,000 were new patients, and village health workers administered nearly 140,000 first aid treatments.

From the standpoint of quality, there was, of course, no absolute standard; however, the general impression of the work of village health workers was that it was remarkably satisfactory. The work of the subdistrict health physicians varied in quality, reflecting variations in aptitude and training. On the whole, however, the training these physicians had received in provincial medical schools was so poor that simple diagnostic procedures became somewhat unreliable in their hands, and asepsis and cleanliness often were neglected. We tried to remedy these deficiencies as we went along, but eventually this proved futile and we had to organize further formal coursework for them.

Furtherance of Sanitation

The value of potable water supplies and appropriate sanitation in disease prevention is immeasurable, but regrettably, rural sanitary engineering was an unexplored field at that time, and we could find no one professionally trained to help us. Nevertheless, we did our best with the limited possibilities at hand.

For example, we decreased contamination in village wells by making two changes. First, we had the farmers raise the level of the mouths of the wells so as to prevent surface water pollutants from draining down into the cavities. Second, we replaced individual family buckets with a common bucket, hung permanently on a hook at the top of the well. Because that bucket never came into contact with contamination from the ground, as had the buckets that family members brought and set down

可观的医疗救助。当年，医院收治患者 600 余人，累计住院天数超过 10 000 天。主治医生们完成了 260 多台手术而无一例患者死亡，外出出诊近 200 次。乡卫生站收治 65 000 多人，其中新增收治患者 15 000 人，村卫生员开展了近 140 000 人次的急救活动。

当然，医疗卫生照护质量并没有绝对的标准；但村卫生员的工作给人的总体印象是非常令人满意的。乡卫生站医生的工作质量参差不齐，反映了这些医生自身能力和接受培训的差异。但总的来说，在省医学院受过培训的医生则更差，他们有时连简单的诊断程序都不能准确地完成，还忽视无菌和清洁的原则。我们虽一直在努力弥补这些缺陷，但最终证明这是徒劳的，因此不得不为他们开设正式课程。

卫生工作的进一步发展

卫生合格的饮用水供应与搞好环境卫生在预防疾病方面的价值是不可估量的；但遗憾的是，当时农村卫生工程还是一个未发展的领域，我们找不到一个专业的人来帮助我们。尽管如此，我们还是在手头有限的条件下竭尽所能。

例如，我们通过利用两种改进措施来减少村内水井的污染。第一个措施，我们让农民提高了井口的高度，以防止地表水污染物流入井内。第二个措施，我们用长期挂在井顶挂钩上的公用水桶代替个人家庭的取水桶。因为公用取水桶不接触地面的污染物，

in the adjacent area while waiting their turns to draw water, this too, decreased pollution to an extent. Compared with the enormous need, our efforts were marginal, but every little bit helped.

Bathing facilities in the village had been nonexistent. It was commonly said at that time that villagers bathed or were bathed only three times in a lifetime: at birth, at marriage, and at death. So we built some communal bathhouses. Our three bathhouses opened 121 times that year, and we noted that 8,500 baths were taken. The schoolchildren and village health workers bathed free of charge; others paid Y0.01 each. This may sound primitive, but it was really an innovation in community life. It was also of great importance in rural China at that time, not for aesthetic reasons alone, but because skin infections, which could be prevented by frequent bathing, were so commonplace.

Control of Communicable Diseases

At that time (mid-1930s), smallpox was still prevalent. Attempts had been made in many parts of the country to prevent its spread by vaccination programs. These failed in most instances because authorities were unable to reach every family, and even among those whom they reached, the issue of who was most at risk by virtue of age was neglected. In Dingxian, however, this was not a question. We could reach a very high percentage of the population at risk, and we got to the children who most needed it; thus, we were able to go a long way in controlling the disease. In time, when smallpox broke out in neighboring areas, it did not appear in ours.

Vaccination against cholera was another success story. In 1934 North China as a whole suffered an epidemic of cholera, but Dingxian and surrounding areas had only a few cases, and even those were successfully treated in our hospital.

而家庭成员带来的水桶在等待轮流取水时常放在附近地上，如此做法也在一定程度上减少了污染。与巨大的需求相比，我们所做的努力杯水车薪，但我们深知，不积跬步，无以至千里。

村里没有洗浴设施。当时人们普遍说，村民一生只洗三次澡：出生、结婚和死亡时。所以我们建立了一些公共浴室。我们的三个浴室那一年开放 121 次，我们记录有 8500 人次洗浴。小学生和村卫生员洗澡免费，其余人每次只付 1 分钱。这听起来可能很原始，但它确实是社区生活中的一项创新。这在当时的中国农村也很重要，不仅是为了洁净，还因为可以通过经常洗澡来预防非常普遍的皮肤感染。

传染病控制

20 世纪 30 年代中期，天花仍然流行。我国的许多地区已尝试通过接种疫苗来防止天花的传播。这些努力在大多数情况下都失败了，原因是当局无法深入到每个家庭；甚至在他们能接触到的人中，也忽视了哪个年龄段的人面临最大的风险。但是在定县，这并不是一个问题。我们可以接触到所有高危人群，而且我们可以接触到最需要接种的儿童。因此，我们能够在控制疾病方面取得显著成绩。当邻近地区天花暴发时，我们地区却安然无恙。

霍乱疫苗接种是另一个成功案例。1934 年整个华北地区暴发霍乱，但定县及周边地区仅有少数病例，且这些患者都收治在我们医院，且诊疗有效。

Health Education

The Department of Rural Health provided health education for all primary-school children and for various adult groups, reflecting the strong belief of its director that general medical work must always be correlated with educational work. We began with the children for several reasons. They were at a receptive, impressionable age when new habits can be formed easily. They attended school for a two-year period at least, which gave us an opportunity to reinforce the teaching over an extended period. Moreover, they could serve as a conduit through which we could indirectly teach something to the older generation.

For our health education program we relied heavily on the primary-school teachers and the school nurse. First, however, we had to teach the teachers. As it was, students in the normal schools received an education heavily weighted toward the theoretical side, emphasizing teaching principles and techniques of administration, and often neglecting practical subject material. We had to convince the teachers both that teaching hygiene was worthwhile and that it was their responsibility. Next, we arranged for a special nurse to prepare a series of textbooks on the subject. To correlate with the lessons, we issued earthenware spitoons, washbasins, and individual drinking cups to be distributed to the children.

The importance of potable water received special emphasis; with the help of village health workers, we constructed many new school wells or disinfected existing ones, or made arrangement to supply boiled water where neither of these measures could be accomplished. We also built latrines.

A nurse visited each school on a regular weekly basis, treating the children for various ear and eye conditions and ringworm of the scalp and referring those with dental problems to a special clinic. Contents of a school first aid box were available to the nurse; such boxes had been supplied at a minimal cost through the MEM. Schools replenished the

健康教育

农村卫生局对所有小学生和各类成年人群提供健康教育，这体现出卫生局负责人的坚定信念：一般医疗工作必须始终与教育工作挂钩。我们从儿童开始进行健康教育有以下几个原因。首先，儿童接受能力强，处于易受影响的年龄段，容易养成新的习惯。其次，他们至少要上两年学，这让我们有机会在更长的时间内加强教育。此外，他们可以作为一个渠道，我们能通过他们间接向长辈们传输知识。

我们的健康教育项目主要依靠小学教师和学校护士。但是，需要先对老师进行教育。事实上，师范学校的学生所接受的教育偏重于理论方面，强调教学原则和管理技术，而往往忽略了实践问题教育。我们不得不说服教师，告诉他们讲授卫生是值得的，而且这也是他们本身的责任。接下来，我们安排了一名专门护士来准备一系列与健康教育有关的教科书。为了配合课程，我们发给儿童陶制痰盂、洗脸盆及个人饮水杯。

饮用水的重要性受到了特别重视。在村卫生员的帮助下，我们新修建了许多学校水井，或对现有水井进行消毒，如果不具备实施上述措施之一的条件，我们安排供应开水。我们还修建了公共厕所。

一名护士每周定期访视每所学校，为儿童治疗各种耳部和眼部疾病以及头皮癣，并将有牙齿问题的孩子转送到专科诊所。护士可以使用学校急救箱中的物品；这个急救箱是通过平民教育运

207

contents at their own expense, amounting to less than Y1.00 annually.

For the adults, I personally revised The One Thousand Characters text of the Adult People's Schools to include eight complete lessons and four references to health in the four-months course. Also, the district health center held an annual health exhibit during Chinese New Year, when thousands of villagers flocked to Dingxian. Staff members distributed health literature and demonstrated proper ways of bathing and feeding children.

Improvement of Maternal and Child Health

Progress in the realm of maternal and child health was impeded by prevailing social attitudes and economic conditions. Maternal welfare was not a subject that elicited much interest or concern in the village. In the rare instances when a case did become an issue, the outcome was often adverse. For example, some pregnant young wives wanted very much to deliver in the district health center under the care of a qualified midwife but were effectively discouraged from doing so by their mothers-in-law, whose ideas carried great weight in the family, and who thought delivery should take place at home.

Our program also included family planning, for which any forward-looking social program should provide. Villagers at that time believed that there was no way of limiting the number of children they might produce. We were among the first, if not the first, group to make family planning services available.

We might have achieved more had it not been for an entangled web of economic circumstances and traditional social values that stood in the way. Among the obstacles was the strong village preference for large families. Sons were especially desired because they were expected to carry on the family line and to increase the prosperity of the family; moreover, there was always an outside chance that a son

动按照最低成本价供应的。学校用自己的经费补充急救箱的物资，每年不到一元钱。

对于成人，我亲自修订了成人学校的千字文教科书，在四个月的课程中包含八节完整的课程，有四课是关于卫生问题方面的。此外，每年春节时有成千上万的村民涌向定县，区卫生中心都要举办一次卫生健康展览。工作人员发放卫生宣传材料，并作正确洗澡和喂食儿童的方法示范。

妇幼卫生的改善

社会风气和经济条件阻碍了妇幼卫生领域的进步。妇女福祉话题难以在农村引起太多兴趣或关注。在少数情况下，当某案例成为普遍问题时，往往会出现负面结局。例如，有些年轻的孕妇非常想在区卫生站在合格助产士护理下进行分娩，但她们的婆婆们不同意这样做，后者的想法在家庭中占有重要地位，她们认为分娩应当在家里进行。

我们的项目也包括了计划生育，任何有远见的社会规划都应当提供这项服务。当时的村民认为，生儿育女的数量是没有办法限制的。即使不是最早，我们也是较早提供计划生育服务的团体之一。

如果不是受经济环境与传统社会价值观的阻碍，我们本可以取得更大的成就。障碍之一是农村强烈的大家族观念。村民们生儿子意愿强烈，因为儿子可以传宗接代，让家族生活蒸蒸日上；

might become famous and add luster to the family name. Another major impediment was the lack of any tested and safe means of contraception, one sufficiently simple and inexpensive for extensive use under rural conditions.

The Department of Health did undertake some successful programs. Seeking to reduce the high rate of infant mortality, we enrolled a number of mothers in short classes for housewives, made many pre- and postnatal visits at home, and persuaded a continually growing number of women to deliver their babies at the district center under qualified care.

In other areas, such as midwifery, we encountered difficulties and made mistakes. Sometimes the solution to a particular problem was so elusive that we were almost inclined to abandon the issue. At that time, child delivery was still in the hands of ignorant old women. So, at first, we brought in a specially trained young midwife, with an experienced physician of obstetrics to back her up.

The villagers would not accept an outsider of only twenty-five years of age as a trustworthy person, however. Moreover, there were so few abnormal labor cases that the back-up physician was a luxury.

So we attempted to retrain the old traditional midwives. This turned out to be difficult for many reasons. Because these midwives were unable to read and write, special instructional materials had to be prepared. Furthermore, the traditional midwives resented the young, unmarried woman we selected as the trainer. She had had advanced training, and they had not. She was relatively well educated, and they were illiterate. Nevertheless, they regarded her as an inexperienced upstart and demonstrated a good deal of jealousy. In any event, we learned that it was very difficult to correct their lifetime habits, even to enforce the practice of cleanliness.

此外，一旦一个儿子功成名就，就可以光宗耀祖。另一主要障碍就是缺乏经过测试的安全的避孕手段，一种简单且价廉能在农村推广使用的避孕方法。

卫生局确实开展了一些成功的项目。为降低婴儿的高死亡率，我们招募了一定数量的承担家庭主妇的母亲开设了短期班，进行了许多围产期家庭访视，并说服越来越多的妇女去区卫生中心在合格护理人员的照护下完成分娩。

我们也在一些工作领域遇到了困难，犯了一些错误。有时，我们对解决某个特定问题无所适从，以至于我们几乎对该问题缴械投降。接生就是问题之一。那时候，接生仍然依赖无知的老年接生婆。所以，一开始，我们请来了一位受过专业训练的年轻助产士，并有一位经验丰富的产科医师为其做后盾。

然而，村民不会信赖一个年仅 25 岁的外来人。而且，难产病例毕竟很少，因而支持助产士的产科医生就成为奢侈的摆设。

所以，我们试图对旧式传统接生婆重新进行培训。由于种种原因，该项举措举步维艰。这些接生婆不会读写，因此必须准备特殊的教学材料。此外，传统接生婆对我们选拔年轻的未婚妇女作为培养对象怨气满腹，因为她们没有像那些年轻的受训者接受过高级培训，她们是文盲，而那些年轻的受训者接受过较好的教育。自然而然，旧式接生婆将年轻的受训者视为无经验的暴发户，并表现出很大的嫉妒心。无论如何，我们认识到，要改变这些接生婆一生的习惯是非常困难的，哪怕是让她们养成清洁的习惯都非常不易。

Eventually, rather than retraining the old midwives, we selected and trained one of their younger relatives, who, as a member of their own family, would receive the older woman's support in her new role. This approach also eliminated the problem of jealousy. We thought that at last we had made an encouraging start. After a time, however, we found that this was impractical; the young woman was usually too busy to fulfill the responsibilities of this extra and irregular work.

This lurching back and forth on such an urgent problem as the need for qualified midwifery was very frustrating, but experience has reinforced our belief that there is no easy solution to this question. Changing attitudes in this area may take more than one generation.

INSTRUCTIONAL ACTIVITIES

By 1935, in just a few short years, our field activities had expanded enormously and, despite many difficulties, we were rendering a great deal of help to the villagers. In relation to these activities, we had organized four different types of training or continuing education. We were now prepared to shift our focus from the various clinical and health education activities to the training programs, whose students included both our own staff members and medical and nursing undergraduates at other institutions.

Our key training program was that provided to the village health workers. The preparation of rudimentarily educated villagers to serve as basic personnel in a three-tiered integrated rural health system had been an exceptional challenge. No one in our country had even conceived of such a program at that time.

 After some discussion, the MEM leadership had agreed with my general plan to provide ten days of training to each worker. I proposed that a group should meet for instruction at some suitable central point, such as a primary school or a subdistrict health station, that each student could reach on foot within an hour or so. This would obviate the expense

最后，我们选择旧式接生婆年轻的亲属接受培训，而且在新的岗位上将会得到旧式接生婆的帮助。这一做法的确消除了旧式接生婆的嫉妒问题，我们认为终于有了一个令人鼓舞的开端，但是，不久之后我们发现这样做是不切实际的，年轻的妇女通常很忙，无法从事这项额外的、不规律的工作。

在像需要合格助产士这样紧迫的问题上来回徘徊非常令人沮丧，但是这些经历进一步启示我们，这一问题不容易解决。在这一地区扭转这类观念可能需要不止一代人的努力。

示教性的活动

到 1935 年，在短短的几年中，我们的现场活动得到了极大的扩展。尽管困难重重，我们还是给村民提供了很多帮助。针对这些活动， 我们组织了四种不同类型的培训或继续教育。现在我们准备把重点从各种临床工作或健康教育活动转移到培训项目，培训的学员包括我们自己的工作人员和在其他机构的医学及护理本科生。

我们的主要培训项目是针对村卫生员的。让受过初等教育的村民成为农村三级卫生体系的基层工作者是一项特殊的挑战。当时，我们国家根本没有人设想过这样的方案。

经过一番讨论后，平民教育运动的领导同意我对每个卫生员提供 10 天培训的计划。我建议小组应设在合适的中心地点进行教学，诸如一所小学或乡卫生站，以便每个学生能在 1 小时

of overnight accommodations. Classes would meet daily on a regular basis.

The Alumni Association would play a sustentative role. It would bear the cost of a free noon meal to each volunteer. More importantly, after training was completed, the association was expected to give continuous moral support to the volunteer so as to nurture continuing interest in the work. Arrangements for words of praise from the magistrate and a small annual "bonus" that could be graded according to definite standards of achievement, for example, provided ample incentive.

Some MEM spokespersons had been skeptical about the proposed length of the training session, thinking that ten days was too short. Experience proved that this was a good decision, however. To be sure, we wanted to avoid at all costs giving the impression that we were training "doctors." In any case, the intent of our training was not so much to convey factual information as it was to institute a good working relationship between the student and the health station physician who would serve as that student's supervisor. We believed in accenting supervised practice rather than classroom explanations as the primary learning method.

As director of the department, I felt that I should train at least the first group of health workers before passing the task along to the subdistrict health station physicians, not because I had experience but because I wanted to experiment to find the best means of doing it. Choices as to what to emphasize had to be made and a syllabus prepared.

In retrospect, it seemed appropriate to concentrate on certain areas: general matters of hygiene, emphasizing cleanliness; birth and death registry; immunization techniques; smallpox control; and measures of prevention for trachoma and skin infections. These choices reflected, in general, the prevailing major health problems in the area and, in particular, the relative simplicity and low cost of eliminating smallpox.

左右步行到达。这样可以不必为住宿支付费用，并且可以每天上课。

校友会起到支持作用，承担每位志愿者的免费午餐。更重要的是，培训完成后，我们要求校友会继续在道义上支持志愿者，以培养对此项工作的持续兴趣。例如，安排地方行政官表彰，以成绩为标准发给少量的年终奖金，对志愿者进行充分激励。

一些平民教育运动发言人对于拟定的培训课时长度持怀疑态度，认为十天太短。但是，实际证明这是一个好的决定。可以肯定的是，我们不惜任何代价避免给人们一种我们是正在培训"医生"的印象。无论如何，我们培训的目的与其说是传达真实的信息，不如说是在学生和作为学生导师的卫生站医生之间建立良好的工作关系。我们相信加强对实践的督导是最主要的学习方法，而不是课堂上的讲解。

作为卫生局负责人，在将此任务交给街道卫生站医生之前，我认为我至少应该先培训第一批卫生员，并非因我已有经验而是我想通过试验找出开展这项工作最好的方法。必须明确重点是什么，并准备好教学大纲。

回想起来，专注于某些领域培训似乎是合适的，这包括：一般卫生知识，强调清洁，出生与死亡登记，免疫接种技术，天花控制，沙眼与皮肤感染的预防措施，这些大体涵盖了该地区普遍存在的主要卫生问题，特别是消灭天花，其工作相对简单和成本

The importance of maintaining a vital statistics registry was evident.

The syllabus, as it evolved, contained seven lessons, to be presented within ten days or less. The first lesson covered general health matters, focusing on infection, treatment of cuts, and use of antiseptics and the importance of cleanliness. We discussed the need to keep the eyes clean to avoid infection that could lead to trachoma and the need to wash clothes to prevent lice infestation. The second lesson, given in two parts, dealt with water supplies and latrine construction and techniques for vaccination against smallpox and cholera. The third lesson offered a review and individual practice in vaccination techniques. The fourth delved deeper into the topics of cleanliness and sterilization, introduced the student to the contents of the first aid box, and addressed the dangers of opium smoking and the hazard of carbon monoxide poisoning. Brief remarks on the disadvantages of large families and some familiarization with quinine suppositories and the metallic cervical ring in this context were also offered. Workers were advised of the value of soybean milk in infant feeding. The fifth lesson provided for practice in bandaging and other first aid techniques. The sixth offered another review, together with instructions for completing simple birth and death forms. We recommended that symptoms of illness be listed where the cause of death was uncertain. The final lesson covered some clinical material and then shifted to regulations concerning the use of certain medications and to procedures for referring patients to the subdistrict stations.

When I turned the training over to the subdistrict health station physicians, I was well aware that the success of the training depended not only on what was taught but also on the personality of the teacher. The instructor had an inherent advantage in that, in our cultural tradition, the teacher-pupil relationship is generally respected. Still, mutual respect and confidence must be developed on an individual basis. So we urged the physicians who trained the villagers to use simple language, avoid the use of technical terminology, and keep their expectations of the students modest.

216

较低。维护生命统计登记的重要性显而易见。

　　教学大纲是逐步完善的，共包含七节课，在十天或更短的时间内讲授。第一节课讲述一般卫生问题，聚焦感染、伤口处理、抗菌剂的使用以及清洁的重要性。我们讨论了保持眼睛清洁对避免沙眼感染的必要性，以及勤洗衣服以预防生虱子的必要性。第二节课分为两部分，涉及供水与公厕的修建以及预防天花和霍乱的疫苗接种技术。第三节课讲述疫苗接种技术概述和个人实践。第四节课深入探讨清洁与消毒课题，给学生介绍急救箱的物品，讲述吸食鸦片的危害和一氧化碳中毒的危害。本节课还简要介绍了传统大家族的不足，在这节课中也让大家熟悉奎宁栓剂及金属宫内节育环。向卫生员讲解豆浆在婴儿喂养中的价值。第五节课提供了绷带和其他急救技术的实习。第六课为再次复习，以及指导填写简单的出生与死亡表格。我们建议对死因不确定的应列出疾病的症状。最后一节课涉及一些临床知识，然后讲述按有关规定使用某些药品以及将患者转诊到乡卫生站的程序。

　　当我把培训工作交给乡卫生站的医生时，我很清楚地意识到，培训成功与否不仅取决于教授的内容，也取决于教师的素质。教师有先天优势，因为尊师重道根植于我们的文化传统中。尽管如此，相互尊重和信任必须建立在个人基础上。所以，我们敦促培训村民的医生使用通俗易懂的语言，避免使用专业术语，对学生的要求不要过高。

Concerning substance, we insisted that they stress proper execution of the task at hand, rather than the acquisition of additional skills. For example, the physician as trainer was to convince the workers of the importance of filling in registration forms completely; of describing symptoms of terminal illness as accurately as possible; of giving vaccinations according to prescribed procedures; of providing additional commentary when handing out health literature; and, above all, of not making their own diagnoses, but rather sending patients to a trained physician at the subdistrict station.

In the final analysis, this phase of our training program was exceptionally successful. The syllabus proved satisfactory, the teachers capable, and the health workers reliable and responsive. Personally, I found the enthusiasm of the village workers really inspiring; they were always enthusiastic and eager to learn, they did not expect too much remuneration, and they were uniformly proud of their ability to assist their fellow villagers.

Experience quickly revealed that the subdistrict station physicians themselves needed more training. We had visualized that when the Dingxian model was adopted throughout the country, in accordance with the 1934 central government recommendation, graduates of provincial medical schools would head the subdistrict health stations, while graduates of the better medical schools would head the district health centers.

Within each of these two categories of medical school, however, there was great diversity in the quality of training from institution to institution; medical education in China at that time had no uniform standard. We had only the broadest of notions of what could be expected of an individual graduate, therefore, and in any event the training of all provincial school graduates was poor. This was apparent in the typical neglect of asepsis among the graduates and their ineptness in diagnosis. Nursing education also was deficient. Moreover, the training students received in clinical medicine and in public health even at the better medical schools was

对于培训内容，我们坚持认为应当着重围绕村卫生员本职工作开展培训，而不是获得额外的技能。例如，作为一名培训师的医生要让卫生员明白完成填写登记表的重要性，学会尽可能准确描述临终疾病的症状；按照规定程序接种疫苗；在分发卫生宣传资料的时候还能够提供自己的讲解；最重要的是，不需要他们做出自己的诊断，而是将患者转诊到乡卫生站受过培训的医生手中。

经过最终的评价，我们这一阶段的培训项目非常成功，教学大纲称心如意，教师材优干济，卫生员干练可靠。在我眼里，卫生员的热情感人肺腑；他们一向热情好学，不期望太多的报酬；他们一致为自己能够帮助村民而感到自豪。

很快，实践表明乡卫生站医生自身需要更多的培训。根据1934 年中央政府的建议，我们曾设想，当定县模式在全国推广时，省医学院的毕业生将担任乡卫生站负责人，而更好的医学院毕业生将担任区卫生中心负责人。

然而，在这两种类型的医学院中，不同学院之间的教育质量存在很大差异；那时，我国的医学教育还没有统一的标准。因此，我们对毕业生的期望只有最笼统的概念。无论如何，所有省级医学院毕业生的教育都很差。明显的是，这些毕业生特别忽视无菌操作且在疾病诊断上也不合格。护理教育也欠缺。此外，即使更好的医学院，学生在临床医学和公共卫生方面接受的教育也很薄

weak. Before we were willing to entrust certain responsibilities to the young physicians, therefore, it was necessary to supplement crucial gaps in their training.

In time, we organized a two-year in-service training program for physicians serving in rural subdistrict health stations. It proved satisfactory, although in developing its curriculum, we had, as in so many other instances, no experience to guide us.

The general plan called for classroom instruction during the first year, with supervised practice in the field. The second year was devoted completely to supervised field practice. This emphasis reflected a strong personal conviction, originating in experience in European and American public health schools, that postgraduate training for technically trained personnel is most effective when founded on participation in responsible activities, under supervision. Inasmuch as the field facilities in Dingxian were well developed and were directly under the control of the Department of Health, the opportunity of developing students by the academically sound technique of "learning by doing" seemed unique.

The classroom discussion component of the program was arranged on a monthly basis. At the outset, in September, there was a two-week opening session devoted to general rural problems. This was followed by regular weekly sessions over a nine-month period, with a special topic addressed each month. From October to June, these were, respectively: (1) asepsis and elementary nursing practice, (2) diagnostic techniques, (3) health education and school health, (4) training and supervision of village workers, (5) rural public health principles, (6) smallpox control, (7) sanitation, (8) rural medical relief, and (9) administrative problems in rural health practice.

Because the students constituted the crucial link between the district and village levels, implementation of rural programs was highly dependent on the ability of these students, and it was essential to prepare

弱。因此，在打算对年轻医生委以重任时，很有必要通过培训补足他们的关键差距。

　　我们及时地为农村乡卫生站服务的医生组织了一个为期两年的在职培训项目。尽管在制定课程时，与很多其他事情一样，我们并没有可借鉴的经验，但此事实证明，该项目是令人满意的。

　　对乡卫生站医生的培训，总体计划要求在第一年进行课堂教学，并在督导下进行现场实习。第二年全部是督导下的现场实习。这样的督导安排源于我对欧美公共卫生学院经验的信念，即：对研究生人员的技术训练只有建立在有人督导负责任的活动中才最有效。因为定县已有了完备的现场设施而且是在卫生局的直接管辖之下。看来，这种"边干边学"的学术方法来培养学生的实践是独一无二的。

　　该项目每月安排一次课堂讨论。在 9 月份开始，有为期两周的上课时间，对一般农村问题进行公开讨论。随后，每周一次定期讲课共约 9 个月，每个月讨论一个专题。从 10 月到 6 月分别为：（1）无菌操作与基础护理实践，（2）诊断技术，（3）健康教育与学校卫生，（4）村卫生员的培训与督导，（5）农村公共卫生原则，（6）天花防治，（7）环境卫生，（8）农村医疗援助，（9）农村卫生实践中的管理问题。

　　由于学生是区、村两级的重要纽带，农村项目的实施高度依赖这些学生的能力，因此对他们的良好培养是至关重要的。他们

them well. Their reaction to the supplementary' program was essentially positive, although initially many objected to being given instruction in nursing techniques. By the end of the month, however, they realized the significance of simple techniques and had developed an appreciation of the nurses' contribution. The sessions devoted to diagnosis, led by senior members of the medical staff, proved to be of special interest to the group.

Rural health nursing represented another locus of training effort. We ran two nursing education programs, one a three-year undergraduate program for young women of the district, the other a six-month program for graduate nurses—all, of course, trained in hospitals in other parts of the country. The graduate nurses were prepared for such tasks as development of school health work, collaboration in communicable disease eradication programs, and supervision of village workers and local midwives. Nothing like this program existed anywhere else in China. Through the undergraduate program, we were hoping to develop a supply of local nurses who would live and work in the area and who were familiar with the problems of rural health practice.

Ultimately, we organized the final component of our system, completing the bridge we had hoped to construct between rural and urban China, giving villagers in a remote rural district access to the most advanced scientific medical knowledge in China. From its inception the MEM had relied on the PUMC for advice and personnel in the medical field. Now we were prepared to offer a valuable resource in return, a rural health field training site.

Once the demonstration course in rural public health had been established at Dingxian, it drew undergraduate and postgraduate students not only from the PUMC but also from Shanghai Medical College and Hu nan-Yale Medical College in Hunan. We devised a similar program for PUMC nursing students as well. The students came in small groups, spending anywhere from three days to four weeks with us, during which

对这个额外的培训项目基本持肯定态度，尽管最初很多人反对学习护理技术。然而，到月底，他们意识到简单技术的重要性，并对护士的贡献表示赞赏。学生对由高级医学专业人员开设的诊断课程特别感兴趣。

农村卫生护理工作是培训工作的另一个重点。我们开设了两个护理教育项目，一个是对区级年轻妇女开设的为期三年的本科课程，另一个是对已毕业护士开设的为期 6 个月的课程——当然，所有护士都在我国其他地区的医院接受过培训。毕业的护士将会从事创建学校卫生工作，合作开展消灭传染病项目以及对村卫生员与地方助产士的督导一类的工作。在我国的其他地方还没有过这样的项目。通过本科课程，我们希望培养一批能够在该地区生活和工作并熟悉农村卫生实践问题的当地护士。

最后，我们如愿以偿，完成了三级卫生体系最后的组成部分，搭建了中国农村和城市之间的桥梁，让偏远农村地区的村民能够获取到中国最先进的现代医学知识。从一开始，平民教育运动一直依赖北京协和医学院在医疗领域的指导和人力。现在，我们准备用农村卫生现场培训基地这一宝贵的资源回报他们。

定县农村公共卫生示范课程一经建立，不仅吸引了来自北京协和医学院的本科生和研究生，也吸引了来自上海医学院、湖南湘雅医学院的在校生与研究生。我们也对北京协和医学院的护士生设计了一个类似的项目。学生组成小组来定县，同我们一起度

time they gained firsthand impressions of conditions in the market towns and villages of an ordinary rural district.

To emphasize the contrast with conditions of practice in urban China and to highlight the harsh realities of rural China's health and medical problems, I always used local examples, as my own public health professor had done. When the students visited the wards, they saw us using locally manufactured equipment and locally constructed facilities as best we could. Before touring the wards of the district center hospital, the students were always furnished with complete records on the patients they saw. Lectures on preventive medicine, highlighting vaccination measures and school health, were reinforced with field trips to the villages, which permitted exchanges on health matters with the local inhabitants.

While all this experience provided a stark realization of the difficulties of providing quality care under such circumstances, it also showed how challenging it could be to formulate inventive solutions to seemingly insoluble problems. Although the clerkship in rural health was rather short, most of the students seem to have been deeply impressed by it and felt that it was a highpoint of their undergraduate education in rural health.

Without an effective field organization, we could never have provided such an experience, of course, and we stressed to each group that wherever they found themselves after graduation, if they went into the public health field, they would also have to devote time and attention to administrative matters. Otherwise there could be no assurance of quality. Technological knowledge alone would not suffice; they also had to become knowledgeable about administration.

Besides giving training to students who came to us, Miss Zhang, the nurse-midwife on our staff, and I did some training on the outside, at the Hubei Provincial Medical School. She conducted a midwifery course,

过三天到四周的时间。在这段时间里，他们对普通农村地区的集镇和村庄的情况有了初步认识。

为了强调与中国城市卫生实践的差别，并突出中国农村的卫生和医疗问题，我则经常仿照我自己的公共卫生教授的经验和当地的实例开展培训。当学生们参观病房时，看到了我们尽可能使用当地制造的设备和当地建造的设施。在参观区中心医院的病房之前，学生总能看到他们所见患者的完整病历。以疫苗接种方法与学校卫生为主题的预防医学讲座，都会辅以农村实地考察，让学生有机会与当地居民交流卫生问题，这无疑加强了培训的效果。

所有这些经验都让人们清楚地认识到，在这种情况下提供优质照护是多么困难，同时这也表明，为看似无法解决的问题提出创造性的解决方案是多么具有挑战性。尽管农村卫生实习时间较短，但大多数学生对此都印象深刻，认为农村卫生是他们本科教育的一个亮点。

当然，没有一个有效的现场组织，我们无法让学生有这样一段经历。我们向每个小组强调，毕业后无论他们在哪里，只要从事公共卫生工作，他们也必须在行政事务方面投入时间和精力，否则就无法保证工作质量。因为仅靠专业技术知识是不够的，他们还必须对行政管理有所了解。

除了对来我们这里的学生进行培训外，我们助产士章女士（章裴成）和我还在湖北省医学院进行了一些外部培训。她开设了助

and I taught a regular four-hours-per-week course in public health for the medical undergraduates. These and other cooperative training and research activities added to the pressures on my time.

The training programs at Dingxian improved the quality of care being administered because the continual influx of outsiders stimulated those directly involved in the training programs to continue to improve their skills. There were broader benefits as well, for the training we provided would have been noteworthy on the basis of the number of persons we exposed to rural health problems alone. Beyond this, we felt we were paving the way for the development of medical education in relation to community needs in other parts of China as well. In that respect it was an important step toward my own personal goal of introducing scientific knowledge gradually, carefully, and continuously among the rural people.

Housing problem

We could look back on our accomplishment at Dingxian with pride. About three years after we had begun, the Dingxian model of community medicine had demonstrated its practicability under prevailing conditions in rural areas of North China. At a minimum it had proved effective in limiting the spread of communicable disease and meeting the most urgent medical needs of villagers, while most agreed that its accomplishments went far beyond that. We had devised a model of rural health care delivery that could be implemented anywhere in our vast and diverse country, linking remote villages to the most advanced technical centers in the cities. Also, while doing so, as Robert S. K. Lim and others noted, we had demonstrated an important principle of medical education, specifically, that it is entirely possible to correlate instruction in public health and clinical medicine in a meaningful way.

Before hostilities with Japan curtailed our experimentation after 1937, we had intended, among other things, to expand our survey field to cover a larger statistical database, and, while doing so, improve the accuracy of reporting.

产士课程，而我则定期为医学本科生开设了一门每周四小时的公共卫生课程。这些合作培训和研究活动，在时间上对我增加了压力。

定县培训项目经由管理的改善，提高了照护的质量，不断涌入的外来者对直接参与培训项目的人继续提高他们的技能形成激励作用。我们对接触农村卫生问题的人所提供的培训是值得重视的，对农民健康也很有益处。除此之外，我们觉得我们也为我国其他地方与社区需求相关的医学教育发展铺平了道路。在这方面，这是朝着我个人的目标迈出的重要一步，即逐步、认真、持续地向农民传播科学知识。

其他问题

我们可以自豪地回顾我们在定县取得的成就。在我们开始工作大约三年后，定县社区医疗模式在华北农村地区普遍推广，这证明了该模式的实用性。事实证明，它至少在控制传染病传播及满足村民最紧迫的医疗需求方面是有效的，而多数人认为它的成就远不止于此。我们设计了一种农村医疗照护模式，它可以适用于我国广袤的国土不同地区，能把偏远的村庄与城市中最先进的技术中心联系起来。此外，正如林可胜和其他人所指出的那样，在我们这样做的过程中，印证了医学教育的一个重要原则，即以一种有意义的方式将公共卫生和临床医学的教学联系起来是完全可能的。

我们曾打算扩大我们的调查领域，以在更广泛区域内建立统计数据库，并同时提高报告的准确性，但 1937 年后，抗日战争爆发，限制了我们这些试验。

Also, we were quite aware that our family planning efforts needed expansion. I had already discussed my conviction that a sound family planning program was crucial to overall health improvement with Dr. Marshall Balfour, who succeeded John Grant as Far Eastern representative of the International Health Division of the Rockefeller Foundation. Few, if any, responsible government officials in China in the 1930s, however, shared my conviction; in fact, some saw no correlation at all between fewer births and improved health. Understandably, therefore, there were no family planning programs of any kind in our country at that time, either public or private. Prevailing social values and economic conditions mitigated against such programs at every turn. This problem was of a greater order of magnitude than the need to expand our sample population, therefore, and single-handedly at Dingxian, we could make only limited progress against it.

Another generalized problem that concerned us at Dingxian was how little the urban-trained medical school graduates actually knew of rural life and how inadequately their training had prepared them for dealing with the problems of the peasants, who, after all, represented the majority of our population. We had begun to address this issue by organizing our rural field training site. We all knew that this was only a start, however. As far as the entire country was concerned, it was urgent that far larger numbers of medical students be given practical experience in the application of scientific knowledge in the countryside.

Economic issues also needed attention. In particular, we had not yet really solved the question of how to remunerate the village health workers. The professional staff at Dingxian were receiving modest salaries out of general funds for the experiment, although they were received less than their peers in urban practice. The village services were to be self-supporting, however, and although the clinics received some income from miniscule patient fees, these funds could not be stretched to provide a salary for the village health workers, and we managed by asking them to volunteer, giving them a bonus and words of praise from

我们也十分清楚，计划生育工作还需要加强。我已经与接替兰安生担任洛克菲勒基金国际卫生部门远东代表的马歇尔·巴尔弗博士讨论了这个问题，我认为健全的计划生育规划对改善健康状况至关重要。然而，在 20 世纪 30 年代，中国拥有实权的政府官员很少赞同我的观点；事实上，有些人认为减少生育与提高健康之间根本无关。因此，可以理解当时在我国没有任何形式的公共或私人的计划生育规划。当时的社会价值观和经济条件在各个方面都对这些项目产生了阻碍作用。这个问题比在更广泛区域内建立统计数据库更具难度。因此，我们在定县单枪匹马工作，只取得有限的进展。

在定县，我们注意到的另一个普遍问题是，在城市接受过培训的医学院毕业生对农村生活知之甚少，已接受过的培训还不足以让他们具备为农民提供照护的能力，而这些农民在我国人口总数占绝对优势。我们已经开始建设农村教学基地来解决这个问题，但是，我们都知道这只是一个开始，就全国而言，迫切需要的是让更多的医学生获得在农村应用科学知识的实践经验。

经济问题也同样需要关注。至今我们还没有真正解决农村卫生员的报酬问题，这尤其值得重视。定县的专业工作人员从实验经费中领取微薄的工资，比他们在城市行医的同行收入要低。然而，农村服务是自给自足的，虽然诊所从微不足道的患者费用中获得了一些收入，但这些资金无法用于支付村卫生员的工资，所以我们设法让他们做志愿者，在年终给予他们一定的奖金和由地区行

the district magistrate at the end of the year. This worked satisfactorily enough, but it was no long-term solution.

A related issue concerned the support of the system in toto. We believed that we had devised a system well within the economic reach of the villages, given that collectively, district inhabitants had been paying about ¥120,000 per year for medical service of one kind or another. The cost of our system would be less than ¥40,000, or Yo.io per person, so there was margin to spare. Nevertheless, the question remained as to how the available resources could be concentrated for collective use. Jimmy Yen and I frequently discussed the possibility that this could be accomplished under government authority; this was why relations between the MEM and the district government were becoming increasingly close. Already the Dingxian district authorities were becoming interested, and whereas they had expended practically nothing for community health in 1932, by 1935 they were pledging ¥12,000 annually to the health system. It was a step toward state medicine, an idea we had been advocating since student days at the PUMC.

OBSERVATIONS OF RURAL HEALTH PROGRAMS ABROAD

While serving as Director of the Department of Rural Health at Dingxian, I personally had many opportunities to meet and talk to other persons working in public health, community medicine, and medical education both at home and abroad. Biennial meetings of the Chinese Medical Association provided one lively forum of interchange. Other opportunities arose in discussion with guest lecturers at the PUMC, foreign and domestic visitors who came to Dingxian, and my own travel abroad. Visitors at Dingxian, for example, included Selskar Gunn of the International Health Division of the Rockefeller Foundation; Marian Yang, a Chinese national and a nurse, who had developed an

政长官授予的表彰。这样做虽尚能令他们满意，但绝非长久之计。

如何将现有资源整合起来造福于所有人仍然是事关整个三级卫生体系成败的问题。我们认为我们已设计的体系是在农村可承担的经济范围之内。当时的情况是：该地区所有居民每年需支付的卫生总费用约为 12 万元，而我们的体系可使成本少于 4 万元，相当于每人支付 0.1 元，这也证明了卫生总费用有可节约的余地。晏阳初和我经常讨论由政府当局整合资源服务公众的可能性；这就是为什么平民教育运动与区政府之间的关系越来越密切的原因。定县的区负责人最终对此事有了兴趣。尽管 1932 年他们在社区卫生方面几乎没有投入任何资金，但到 1935 年，当局承诺每年拨款 12 000 元给卫生系统。这是走向国家医学（公费医疗）的一步，这也是我们在北京协和医学院当学生时就一直提倡的想法。

国外农村卫生规划观察

在担任定县卫生局负责人期间，我个人有许多机会与国内外从事公共卫生、社会医学和医学教育工作的人会面和交流。中华医学会每两年一次的论坛为大家提供了一个畅所欲言的平台。另外一些机会是与来自北京协和医学院做报告的学者、来定县的国内外参观者讨论，以及我自己出国考察。例如，来定县的参观者包括洛克菲勒基金国际卫生部的塞尔斯卡·冈恩；一名中国医务工作者杨崇瑞，她曾在北京市卫生站开展了一个创新项目，在城市条件下对旧式接生婆进行再培训；以及安准加·斯坦帕尔博士，

innovative program at the Peking Urban Health station for retraining traditional midwives under urban conditions; and Dr. Andrija Stampar, a public health physician from Yugoslavia and highly respected figure in eastern European social medicine, whom we enjoyed especially. Both individually and collectively, these experiences taught me that a great deal of understanding and appreciation derives from free exchange of ideas among persons of various backgrounds.

My main experience in the context of international exchange during the 1930s was an extended study trip abroad in 1935, which included visits to the Soviet Union, Yugoslavia, and India. It was on Stampar's recommendation that the Ministry of Health and the League of Nations arranged for my visit to these countries. Because of the article on proteolytic enzymes that I had written as a PUMC student under Robert S. K. Lim, I traveled to the Soviet Union with a group of physiologists, who, with Lim as head, were to attend an international conference on physiology in Leningrad.

On the way to the Soviet Union, the delegation traveled by rail through Manchuko (Manchuria), which at that time was already under Japanese occupation, although open war would not break out between our two countries for two more years. The journey by train from Beijing to Moscow took ten days. At Mukden, the Japanese confined us to the train, not even allowing us to step down onto the platform. Farther north, at Harbin, we changed trains and headed for Manchouli, on the Siberian border. There I had the terrible experience of seeing a young Japanese railroad officer brutally cuff an old Chinese peasant across the face, as well as kick him violently. The old man dared not cry, and the people around him remained silent. I was indignant and ashamed, but I could not help that poor fellow.

In Moscow, official interpreters met our train. Although I was to learn Russian fifteen or so years later, I did not speak the language at that time, nor did anyone in our group. We shared a Ford taxi to our hotel with two

一位来自南斯拉夫的公共卫生医生，在东欧社会医学方面一个受人尊敬的人物，我们尤其欣赏他。我本人和所在集体的经历都让我认识到，不同背景的人之间自由交流意见可以让彼此了解对方的工作并相互欣赏。

我在 20 世纪 30 年代国际交流方面的主要经历是在 1935 年的一次出国，对多个国家进行了考察。这次考察包括访问苏联、南斯拉夫和印度。在安准加·斯坦帕尔的推荐下，卫生部和国际联盟安排了我对这些国家的访问。我在北京协和医学院师从林可胜时写过一篇关于蛋白水解酶的论文，让我获得与林可胜带队的一批生理学家一起访问了苏联，参加在列宁格勒举行的一次国际生理学学术会议。

抗日战争在两年后才爆发，但那时东北三省已被日本占领，我代表团乘火车经过这一地区。从北京乘火车到莫斯科要花十天。在沈阳，日本人把我们软禁在火车上，甚至不许我们走上站台。再往北，我们在哈尔滨换乘火车，前往与西伯利亚边境接壤的满洲里。在那里，我有一次可怕的经历，我看见一个年轻的日本铁路官员残酷地打一个中国农民的耳光，还狠狠地踢了他一脚。这位老人不敢哭，围观的人们都不敢作声。我既气愤又羞愧，但也帮不了这个可怜的人。

在莫斯科，官方翻译来车站迎接我们。在当时我和我们组里的人都不会讲俄语，我是在此之后的 15 年左右才学习了俄语。我们与两位美国人共乘一辆福特牌出租车去宾馆，两位美国人低

Americans, who complained under their breaths at the slowness of the vehicle. Their English was not lost on the driver, however, who turned to the surprised passengers in the rear of the cab and remarked, for their benefit, "Nothing in the world can be done without patience."

At the hotel, several young, well-dressed, English-speaking women arranged our travel plans. They assigned me to a sparsely furnished room that I shared with Dr. Hou Zonglian, who some years hence would become dean of the Shanxi Provincial Medical College. Later I met some old friends, including an Austrian physician who had once visited Dingxian, and Hilda Yen, niece of Dr. W. W. Yen, China's ambassador to the Soviet Union, with whom she was staying. The ambassador welcomed the Chinese delegation with a banquet at the embassy. Later in Leningrad, we were entertained by the Russians as well. There we attended a large reception replete with an elaborate buffet and many vodka toasts.

Our general impressions were limited, as we were not free to stray far from the hotel. The people we observed on the surrounding streets were quite simply dressed in contrast to our hotel guides, and we saw few smiling faces. We were told that there was a thriving black market. The subway trains were clean and comfortable, and the tunnels were paved with marble and decorated with large wall paintings.

Transportation and hotel accommodations in Leningrad were better than those in Moscow. The conference of physiologists was held in the hall of a great palace built before the Revolution. Foreign Minister I. V. Molotov addressed the group. The size and scale of the conference was impressive as there were hundreds of delegates from all over the world. Disappointingly, however, there were few small group discussions. We met the over-80-year-old, world-renowned physiologist Ivan Pavlov, who walked with a cane and had little to say. Assistants demonstrated his experiments with the conditioned reflex in a small laboratory, which was simply equipped and somewhat outmoded. Nothing was mentioned of his

声抱怨车开得太慢。但是这没有瞒过那位懂英语的司机，只见司机转过头，对着车厢里那些吃惊的乘客说："在这个世界上，没有耐心什么事情也做不成"。

在宾馆内，几个衣着考究的会讲英语的年轻女士安排我们的访问计划。她们给我安排了一间陈设简陋的房间，我与侯宗濂医生同住；几年以后，侯宗濂医生出任西安医学院院长。后来我遇到了一些老朋友，包括一位曾经访问过定县的奥地利医生及与她同在一起的颜女士，她是我国驻苏大使颜惠庆博士的侄女。在大使馆，大使设宴欢迎中国代表团。后来在列宁格勒，我们也受到俄国人的款待。我们参加了盛大的宴会，享用了精致的自助餐和伏特加酒。

我们不能离开宾馆太远，所以对这座城市的总体印象有限。我们看到周围街道上的人们衣着朴素，不苟言笑，与宾馆的导游形成鲜明对比。我们听说有一个繁荣的黑市。地铁车厢干净舒适，隧道铺着大理石，墙上挂着大型壁画。

列宁格勒的交通和酒店住宿都比莫斯科好一些。生理学家会议是在十月革命前修建的一所巨大宫殿的大厅里举办的。外交部长莫洛托夫向大家致辞。由于有数百名来自全世界的与会者，此次会议的规模与水平都令人难忘。不过会议只安排了少数小组讨论，空留遗憾。我们与80多岁的世界闻名的生理学家伊万·巴甫洛夫会面；他拄着拐杖走路，很少发言。助手们在一个小实验室里演示了他的条件反射实验，该实验室装备简单，有些过时。

world-famous work on gastric-juice secretions.

Local tours in Moscow and Leningrad included visits to a teaching hospital in a medical school, a tuberculosis santitarium for children, and an abortion hospital. The teaching hospital was an old, rather decrepit building. My guide, a middle-aged woman who spoke fairly good English, took me only to wards containing ten or more patients. They were not entirely clean. To my surprise, an elderly professor of gynecology commented to me privately: "No drugs. No equipment. I wish I could work in another country." At the tuberculosis sanitarium children of all ages were being treated with sunbathing and special diets. The institution itself appeared to be well managed, but nothing was mentioned about diagnostic techniques or patient recovery rates.

While it was to reverse its policy after World War II, the Soviet Union was concerned at that time about a problem of overpopulation, and Moscow alone had four hospitals devoted exclusively to performing abortions. While I was able to visit one such hospital, I was never able to learn exactly how many beds were available for this purpose. I watched one abortion being performed, an unpleasant experience in that it was done with a special long spoon and no anesthesia, and my impression was that it was quite hard on the patient. The patient made no complaint but frowned as she walked away from the surgery, disregarding other young women in the room who were laughing under their breaths, seemingly because they found her discomfort amusing.

The same interpreter accompanied me to Kiev, in the Ukraine, and thinking about the incidence of abortion, I discussed the issue with her. She was willing to talk at length on the subject, emphasizing that there was great public resistance to contraception, especially on the part of men, who were generally unwilling to use condoms. In Kolkhis, we visited a collective farm to view its nursery. There, two elderly women were caring for about twenty infants. The children were fed unpasteurized

在那次会上没提到巴普洛夫举世闻名的胃液分泌的研究工作。

在莫斯科与列宁格勒考察期间，我们参观了一所医学院的教学医院、一所儿童结核病疗养院和一所人工流产医院。教学医院是一个古老而相当破旧的建筑。我的向导是一位讲一口流利英语的中年妇女，她只带我参观了一个住着十几人患者的病房。这些病房都不太干净。令我惊异的是，一位年长的妇科教授私下对我说："没有药品，没有设备，我希望我能在别的国家工作"。在儿童结核病疗养院，所有年龄段的儿童都接受日光浴和特殊饮食治疗。看来该机构本身管理良好，但没提及医院的诊断技术或患者康复率。

第二次世界大战后，苏联调整了政策。当时的苏联担心人口过剩的问题，仅在莫斯科就有四家专门从事人工流产的医院。我当时参观了其中一所，但我不清楚有多少张病床用于人流手术。我观看了一次人工流产手术，这是一次不愉快的经历，因为手术是用一根很长的刮匙在没有麻醉的情况下进行的，在我的印象中，这对患者是很痛苦的。患者没有任何抱怨，只是皱着眉头离开了手术室，全然无视房间内的其他妇女正在低声发笑，她们显然对她的不舒服觉得很有趣。

同一位翻译陪我去了乌克兰的基辅，我和她讨论了人工流产发生率这个问题。她也愿意详细讨论这一话题，并强调公众对避孕的强烈抵制，尤其是男性，他们通常不愿意使用避孕套。我们参观了一个集体农场的托儿所。那里有两个老年妇人照看着大约

milk and there was apparently no trained medical attention available. The place was unclean and fly-infested.

Border officials permitted me to retain the many articles on health in the Soviet Union that my interpreter provided, so I was able to bring them home. In Geneva, where I met with League of Nations officials, I was asked my impressions of the visit. The Soviet Union, I answered, was ahead of many countries in practicing state medicine, but the quality of its service had to be improved.

Subsequently I visited Yugoslavia, where I found conditions to be quite different and much more interesting. Dr. Borislav Borcic, who for two years had served the Chinese Ministry of Health in an advisory capacity, had arranged for me to visit rural health care facilities in the Croatian region of the country. Accompanied by two sanitary engineers, a Mr. Petrik and a Mr. Tedorovitch, I traveled extensively through this area for three months in a motor vehicle equipped for rough terrain.

Their rural health program had two chief components, a system of small health centers and a project to improve rural water supplies. An experienced nurse administered each health center and was responsible for teaching hygiene to children and adults, stressing personal cleanliness and protection against infectious disease. She also gave some first aid treatments. The centers were quite numerous but, in contrast to village health stations in China, had no apparent link to any agency offering medical relief under a trained physician. Moreover, I saw no other evidence of any systematic effort to apply scientific medical knowledge, preventive or curative, in rural areas.

As to the provision of potable water in the rural areas, a really remarkable number of wells had been constructed. While some were rather shallow, all had been protected with a cover as well as supplied with a pump. The pumps were not the usual pressure type; rather, they had a series of metal cups, which functioned generally like windmill

20 名婴儿。婴儿喝的牛奶未经消毒，显然这里缺少训练有素、能够提供医疗照护的人。该地方卫生很差且苍蝇群集。

边境的官员允许我保留翻译提供给我的许多关于苏联卫生的文章，因此我能够将它们带回国。在日内瓦，我会见了国际联盟官员，他们问及我对这次访问的印象。我回答说，苏联在实行公费医疗方面领先于许多国家，但照护质量有待提高。

随后我访问了南斯拉夫，我发现那里的情况大不相同，且更令人感兴趣。博维斯拉夫·博西克医生曾以顾问身份在中国卫生部工作了两年，他安排我访问了该国克罗地亚地区的农村卫生保健机构。在两位清洁工程师皮特克先生和特多罗维切先生的陪同下，我花了三个月乘坐一辆能够在崎岖路面行驶的汽车走遍了整个地区。

他们的农村卫生规划有两个主要组成部分，一个是小型卫生中心系统，另一个是改善农村供水的项目。每个卫生中心由一名经验丰富的护士管理，并负责对成人和儿童进行健康教育，主要内容是个人卫生及传染病预防。这位护士也进行一些急救。这些中心数量众多，但与中国的农村卫生站相比，这些中心没有与那些由训练有素的医疗工作者主导的医疗机构建立协作关系。此外，在那里我没有看到系统地将现代医学知识（预防或治疗）用于农村地区的任何证据。

当地已经建造了大量水井在农村地区供应饮用水。有些井很浅，但所有的井都有井盖保护，并配备一个水泵。这种水泵不是常见的压力型，而是有一串金属杯，它们的功能通常就像风车的

buckets, continuously dipping water from the well and channeling it into a pipe, from which there was a perpetual flow of fresh water. The device was much less expensive than a pressure pump and relatively easier to repair in case of damage.

These wells were distributed throughout the rural areas, providing the villagers with easy access to fairly clean drinking water. They could also use the water for washing, as it was quite abundant. There was also a minor program of school health, directed by Andrija Stampar's wife, about which I heard when I had dinner with them in their home one night.

In Zagreb, the Croatian province capital, my hosts took me to the Rockefeller Foundation-supported institute of hygiene, which, not unlike the MEM, advocated an integrated approach to the solution of rural problems. The range of interest of this institution was broader than ours, however, and its faculty and staff included, in addition to medical personnel, sanitary engineers, agronomists, and specialists in veterinary medicine. I sat in on a discussion of modern storage of livestock feed. This was quite unlike the institutes of hygiene and schools of public health that I knew of elsewhere at the time. Those I was familiar with in the United States seemed to be concerned more with theoretical knowledge and scientific research than with the practical application of scientific knowledge for the benefit of the general population. Regrettably, decades later public health professors in the West seemed to be encouraging graduate students along the same lines.

My country, I later noted, was relatively deficient in developing a potable water supply system and in implementing sanitary engineering as a major part of the public health service. Economic conditions would have made it very difficult to construct wells of the type found in Yugoslavia, however. Moreover, China had few sanitary engineers and only one small department of civil engineering at Qinghua University that concerned itself with sanitary engineering and whose cooperation, in any event, was difficult to secure on projects such as Dingxian.

提桶，不断从水井中汲取水，然后把水引入一根管子里，水管中就不断有新鲜水流出。这种装置比压力泵便宜得多，而且在损坏时也相对容易修理。

这些水井遍布农村地区，为村民提供了相当干净的饮用水。由于水量充足，村民也能用这些水洗澡。有一天晚上，我在斯坦帕尔家中做客，还了解到他的妻子在当地领导着一个小型的学校卫生项目。

在克罗地亚省的省会萨格勒布，接待方带我去洛克菲勒基金资助的卫生研究院；该研究院与平民教育运动一样，提倡采用综合方法来解决农村问题。但是，这个研究院关注的范围比我们更广泛，教职员工除了医学人员之外还包括卫生工程师、农学家及兽医专家。我参加了一场关于现代化家畜饲料储存的讨论。这与我知道的当时其他任何地方的卫生研究院和公共卫生学院很不一样。我在美国所熟悉的是他们更关心理论知识和科学研究，而不是造福大众的科学知识的实际应用。令人遗憾的是，几十年后的西方公共卫生教授仍然鼓励研究生沿袭这一路线。

我后来指出，在发展饮用水供应系统和将卫生工程应用于公共卫生服务方面，我国做得仍还不够。然而，经济条件并不允许建造像南斯拉夫那种类型的水井。而且，中国的清洁工程师很少，只有清华大学一个很小的土木工程系关注清洁工程；而在这样的项目上，定县也很难获得与他们合作的机会。

The final visit of the journey, to India and Ceylon, was a disappointment. Most of the time was spent in Colombo and the surrounding regions of what is now Sri Lanka. I saw only some hookworm control clinics, where the part-time physicians failed to make careful examination of patients, and where laboratory evidence was generally lacking. The attitude of the physicians toward the poor peasants suffering from disease was quite unpleasant; for example, they reprimanded even seriously ill patients for not following directions properly.

India's vertical approach to health care disturbed me because I believe so strongly that health improvement cannot be achieved without concurrent progress in in other socioeconomic areas. A minority of Indians seemed to enjoy all the advantages of modern science in Western civilization, while the vast majority had very little; food, clothing, and shelter were critical problems. I have no firsthand knowledge of the situation at present; it may be much better.

Of all that I had seen, I was most impressed with work being done among the peasants in Yugoslavia. On the whole, I came away more certain than ever that we were on the right path of rural health experience with the Dingxian model, as it was based on working closely with the villagers in helping them solve their problems. I returned to work with heightened enthusiasm and was able to continue for two more years before the Sino-Japanese War began in 1937.

这次考察的最后一站印度和锡兰（现在叫斯里兰卡）令人失望。大多数时间是在科伦坡及其周边地区考察。我只看到一些钩虫病防治诊所，在那里兼职的医生不对患者做细致的检查，而且普遍缺乏实验室证据。医生对患病的贫苦农民的态度很不友好，例如，他们甚至责备重症患者没有正确遵循他们的医嘱。

印度的垂直医疗模式也令我困扰。因为我坚信，如果没有其他社会经济领域的同步进步，就不可能改善健康状况。西方文明中的现代科技带来的便利是少数印度人的特权，绝大多数人则被拒之门外；食物、衣服和住所都是严重的问题。我没有他们现今情况的第一手材料，可能现在已经改善了很多。

在我所看到的一切中，最令我印象深刻的是在南斯拉夫农民中所做的工作。总的来说，我比过去任何时候都更加确信我们走定县模式的农村卫生模式这条路是正确的，因为它是建立在与村民密切合作、以帮助他们解决问题的基础上。我以极大的热情重返工作岗位，并继续工作了两年，直至 1937 年抗日战争爆发。

译者：佟训靓，冷志伟

Chapter 4

Medicine and Health Under Wartime Conditions

While the work at Dingxian had been going on, the Japanese had been pushing further into North China and along the coastal provinces. In mid-1937, open, although undeclared, war broke out between the two countries, making it impossible to continue our field training. For nearly thirteen years thereafter, China knew hardship and chaos, caused partly by Japanese aggression and partly by the corruption of the Nationalist regime, whose indifference to the concerns of the people in the end left broad segments of the population, including many intellectuals, disdainful of its leadership.

Shortly after we were compelled to discontinue the Dingxian experiment, I left Beijing to do war relief work in South China, initially joining Robert S. K. Lim in Changsha, in Hunan Province. Not long after, I was asked to lend help in my native city of Chengdu, in Sichuan Province, which was being heavily bombed by Japanese warplanes. So I returned home in May 1939.

There, aside from organizing relief for the wounded, I taught public health in two local universities and in the early 1940s, notwithstanding the ongoing conflict, in my capacity as provincial commissioner of health, organized a provincewide system of state medicine, based on the Dingxian model. The Sino-Japanese War ended in 1945, and in 1946, I was invited to Chongqing, another major city in Sichuan Province, to

第 4 章

战时的医学与卫生

我在定县工作正在进行的同时，日本侵略军向华北和沿海数省推进。1937 年中期，虽未正式宣战，但两国间爆发了战争，我们的现场培训不能再继续下去了。在此后将近 8 年的抗日战争期间，我国经历了苦难和混乱，部分原因是日军的侵略，部分原因是国民党政权的腐败。国民党政权对人民所关切的事漠不关心，最终导致包括许多知识分子在内的广大民众对其领导彻底失去信心。

在我们被迫中断定县实验后不久，我就离开了北京，到华南进行战时救援工作，最初在湖南长沙参加林可胜的工作。此后不久，我被要求去我的家乡四川工作，那里被日本战斗机肆虐轰炸。我于 1939 年 5 月回到家中。

在成都，除了组织对伤员的救助外，我还在两所当地大学教授公共卫生课程；在 20 世纪 40 年代初，尽管战争仍在继续，我还是基于定县模式，以省卫生专员的身份组织了一个全省范围的公立医疗体系。1945 年抗日战争结束，1946 年，我应邀到四川

establish a new medical college. Once the medical college at National Chongqing University became operational, I served as its dean and as a professor in its School of Public Health until 1952. While these experiences were of an order different from that at Dingxian, they, too, provided valuable insights that furthered my evolving views on rural health, community medicine, and medical education.

PRELIBERATION CHINA: 1937 TO 1949

Meanwhile, in the enemy-occupied heartland of China, the Guomindang and its Western allies and the Chinese Communist party (CCP) were collaborating in a show of internal unity against external danger to try to oust the Japanese. Notwithstanding a barely concealed mutual emnity, the uneasy alliance between the Guomindang and Communists was maintained throughout the war years. After Japan's surrender in 1945, the united front predictably broke apart, revealing a nation that was in fact politically divided and economically in ruins.

Support for the Guomindang had eroded widely. In the interim the CCP not only had amassed a broad base of peasant support but also had gained the allegiance of many urban intellectuals, including some medical specialists. Disillusioned by the failures and the excesses of the Guomindang, this educated group was now pinning its hopes for the country's future on the Communist leadership and the ideological commitment of that leadership to socialist principles. To them, the party commitment to the well-being of the common people seemed to proffer hope for a better country and, with it, the prospect of health protection for all.

The civil war that broke out in China after the close of the Sino-Japanese War spanned four more years and exacted a high price in lives and human suffering. Those who supported the CCP were rewarded with victory at last in 1949, however, with the flight of Chiang Kai-shek and his supporters to Taiwan Province and the proclamation of the People's Republic of China in Beijing in October of that year.

省的另一个大城市重庆去创办一所新的医学院。从国立重庆大学医学院创办伊始直至 1952 年，我一直担任医学院的院长和公共卫生系教授。尽管这些经验与定县不同，也为我提供了宝贵的见识，开阔了我在农村卫生、社区医学和医学教育方面的眼界。

解放前的中国：1937 年至 1949 年

与此同时，在被敌军占领的中国腹地，国共统一战线形成，内部合作，一致反抗日本侵略者。1945 年日本投降后，统一战线破裂，内战爆发。

人民对国民党的拥护普遍有所下降。共产党不仅拥有广泛的农民支持基础，而且获得了包括一些医学专家在内的许多城市知识分子的支持。国民党的失败和暴行使这些受教育的人醒悟了，他们把对国家未来的希望寄托于共产党的领导层以及其对社会主义原则的思想信念上。对他们来说，党对普通民众福祉的承诺似乎为构建一个更好的国家带来了希望，有了这些，全民保健才有希望。

抗日战争结束后，中国爆发了长达四年多的内战，付出了生命和人类苦难的高昂代价。终于，中国共产党带领广大人民在 1949 年获得胜利；同年 10 月中华人民共和国在北京正式宣告成立。

HEALTH DEVELOPMENT AND MEDICAL EDUCATION IN SICHUAN PROVINCE

What I am able to add to an account of the Chinese experience in rural health development during the Sino-Japanese War and there after until 1949 is limited to what I knew through my immediate personal experience or through personal contacts in southwestern China. In that part of the country, which felt the impact of the hostilities but managed to evade occupation, medical personnel stayed in touch as best they could and functioned in their roles wherever they found themselves.

Quite a few modern-trained physicians left their native cities in the Japanese-controlled northern and coastal regions or the central Yangtze River valley and resettled farther in the interior. There they convened on several occasions at general meetings of the Chinese Medical Association (CMA), called by its president, P.Z. Jin. Jin, who had been elected to his office just before the war, retained oversight of CMA affairs during this period. The meetings in both Kunming in 1940 and Chongqing in 1943 were relatively well attended considering that a major war was under way. Some 500 members attended the first postwar meeting, held in Nanjing, and twenty-five papers were presented. Dr. Zhu Zhanggen was elected to the presidency in 1947.

The Dingxian experiment, which had just begun to gain national and international recognition, ended shortly after the incident at the Marco Polo bridge on July 7, 1937. Japanese forces soon occupied Beijing, and it became impossible to offer systematic field training at the Dingxian site. Many staff members left at once. A few subdistrict personnel and village health workers remained but by the following year operations had terminated entirely.

For the moment, my personal future remained clouded. Two years earlier, in 1936, I had been appointed superintendent of both the Peking First Health Station and the Dingxian Rural Health Station. Earnings

四川省卫生事业的发展和医学教育

对有关中国农村卫生在抗日战争开始直到 1949 年之间发展的经验，我所能补充的内容只限于我个人的直接经历或来自我在西南接触到的其他人。在西南地区可以感觉到战争的冲击，但都在想方设法地避免被占领，医务人员尽可能保持联系，并随时随地发挥自己的作用。

相当多经过现代培训的医生离开了他们在日本控制的北部和沿海地区或长江流域中部的家乡，在更远的内陆地区定居。在内地，由中华医学会会长金宝善召集了几次全体会议；金宝善在战前才当选这一公职，在此时期他一直悉心照管着中华医学会的事务。由于处在战争时期，只有 1940 年在昆明和 1943 年在重庆举办的两次会议出席率比较好。约有 500 名成员参加了在南京召开的第一次战后会议，发表了 25 篇文章。1947 年，朱章赓博士当选为会长。

1937 年 7 月 7 日卢沟桥事变后不久，刚开始得到国家和国际认可的定县实验就中止了。日军很快占领了北京，因此我们已不可能在定县提供系统的现场培训。许多工作人员立即离开了定县。一些街道工作人员和村卫生员仍然留在那里，但到第二年这项工作就彻底停止了。

那时，我个人的前途未卜。两年前，即 1936 年，我被任命为北平第一卫生事务所和定县农村卫生站的负责人。我在不同岗

from my various posts allowed me to provide comfortably for my family, and medical officers of the Japanese occupational forces expressed interest in, and respect for, my work.

Without sovereignty, however, it was useless to attempt constructive activities. Moreover, the brutality of the Japanese militarists toward the defeated Chinese seemed unconscionable to me; their behavior reignited the intense Nationalist sentiments I had experienced as a medical student during the anti-British protests of 1925. It became impossible to remain closeted within the walls of academe at such a time. Indignation and patriotism compelled me to find some alternative, some way to apply my medical training on behalf of my compatriots.

So, in May 1938, at my own expense, I left Beijing in great secrecy to join Professor Robert S. K. Lim, in war relief work in South China. Lim meanwhile had been appointed director of the Chinese Red Cross, whose headquarters were at Changsha, capital of Hunan Province. My departure from Beijing was so secret that neither the medical college nor the staff of the Peking First Health Station had been informed of my intention to leave.

In a very roundabout journey, I made my way to Changsha in South China. Fang Shih-san, a returned student from Japan and a member of the PUMC Board of Trustees, had been able to secure a permit for me to travel via Tianjin and Shanghai. So I followed that route and then took an ocean liner to Hongkong and from there a plane to Changsha to join Lim.

By the time I arrived at Changsha, Japanese forces were already pushing very close to the city and Cuomindang forces were retreating. The Chinese Red Cross had withdrawn farther into the interior, southwestward some 400 miles, to Guiyang, capital of Guizhou Province. Pressing on to Guizhou, I found the Chinese Red Cross there inadequately organized to work efficiently, so I had to abandon plans for useful activity through that channel.

位上的收入使我能够轻松地养家糊口，日本占领军的军医官对我的工作表现出兴趣和尊重。

然而，在失去主权的情况下想要搞建设性的活动是徒劳的。日军对战败的中国人的暴行令人发指；他们的行为重新点燃了我在 1925 年中英对抗时，作为一名医学生所经历过的强烈的民族主义情绪。在这种时候我不可能继续留在医学院的围墙内空谈。愤怒和爱国热情激发我做出其他选择，为了我的同胞而继续开展医学培训。

因此，我于 1938 年 5 月十分秘密地自费离开北京，参加了林可胜教授主持的华南战地救援工作。当时林教授已被任命为中国红十字会会长，总部设在湖南省省会长沙。我是秘密离开的，所以医学院和北京第一卫生事务所的职员均不知晓我的离京意图。

我在十分波折的旅行中向南方的长沙前进。一位日本回国留学生同时又是北京协和医学院董事会的成员方石珊为我拿到一张途径天津和上海的许可证。于是我沿着此路线乘船到香港，然后由香港乘机到达长沙与林可胜汇合。

我到达时，日军已逼近长沙，国民党军队正在撤退。中国红十字会已撤至内地，离贵州省会贵阳西南方向约 300 公里处。我加紧赶往贵州，发现那里的中国红十字会组织不当而不能有效地工作，因而我不得不放弃经由这一渠道开展有益活动的计划。

In the same province, however, I found an opportunity for constructive action through the North China Council of Rural Reconstruction. The council had recently transferred its operations to Guizhou Province from Shandong Province, which had been one of the first areas occupied by the Japanese. Like the PUMC, the North China Council of Rural Reconstruction was a Rockefeller- supported program, but its objective was developmental rather than educational. Broadly stated, its principal goal was national reconstruction with special reference to rural problems;1 it offered experimental training to university students in public health, agriculture, and other fields. I became head of its Health Department and acting director of its Rural Institute.

The field activities of the council were based in Dingfan District, some twenty miles from Guiyang, a rural area not unlike Dingxian. Soon after my arrival, arrangements were concluded for Dingfan to become a site for field training in community medicine for senior medical students from Guiyang Provincial Medical College, just as PUMC and other students in North China had been sent to Dingxian. One of my students there later became dean of the School of Public Health of Kunming Medical College.

Organizing Wartime Medical Relief

At this moment the provincial government of Sichuan was reorganized under a new secretary-general, and I was asked to return to Chengdu, the city where I had been born, to organize a medical relief program. Up to that time the government had made no provision for war victims, and such provision was badly needed. Japanese bombs were wounding and killing inhabitants of the city every day. My father, who was still living at the time, urged me to return home.

Although I was reluctant to return for several reasons, I finally decided to do so, compelled by the dire need of the local inhabitants. My hesitation arose partly from reluctance to leave newly assumed

然而，还是在贵州省，我发现了一个通过华北农村建设委员会开展建设性活动的机会。该委员会把被日本人最早占领的山东地区的工作转移至贵州。华北农村建设委员会如同北京协和医学院一样，也是洛克菲勒基金会支持的项目之一，但其目的是发展而不是教育培训。总的来说，其主要目标是国家建设问题，特别是农村建设问题，它给大学生提供公共卫生、农业和其他方面的实验培训。我当了卫生部门的负责人及农村研究所的代理所长。

该委员会的现场活动建立在离贵阳30公里的定番州，一个与定县相似的农村地区。我到达后不久，就决定把定番州作为贵阳省立医学院高年级医学生进行社区医学现场培训基地，就像北京协和医学院和华北的其他学生被送往定县一样。我在那里的一位学生后来成为昆明医学院公共卫生学院的院长。

组织战时医疗援救

此时，一位新秘书长重组了四川省政府，我被邀回到我出生的成都市去筹建医疗援救项目。直到那时，国民党政府还没有为战争受害者提供任何援助，然而这种援助是人民急需的。日军的炸弹每天都在伤害这座城市的居民。家父那时仍健在，也极力主张我回去。

尽管出于多方面的原因我不愿意回去，但鉴于当地居民的迫切需要，我最终做出了回去的决定。我的犹豫一方面是因为我不

responsibilities with the North China Council of Rural Reconstruction and partly from my hesitation to undertake a program that was to receive practically nothing in the way of support. Even with the best financing, it would have been difficult enough to organize and run such a program. But I was to be given only ¥3,000 to start operations, the equivalent of the cost of 800 to 1,000 pounds of rice. That was all, nothing else; no equipment, no building, no staff; however, these two reasons for my reluctance paled before a third, and personal, concern, the plight of my family, left behind in Beijing. If I went to Chengdu, the distance between us would increase even further. Still there was nothing to do but try to do my best for the bombing victims, and so in May 1939 I left Guiyang for Chengdu.

In Chengdu I found that no progress in health matters had been made during my sojourn of eighteen years outside the province. The missionary schools and hospitals had influenced the health status of the people to some extent, but their work was largely philanthropic and the Chinese themselves had made no serious attempt to promote public health.

I began to organize medical relief for the hundreds of wounded immediately on my arrival. There was no government hospital in Chengdu at the time. Therefore, my approach was to enlist the collaboration of the missionary hospitals and the medical schools of the West China Union University, which at that time was an amalgamated institution embracing the faculties of several other universities that had had to close down because of the war. The university had been established in the early 1900s by Protestant missionaries from Canada; hence, its original faculty was predominantly foreign. In 1939 many Chinese were also enrolled at the University, including one group from Chilu University in Shandong Province, another group from National Central University in Nanjing, and a few former students at St. John's College in Shanghai. The amalgamated institution was quite willing to cooperate in a program to assist the wounded.

愿放弃刚刚接受的华北农村建设委员会的职务，另一方面是不愿意接受一个几乎得不到任何支持的项目。即使有充足的资金，要筹建和进行这样的项目也相当困难。可是只给我 3000 元，相当于 500 千克大米的价格，去创办医疗援助项目。就这些钱，其他什么也没有；没有设备、没有房子和职员；然而，这两个让我不情愿的原因在第三个之前就显得黯然失色，第三个原因涉及我留在北京的家庭困境。假如我去成都，我与我家庭的距离会更远。然而我没有别的办法，只能尽全力去帮助战争的受害者，因此我于 1939 年 5 月离开贵阳前往成都。

回到成都我发现，在我旅居在外的 18 年中，成都的卫生状况没有任何改善。教会学校和医院对人民的健康情况有一定程度的影响，但主要是慈善性工作，而中国人自己并未真正努力改善公共卫生。

我到达后立即为数百名伤员组织医疗援救。当时成都仍没有公立医院。因而，我设法取得教会医院和华西协合大学医学院的合作；当时，华西协合大学是一个联合大学，包括其他几所因战争而不得不关闭的学院。这所大学在 20 世纪早期由加拿大的新教传教士所建立，因而最初教职工主要是外国人。1939 年，许多中国人也被该校录取，包括一批来自山东省齐鲁大学，另一批来自南京国立中央大学的人员和少数过去是上海圣约翰学院的学生。联合大学非常愿意在一项救助伤员的项目上进行合作。

Medical relief work occupied me more or less full time until early 1941, when I was able to give some attention to organizing a six- month field training program for rural health instruction of medical and nursing students. With the help of the medical schools of the amalgamated university group, we developed a health service in Wenjiang, a town and district of the same name, near Chengdu, as the teaching facility. A former PUMC student, Li Ting-an, took charge of the program.

After the United States declared war against Japan, an American airbase was established at Chengdu, and antiaircraft equipment was brought in. In time, as resistance against the Japanese stiffened, the bombing attacks became less frequent and finally stopped. We were then able to begin to turn our attention primarily from medical relief to the establishment of a provincewide network of health services.

Developing Urban and Rural Health Services

Meanwhile, I had been appointed Professor of Public Health at the the medical school of the West China Union University as well as commissioner of health for Sichuan Province, a huge and populous province that extended some 700 miles from north to south and some 500 miles east to west. At the time of my appointment there was no public health organization of any kind in the province. Even the city of Chengdu, the provincial capital, had no health department.

A framework of public health service had already evolved in connection with our medical relief work, however. The temporary hospitals for the wounded; the isolation hospital; various maternal and child care clinics; and a training center for nurses, midwives, and public health personnel, as well as the rural teaching facility had all been organized. In addition, there were antiepidemic mobile medical corps.

We next began to develop municipal health services in Chengdu and district-run health services in the rural districts. By the time I resigned at the close of the Sino-Japanese War, there were more than eighty health

医疗援救工作几乎占据了我全部的时间，直到 1941 年年初，我才有余力为医学生和护理学生组织一项六个月的农村卫生教育现场培训。在联大医学院同事的帮助下，我们在成都附近的一个城镇和区同名的地区——温江，建立了一个卫生服务中心作为教学机构。北京协和医学院的毕业生李廷安负责此项目。

美国对日宣战后在成都建立了美国空军基地，并引进了防空装备。随着对日反抗的加强，轰炸袭击变得不那么频繁，并最终停止。于是我们才能开始将主要精力从医疗援救转向建立一个全省范围的卫生服务网络。

开展城乡卫生服务

与此同时，我被委任为华西协合大学医学院公共卫生学教授和四川省卫生专员；四川是一个地大而人口众多的省份，南北绵延约 1100 公里，东西绵延约 800 公里。在我上任时，省内没有任何类型的公共卫生组织机构。即使在省会成都市也没有卫生部门。

然而，我们已经形成了一个与医疗救援工作有关的公共卫生服务框架。伤员的临时医院、隔离医院、各种妇幼保健诊所、农村教学机构都已建成。以及护士、助产士和公共卫生人员培训中心，此外，还有流动的抗疫医疗队。

接下来，我们重新在成都开展城市卫生服务，并在农村地区开展以区为级别的卫生服务。到抗日战争结束前我辞职时，四川

centers in the majority of the districts of Sichuan Province. Well-trained technicians and professionals to staff these units were relatively scarce, of course, but essentially the demand was met. Sources of trained personnel included recent graduates of provincial medical colleges and the medical schools of West China University, as well as some older physicians who had come to Sichuan to escape the fighting but who stayed on permanently at the conclusion of hostilities.

With such a large number of rural health centers in Sichuan operated under district government auspices, I felt that during my tenure as commissioner of health, we had made a significant start in the inauguration of state medicine on a provincewide basis. No other province at the time had anywhere near as many rural health centers as had Sichuan.

In addition, total public expenditures for health had increased many times over between 1939 and 1946. Most of the increase reflected expenditures at the local level by district authorities eager to have a health facility in their own jurisdiction for the first time. The provincial budget increased as well, however—exponentially, in fact. In part, the increase was real, indicative of the secretary- general's growing confidence in our program. In part, however, it was attributable to spiraling inflation, which was already terrible, and in the postwar years would reach devastating proportions. From the original ¥3,000 our annual operating budget had increased to more than ¥10 million.

From this experience in wartime Chengdu, I gained some valuable insights. I saw that it was possible to make substantial progress in developing rural health care delivery, even with very limited economic resources and under very trying conditions, provided the support of government officials and medical college administrators could be enlisted. Also, I acquired additional experience in medical education, teaching quite a number of medical and nursing students who later worked in the provincial municipal and district health organizations. That experience reinforced my belief in the crucial role of practical field

省大部分地区已分布有 80 多个卫生院。当然，这些单位配备的受过良好培训的技术员和专业人员仍比较少，但基本能满足需要。这些经过培训的人员来自省立医学院和华西协合大学医学系毕业的学生，以及为躲避战争而来到四川并在战争结束后定居下来的一些年长的医生。

在我身为卫生专员期间，我认为在四川省能有这么多农村卫生中心在区政府的领导下工作，表明我们在一省范围内已为国家的卫生保健体系创立了良好的开端。那时没有哪个省份像四川那样拥有如此多的农村卫生中心。

此外，1939—1946 年期间，四川政府用于卫生的公共支出增加了许多倍。这种支出的增加大部分反映出地方领导开始渴望在自己管辖范围内建立卫生机构。省里的预算也增加了，事实上预算呈指数性增长。有一部分增加是真实的，表明省秘书长对我们的项目越来越有信心。然而，还有部分原因是已经很可怕的通货膨胀，且在战后几年达到毁灭性的程度。我们的年度预算从每年3000 元增加到超过 1000 万元。

从战时成都的经历我得到一些宝贵的见解。我认为即使在极有限的经济资源和极困难的处境下，只要能争取到政府官员和医学院管理人员的支持，仍有可能在农村卫生保健服务的发展上获得实质性的进展。我也从对大量医学生和护士的教学中得到了医学教育方面的额外经验，这些学生后来都在省市和区卫生机构工作。这种经历使我更加相信，现场实地培训对公共卫生人员起着

training for public health personnel.

The support we had received from the provincial government in Sichuan throughout this period was attributable in part to two related personal experiences. First, the provincial governor had become ill. He registered a high fever, and his personal physician had begun treatment with sulfa drugs. The fever of the stricken official decreased, but he then developed conjunctivitis in both eyes. At that time, I was called in for an opinion and, after examining him, attributed his optic condition to sensitivity to sulfa. My advice was to discontinue use of the drugs. Twenty four hours later the conjunctivitis had subsided markedly. The governor and his family concluded that I was a "better" physician than the highly respected person who treated him regularly.

Next, the mother-in-law of the governor developed lobar pneumonia. The same respected physician initially treated her—successfully/ at first, but subsequently she developed an arrhythmic heartbeat. Again I was called in as a consultant and found that her physician had used digitalis, which can cause arrhythmia. Treatment with digitalis was discontinued, and her heartbeat soon returned to normal.

These incidents are recounted as evidence, not of my personal skills as a physician, but underlining that sound clinical training is as important for a public health physician as for any other. In this case, the individual patient benefited from not only my clinical consultations but also the public at large, since shortly thereafter the governor approved a substantial increase in the budget of the provincial health commission, which I headed at the time.

Establishing a National-Level Medical College

After the cessation of hostilities in 1945, that same governor joined the Nationalist central government when it moved eastward from Chongqing back to Nanjing. For the time being, I retained my teaching and administrative posts in Chengdu. In 1946, however, I moved to Chongqing, where I had been asked to establish a medical school at

至关重要的作用。

这一阶段我们从四川省政府得到的支持可部分归功于两件与我相关的个人经历。第一件事是时任省长生病了。病历记录为发高烧，他的私人医生开始用磺胺类药物治疗。省长退烧了，但接着出现了双眼结膜炎。我被叫来会诊，经检查后我认为他的结膜炎是由磺胺类药物过敏所致。我建议停用该药。24 小时后结膜炎明显消退。省长及其家人认为我比经常给他治病的那位备受尊重的私人医生"更高明"。

第二件事是省长的岳母患了大叶肺炎。开始仍是那位受尊重的医生给她治病；最初治疗有效，但随后患者出现了心律不齐。我作为医学顾问再次被请来会诊，发现她的医生给她用了会导致心律不齐的洋地黄。停用洋地黄后她的心律很快恢复正常。

列举这两件事不是为了证明我个人的医术，而是强调正规的临床培训对公共卫生医生和对其他医生一样重要。在这种情况下，不仅患者个人可以从我的临床咨询中获益，广大普通群众也可以受益，因为在这之后不久，省长批准大幅增加省卫生委员会的预算，那时我正是该委员会的主任。

建立一个国家级的医学院

1945 年抗日战争结束后，这位省长在国民党中央政府从重庆东迁回到南京时加入了中央政府。我暂时保留了在成都的教育和行政管理职位。然而，1946 年我被要求搬到重庆，在国立重庆大

National Chongqing University. Once the medical college became operational, I served as its dean and as professor of public health until 1952. The new institution would be effectively the first regular government medical school in a province of 70 million people.

I had to start from scratch, just as I had done in 1939 in organizing the first provincial health administration in Sichuan. Before taking up my new responsibilities, I made a brief trip to the United States. The Japanese had closed down the PUMC in 1942, and now it was to be reopened. I had been asked to serve on its Board of Trustees, and made the trip in that capacity. In the United States, I took the opportunity to visit Harvard, Cornell, and Western Reserve Universities to examine the public health education programs they were setting up in the postwar era.

Returning to China in early 1947, I went to Chongqing and immediately began to establish the preclinical departments of what was to be the Medical College of National Chongqing University, using a rented building for classroom space. At the same time I was appointed superintendent of two teaching hospitals.

The most immediate and urgent problem was inflation. The allotment with which we had undertaken to establish the medical college had been very small to start, but runaway inflation soon decreased its true value further. Many colleagues thought it would be impossible to organize the college because one could not find faculty even for the preclinical departments who would be willing to work for the small salaries we would offer. In a situation of rampant inflation, everyone was quite understandably concerned about nurturing their economic resources, and clinicians could earn far more in private practice than we could pay.

The solution I decided on was to hire promising young medical school graduates, whose immediate earning potential was less than that of older colleagues, and to give them, in place of a high salary, responsibilities and opportunities for professional growth they could

学筹建医学院。医学院从一开始运作直到 1952 年，我都担任其院长和公共卫生教授。新学院实际上是这个有 7000 万人口的省份里第一所由政府办的正规医学院校。

正如 1939 年我在四川筹建第一个卫生院时一样，我不得不从头开始。在就任新职前，我去美国做了一次短暂的旅行。那时，被日本人在 1942 年关闭的北京协和医学院复校了，我被邀请成为其董事会成员，这次我即以此身份进行了这次旅行。在美国，我借机访问了哈佛、康奈尔和西储大学，考察了他们在战后年代建立的公共卫生教育项目。

1947 年初回国后我回到重庆，并立即开始建立国立重庆大学医学院的医学预科部，租用一幢楼做教室场地。同一时期我被任命为两所教学医院的院长。

通货膨胀是最现实和紧迫的问题。拨给我们建立医学院的经费本就少到难以起步，不久无法控制的通货膨胀又进一步降低了经费的真实价值。许多同事认为不可能组建医学院，因为甚至都难以找到医学预科部的教职工，没有人愿意为我们所提供的微薄薪水工作。在通货膨胀猖獗的情况下，很容易理解每个人都关心如何增加自己的收入，而临床医生在私人诊所赚的钱比我们能支付的要多得多。

我采取的办法是任用有前途的、但眼前挣钱的能力比不上老同事的医学校毕业生，我以给他们负责任和专业培养发展的机会

not obtain elsewhere. One of these opportunities was the possibility of a fellowship for advanced training abroad, funded by the American Bureau for Medical Aid to China, a privately sponsored group involved in postwar reconstruction, in whose leadership J. Heng Liu, former Minister of Health, played a prominent role. Through this program, for example, we sent a pathologist, a bacteriologist, and several physiologists to universities in the United States for advanced training.

I selected these prospective faculty members with utmost care, and in time was able to gather a highly qualified faculty, composed of enthusiastic and innovative young clinicians. Only two held the rank of full professor, however, one in biology and the other in pathology. With this faculty assembled, we organized a full six- year medical curriculum, including a one-year internship.

Spiraling inflation, however, continued to threaten the fledgling institution throughout the remainder of Nationalist rule. At one point the equivalent of my entire annual salary was needed to feed my family for just one week, which indicates the severity of the situation. Everywhere people were fighting for food, as the price of rice skyrocketed, not so much because there was a real shortage as because merchants with ties to the Guomindang had stockpiled it to create artificial scarcities. Warlords and landlords in Sichuan Province in particular were making life hard for the peasants, who were preoccupied with a day-to-day struggle for survival. Villages were being emptied as the farmers and their families succumbed to nutritional edema. In the cities, salaried people felt the impact, in particular, and were driven to selling furniture and other family heirlooms to prevent starvation.

Somehow, though, despite the destructive consequences of inflation, the medical college was able to survive and prosper during this difficult period, when the country's resources had been depleted to almost nothing after decades of war, disillusionment, and corruption. We managed by judicious hiring of personnel; by economy in the use of equipment, some

来代替高工资，而这些是他们在其他地方难以获得的。其中一个机会是获得出国进修的奖学金；由美国援华董事会提供资助，该援华会是一个私人赞助的参与战后重建的组织，在原卫生部长刘瑞恒的领导下发挥了突出作用。举例来说，通过这个项目我们派了一名病理学家、一名微生物学家和几名生理学家到美国的大学进修。

我精心挑选了这些有前途的教职工，并及时聚集了一批由高素质、具有热情和创新精神的年轻临床医生组成的教职工团队。可是，只有两个人有正教授头衔，一名是生物学家，另一名是病理学教授。由这样的人员配备，我们建立了包括一年实习期在内的六年医学课程。

然而在整个国民党统治的后期，不断恶化的通货膨胀继续威胁着这个羽翼未丰的学院。从一点上可看出情况的严重性，有一段时间我全年的工资收入只够养活我家人一周。米价飞涨导致人们到处在为食物而战。而米价飞涨与其说是因为真的短缺，还不如说是因为商人与国民党勾结屯积粮食，人为造成的缺粮。尤其是四川的军阀和地主，使得农民生活变得困难，农民每天都在为生存而挣扎。农民及其家庭成员因营养性水肿死亡，村庄逐渐荒芜。在城市中，领工资的人特别能感到这种冲击，他们被迫出售家具和其他传家宝以避免挨饿。

尽管通货膨胀带来了致命的后果，且经历了几十年的战争、贪污腐败而导致国家资源几乎耗尽的困难时期，医学院仍然能够

of which we shared with other university departments; and by other careful administrative decisions. We had even begun to develop a rural field training site in the Beipei area, about two hours distant from the campus; however, this program had to be discontinued with the escalation of Communist efforts to oust the discredited regime. Aside from having to abandon our field training program, however, we felt we had made credible headway in the 1946-1949 period, overcoming not only the financial problems but also the many academic and other difficulties that inevitably arise in the course of such an undertaking.

Late in 1949 the struggle to liberate the country had reached a climax, and tension among the local inhabitants in Chongqing was running especially high. Corruption and the accompanying political and economic chaos had taken their toll on the city's inhabitants, and rampant inflation had sent morale plunging within the teaching profession.

In November the Guomindang troops based at the Chongqing airfield had fled. Some workers at the medical school and the affiliated teaching hospitals, too, were on the verge of flight. The situation climaxed on the 29th of that month with the triumphant entrance of the People's Liberation Army (PLA) into the city that had once been the wartime capital of the Nationalist government.

生存下来并茁壮成长。我们通过合理使用人员，节约设备开支，有些设备与其他大学的教研室合用，以及其他谨慎的行政决策来管理学院。我们甚至开始在离学校约两小时路程的北碚地区开展农村现场培训基地。后期，由于政局变化，这一项目不得不终止。但是，除了不得不放弃现场培训项目外，我们认为在 1946 年到 1949 年期间，我们取得了明显的进展，不仅克服了经费的问题，而且克服了从事这一工作中难以避免的许多学术和其他困难。

1949 年解放全国的斗争达到高潮，重庆当地居民的紧张局势也达到顶点。腐败和随之而来的政治、经济混乱给居民带来了损失，而猖獗的通货膨胀使教师的职业道德也下降了。

11 月，驻扎在重庆机场的国民党军队逃跑。一些医学院和附属教学医院的工作人员也随之外逃。当月 29 日随着解放军胜利进驻曾经是国民党政府首都的重庆市，国民政府彻底结束了在四川的统治。

译者：贾萌萌，冷志伟

Part 2

Postliberation China

**Medicine in Rural China
A Personal Account**

解放后的中国

中国农村之医学
——我的记述

Chapter 5

The Health Experience From 1949 to 1976

Liberation in 1949 found me at National Chongqing University, in Chongqing, serving as dean and professor of public health at its Medical College, which I had organized and established in 1946. That moment in history was one of great optimism in our country, as the Chinese Communist Party (CCP) prepared to assume leadership of the newly established People's Republic of China, proclaimed by Party Chairman Mao Zedong in Beijing in October of that year.

The fundamental commitment of the CCP to the well-being of the common people provided the basis for a vision of a strong, new China, shared by members of the party, intellectuals such as myself, and other segments of the population. Rid of the Nationalist regime, which had sapped the country of its human and material resources, we could at last realistically once again cherish the hope of building a new society. Inflation, hoarding, and speculation, we expected, would soon also disappear, and efforts could be waged to counter the poverty, ignorance, and disease that had so long beset most of the population. As a physician with strong patriotic feelings, I looked forward to contributing to health improvement in the new socialist society.

Like other medical scientists, however, I was not able to contribute much to health development between liberation in 1949 and the death of

第5章

卫生事业发展历程

1949 年中华人民共和国成立前，我在重庆的国立重庆大学任教，并担任我于 1946 年组织成立的重庆大学医学院院长兼公共卫生学教授。10 月 1 日，毛泽东主席在北京宣布，中国共产党领导下的中华人民共和国成立。

中国共产党承诺为广大老百姓带来福祉，这为由党员、像我这样的知识分子和其他群体共同建立强大新中国的愿景奠定了基础。在摆脱浪费国家人力物力的国民党政权之后，我们终于可以真正地重拾建立新社会的希望。我们盼望通货膨胀、囤积和投机现象很快消失，长期困扰广大群众的贫困、落后和疾病等问题也会通过各项措施得以解决。作为一名具有强烈爱国主义情感的医生，我期待为社会主义社会、为改善卫生事业做出贡献。

但是，与其他医学研究者一样，从 1949 年解放到"打倒四人帮"期间，我未能对卫生事业发展做出太多贡献。1957 年之后，

the party chairman in 1976 and the subsequent overthrow of the radical Gang of Four. In the aftermath of party moves that silenced intellectuals and discouraged their initiative after 1957, became impossible for me to pursue my personal interest in enlarging the arena of scientific medical activity in rural China. Less than ten years later, the Cultural Revolution in 1966, with its tumultuous impact on the national life, especially in the scientific and academic spheres, still further circumscribed my activities.

In those years, party policy toward intellectuals as a group underwent a series of tortuous ups and downs, and to a large extent my own fortunes mirrored those shifting positions. Still, I fared better than some others. Political authorities permitted me to perform medical relief in the rural areas from time to time. In addition, I was fortunate to be able to continue teaching public health or directing research at a key medical college throughout a part of that period.

Meanwhile, China had advanced toward party goals on many fronts. Overall, progress in health care delivery had been very great. Between 1958 and the late 1960s, the party had succeeded in coordinating the establishment of a rural health care system that extended throughout the country. Given the numbers of people covered, the distances that separated them, and the dearth of resources—both human and monetary—the building of so extensive a system in so rapid a time was an impressive achievement. That feat, in turn, permitted significant strides in the control of epidemic diseases through massive immunizations of the farmers.

The rapidity with which this was accomplished, nonetheless, precipitated uncertainty among some experienced physicians about the quality of patient care, especially at the village level. The great majority of new recruits had had little or no formal education. Thus they entered the system typically lacking a sound grasp of human physiology and of the scientific basis of disease prevention and treatment. Their medical training was brief and unsystematic, not likely to fill in many of these gaps. There seem to have been no definite standards applied, and training

运动的余波使知识分子沉默下来，我也无法再追求我的个人理想，即扩大中国农村科学医疗活动的舞台。1966 年后国民生活动荡，特别是科学研究停滞，进一步限制了我的活动。

那个年代，我自己的命运在很大程度上映射了曲折动荡的环境。尽管如此，我还是比其他人更幸运一些。政府允许我不定期地在农村地区开展医疗救治。此外，在那段时期，我很幸运地能够在重点医学院继续教授公共卫生课程或指导研究。

与此同时，新中国在许多方面都朝着党确定的目标前进。总体而言，医疗保健工作取得了很大的进展。1958 年至 20 世纪 60 年代后期，党成功地协调建立起遍布全国的农村医疗保健制度。在覆盖人数众多、间隔距离较大以及资源（人力和财力）匮乏的情况下，能够如此快速地建立完善的医疗保健系统确实值得称赞。通过对农民进行大规模的免疫接种，这一系统在控制传染病流行方面取得了显著进展。

然而，由于这一目标的实现速度很快，一些经验丰富的医生对当时医务人员诊治患者的质量持怀疑态度，尤其是在村一级医务人员。绝大多数新工作的医务人员很少或没有受过正规教育。因此，他们在进入系统时，通常缺乏人体生理学以及疾病预防和治疗的科学基础。他们的医学专业教育简短且不系统，无法填补其中的很多差距。当时似乎也没有提出明确的标准，培训也因地点和个人而大相径庭。对新医务工作者的工作进行严密监督本可

varied considerably from place to place and individual to individual. Close supervision of the work of the new recruits could have alleviated some of these problems, but the system had not yet evolved to that point.

In a number of cases the training of even fully credentialed physicians educated in the 1949-1976 period was less than optimal, if only because it had been cut short in midstream. Over much of the period, intellectuals had lost favor, and "expertise" was dis dained. Medical studies were shortened and simplified. Often the teachers who taught these abbreviated programs were products of these curtailed programs themselves.

Another feature of the health experience of the 1949-1976 period that had an enduring impact on health in China was the adaptation of Soviet patterns in scientific organization and research, in line with a foreign policy that called for "leaning to one side" in the global struggle between the superpowers.1 The consequences were particularly significant for public health as a discipline, diverting it from the mainstream of general medicine. From the mid-1950s, public health no longer embraced a broad field of population-based issues but was confined to a narrow set of technical research topics, with emphasis on laboratory experimentation.

Overall, the 1949-1976 period had brought evident progress in health in some respects, while in others the results were less clear. Future years would provide plenty of time for reflection and stocktaking. One issue that seemed likely to be raised at some later date was whether, in the rush to expand the rural health infrastructure after 1958, considerations of quality had been kept in balance with those of quantity.

POSTLIBERATION CHINA: 1949 TO 1976

The well-known political campaigns of this period had major social and economic repercussions, including direct and indirect consequences

以解决其中的一些问题，但该体系尚未成熟。

在许多情况下，即便是那些在 1949 年至 1976 年间接受教育的、获得资质文凭的医生，他们也未能接受最佳的培训，原因之一是其学业经常被打断。在很长一段时间里，知识分子处境尴尬，"专长"得不到重视。医学研究也被缩短和简化了。那些教授简化课程的老师，自己也是这些简化课程的受害者。

1949 年至 1976 年间，我国在科学组织和研究方面采用了苏联模式，这符合当时的外交政策，即在超级大国的全球斗争中"一边倒"，这一卫生事业发展历程特征对中国的卫生事业产生了深远的影响。其结果对公共卫生学科而言尤为显著，使其脱离了医学的主流。从 20 世纪 50 年代中期开始，公共卫生不再包含基于人群问题的广泛领域，而是局限于一系列细分的技术研究主题，重点是实验室实验。

总体而言，1949 年至 1976 年间，卫生事业在某些方面取得了明显进展，但在其他方面的结果还不甚明朗。在未来，将有充足的时间对此进行反思和评估。在未来可能会提出一个问题，即在 1958 年之后急于扩大农村卫生基础建设的过程中，在质量与数量上是否得到了平衡。

解放后的中国：1949 年至 1976 年

在这一时期，众所周知的政治运动对社会和经济产生了重大

for health development. The first of these was the so-called antirightist movement that followed on the Hundred Flowers Campaign in 1956/57. In the Hundred Flowers interlude, intellectual leaders in many fields, including medicine, had been encouraged to speak openly and to evaluate progress and programs under CCP rule. Initial response had been cautious, but the invitation in due time produced a wave of comment and suggestion that the party chairman must have found decidely unwelcome for shortly thereafter the CCP launched an antirightist movement, vilifying those who expressed opposition to party policies and effectively discouraging any further rendering of critical views. Scientifically trained physicians and even some traditional scholar-physicians were included in the group that was rendered mute by the antirightist movement. With those persons silenced, medicine and public health thereafter were largely deprived of the influence of technically trained leadership.

The party launched the "Great Leap Forward" in 1958, emphasizing mobilization for acccelerated economic growth, under an ideological banner featuring themes of national self-sufficiency and labor-intensive production. In the countryside the agricultural cooperatives were organized into still larger socialized collective units—the communes. The communes had both economic and government functions, and their administrative committees were accountable to authorities at the county level. Members of communes were subdivided into brigades and work teams. Farmers were encouraged to have large families as a means of increasing agricultural production.

The interlude was short-lived, however. With respect to science and technologically advanced education, its negative effects were especially felt; medical science had been no less affected than other fields.

影响，也直接和间接地影响了卫生事业的发展。其中，第一个是
1956—1957 年的"百花齐放、百家争鸣"运动之后的"反右派运
动"。在"百花齐放、百家争鸣"期间，鼓励包括医学在内的许
多领域的知识领袖公开发言，并对政府的计划和进展进行评价。
此后不久，"反右派运动"对那些表示反对政策的人进行指责，
并阻止他们进一步提出批评意见。受过科学培训的医师，甚至一
些传统的儒医也未能幸免。随着这些人的沉默，受过技术培训的
领导层对医药和公共卫生事业的影响也大大减弱。

1958 年，党在以国家自给自足和劳动密集型生产为主题的思
想旗帜下，发起了"大跃进"运动，旨在动员加快经济增长。在
农村，农业合作社被组织成更大的社会化集体单位——公社。公
社既有经济职能，又有政府职能，其行政委员会对县级政府负责。
公社成员被细分为大队和工作小组。鼓励农民多生孩子、扩大家
庭规模，以此来增加农业生产。

几年后，"大跃进"停止了。随后是一段相对平静的政治时期，
在此期间，领导层中温和派的观点明显占了上风，知识分子的地
位有所提高。

然而，这一间歇期很短， 1966 年之后十年的混乱和苦难状
况已经有很多著述；在科学和技术的高等教育方面，尤其能感受
到负面影响；医学科学受到的影响不亚于其他领域。

HEALTH DEVELOPMENT BEFORE 1958

Immediately after liberation in 1949 the CCP made clear that its approach to health care would contrast markedly with that of the Guomindang. In accordance with socialist ideology, health protection for the entire population would be a central pillar in the new China. Whereas the Nationalist Ministry of Health had been quite powerless, given as a sop to a loyal party supporter and largely ignored by the inside leadership, CCP members immediately be low the top-ranking echelon stepped in to run the new Ministry of Health themselves. Its authority was immense, and it began early to plan for a centralized health program under state control.

In 1950 the health director for Southwest China Regional Administration summoned me to his office for a face-to-face discussion of health plans. He indicated that he expected soon to institute a health program in our region, under which everyone would have access to free medical care. I was interested to see how that would be accomplished.

That same year, the government held a National Conference on Health in Beijing, which physicians and other health leaders from across the country, including myself, were invited to attend. Premier Zhou Enlai delivered a six-hour speech containing many allusions to the CCP commitment to work for the people and urging the medical profession to devote itself to serving the country. Four slogans greeted the conferees and suggested the future direction of health policy: "Prevention first; serve workers, farmers, and soldiers; combine traditional and Western medicine; mobilize the masses."

Overall, there seemed to be reason for optimism. The health director for our part of China was endorsing state medicine, and at the national level, officials were talking "prevention first." It seemed as if public health teaching would receive strong support and that attention would be given to control of infectious diseases. Regarding the call for combining traditional and Western medicine, although the party chairman had clearly

1958 年之前卫生事业的发展

1949 年中华人民共和国成立后不久，中国共产党明确表示，新中国的医疗保健工作方针将与国民党形成鲜明对比。按照社会主义的理论，全民健康保障将是新中国卫生事业的中心支柱。国民党卫生部被安置了大量非专业人员且被领导层极端忽视，导致其相当无能。相比之下，中国共产党立即派遣高层领导管理新的卫生部。他们具有极大的权威性，并且很早就开始规划国家领导下的中央卫生计划。

1950 年，西南地区管理局卫生局长通知我到他的办公室，面对面地讨论卫生事业规划。他表示很希望在该地区建立一项卫生项目，每个人都可以获得免费医疗。我对此项目很感兴趣。

同年，政府在北京召开全国卫生大会，来自全国各地的医疗卫生工作者和相关领导（包括我本人）都应邀参会。周恩来总理发表了长达六个小时的讲话，其中包含对中国共产党致力于为人民服务的许多典故，并强调医学界要致力于为国家服务。会议确定了卫生工作四项原则："预防为主、面向工农兵、团结中西医、卫生工作与群众运动相结合"。

总体来说，前景乐观。西南卫生局长赞成国家医疗制度，国家级层面的官员们正在谈论"预防为主"。看来公共卫生教学将得到大力支持，传染病控制也将受重视。关于团结中西医的号召，虽然毛泽东主席明确表示将全力支持这一概念，但这究竟预示着

put his power and prestige on the line in support of the concept, what that might portend precisely we could only speculate. Like most of his comrades, he had spent much of his life in rural areas, where traditional medicine was the common form of medical relief and probably had a considerable amount of confidence in its efficacy. Still, he had also had some experiences that disposed him favorably to scientific medicine. One of the modern physicians attached to the PLA in the preliberation period—missionary-trained Fu Lianzhang, for example, had treated the party chairman successfully for malaria. Fu Lianzhang was later assigned to a high-ranking post in the Ministry of Health. The PLA as a group, in fact, had been generally impressed with the surgical skills of the modern physicians who served with them.

As it turned out, initially the party treated the two systems of medicine rather equitably. As the health bureacracy filled with cadres of rural origin, creating a natural constituency for indigenous medicine, however, there soon were signs that it would receive special attention.

In time, deliberate steps were taken to promote traditional medicine by broadening knowledge of it among modern physicians and by increasing the number of formally educated practitioners. Short courses in traditional medicine were introduced into the modern medical curriculum, and new colleges of traditional medicine were established in many cities. Terminology adapted from modern medicine began to infiltrate the lexicon, possibly to give it added legitimacy for scientifically oriented persons.

Party support for traditional medicine was troubling to a few modern physicians at that time. For anyone wrestling with the health problems prevailing in rural areas of our country in the 1950s, however, it was a pragmatic and not unrealistic policy. The rural population did not have access to any other form of relief, and to undermine its confidence in the traditional system under those circumstances would have been an irresponsible action.

什么，我们只能猜测。与大多数同志一样，他一生大部分时间都在农村地区度过，在农村地区，传统医学是医疗救助的常见形式，所以可能他对其疗效有相当大的信心。尽管如此，他也有一些经历，使他对科学医学产生了有利的影响。解放前，曾接受过传教士培训的一位现代医师傅连璋加入了解放军，曾成功地为毛主席治疗了疟疾。傅连璋后来担任卫生部高级官员。总体上，让解放军印象深刻的是与他们共事的现代医师的外科技术。

起初，党相当公平地对待这两个医学体系。然而，由于卫生系统多为农村出身的干部，为本土传统医学创造了天然优势。很快就有迹象表明，传统医学受到特别关注。

随着时间推移，政府通过一系列针对性措施来推广传统医学。包括扩大现代医师对传统医学知识的了解，增加受过正规教育的从业人员数量等。现代医学课程中引入了传统医学短期课程，许多城市建立了新的中医学院。从现代医学改编的名词术语开始渗透到传统医学词汇，使其在以科学为导向的人群中增加了其合法性。

当时，党对传统医学的支持令一些现代医生感到不安。然而，对于要解决 20 世纪 50 年代我国农村地区普遍存在的卫生问题，利用中医是一项务实而非不切实际的政策。农村人口无法获得任何其他形式的医疗，在这种情况下削弱农民对传统医学的信心是不负责任的行为。

Many of the new functionaries of the Ministry of Health had at one time been PLA medical workers. Some of them had received instruction in surgery or other areas essential to keeping an army healthy and on the move. By and large, however, their opportunities for formal education had been few and far between; what they knew came mainly from experience gained in the field.

Underpinning operations in the new health administration were two important working principles: (1) scientific work could, and should, be centrally controlled; and (2) in the framework for control, scientists themselves would be responsible to government and party functionaries who would make the policy decisions. Those functionaries, of course, were, in turn, responsible to the high- ranking officials in their own institutions for program development and execution. Many physicians—chiefly those with modern training, but also including a few scholar-physicians—failed to understand this new arrangement of working within a bureaucratic framework under administrators with little or no formal medical training.

In this context the reconstituted Chinese Medical Association, of which I served as vice president from 1951 to 1956, naturally exercised little voice in health at fairs. It conducted business as usual for a few years, experienced a short-lived merger with an association of scholar-physicians, and then was placed under the direction of the Ministry of Health. Members of the board, formerly appointed, were henceforth chosen by the ministry. Once subsumed under the ministry, however, the CMA had little influence, functioning mainly to support the execution of policies formulated by administrators.

Even at the start of Communist rule, when the CMA had had some autonomy, it exerted only a minimal influence on general medicine and public health. The only subject that seemed to arouse much interest within the CMA, or from those responsible for its activities on the outside, was surgery. This held particularly true when it came to representing our country at international conferences, most of which were held in Soviet and eastern

卫生部的许多新公务员曾经是解放军的医务工作者。他们中一些人接受过专业训练，包括在外科手术以及维护军人健康和战斗力的其他关键技术。但总的来说，他们接受正规教育的机会很少且远远不够，其知识主要来源于战地的实践经验。

新的卫生行政机构基本运作有两个重要的工作原则：（1）科学工作应该集中管理；（2）在管理框架内，科学家本身也应对政府和决策制定的党内工作人员负责。当然，这些党内工作人员反过来又对机构内开展和执行项目的高层官员负责。许多医生——主要是受过现代培训的医生，也包括一些儒医不能理解这种几乎没有受过正规医学培训的行政人员在官僚框架内的新工作模式。

在这种情况下，重组后的中华医学会（1951 年至 1956 年我担任副会长）自然对卫生事务几乎没有发言权。此后几年，中华医学会一如既往地开展业务，经历了与儒医协会的短暂合并，然后隶属于卫生部。以前被任命的委员会成员，此后由卫生部遴选。隶属于卫生部后，中华医学会影响减弱，主要职能是支持卫生部制定的政策的执行。

中华医学会在建国初期有一定的自治权，但它对全科医学和公共卫生的影响微乎其微。外科是唯一引起中华医学会内外极大兴趣的学科，这特别明显地表现为外科医生代表我国出席大多数在苏联和东欧国家举行的国际会议。典型的例子就是外科医生被

European bloc countries. Typically, it was surgeons who were sent to publicize medical advances in the new China to the outside world. It was not without irony that many of surgeons representing China had been trained at the PUMC, which in the light of its former foreign connections was being subjected to voluminous criticism by Chinese authorities at the time.

Strengthening its ties to other socialist countries, and seeking to learn from them, China was heavily engaged in remodeling its medical education and research organizations. Health and medical resources were being tunneled into the construction and development of large urban hospitals, teaching institutions, and research organizations. Many high-ranking officials were sent abroad on study tours, while lower-ranking functionaries were brought together at locations in China.

I, myself, was sent to the Northeastern Provinces to study Russian models in public health training. Having taught myself the Russian language, I was asked to translate a public health text for use in the secondary medical schools that were operated by provincial government authorities.

In the early 1950s, China critically lacked physicians. Qualified medical school instructors were even more scarce. Accordingly, under a new policy in effect with the academic year 1952/53, the medical school studies program was reduced from six to four years for the sake of rapid turnout. As a solution to the shortage of faculty, a number of relatively inexperienced young instructors were recruited and given short, supplementary medical courses intended to compensate for the deficiencies in their backgrounds. Older professors had trouble adapting their instruction to the new simplified program, which bypassed much of the clinical material and laboratory experimentation of an earlier period.

The policy was modified after only one year amid fears about the quality of future health care expressed by the general public as well as by physicians. Another year was added to the medical curriculum, bringing the total to five. This arrangement remained in effect until 1958.

派去向外界宣传新中国的医学进步。具有讽刺意味的是，这些代表中国的外科医生中许多都曾在北京协和医学院接受过培训，鉴于该校以前与海外的联系而曾受到过多次批评。

通过加强与其他社会主义国家的联系和学习，中国积极重塑医学教育和研究机构。大量卫生和医疗资源不断投入建设和发展大型城镇医院、教学机构和研究机构。许多高级官员被派往国外考察，而一般工作人员则被派往各地集中培训。

我本人被派往东北部省份，在公共卫生培训中研究苏联模式。在自学俄语后，安排我翻译一本公共卫生教科书，供省政府创办的中等专科医学校使用。

20 世纪 50 年代初，中国严重缺乏医师，而医学院里合格的教员更加匮乏。因此，根据 1952—1953 学年生效的一项新政策，医学院学制从六年减少到四年，以便尽早参加工作。为解决教员短缺问题，学校招募了一些相对缺乏经验的年轻教员，并开设了简短的补充医学课程，以弥补其背景的不足。年长的教授们艰难地适应新的简化教学程序，该程序绕过了早期的许多临床和实验室教学内容。

由于公众以及医生对未来医疗质量感到担忧，该政策在实行了仅一年后就进行了修改。学制又增加了一年，使总数达到五年。1958 年之前，一直遵循这一安排。

Medical school programs addressed the needs of students preparing for clinical work in urban or county hospitals or research institutions, and attention to the public health content of the curriculum soon became quite perfunctory. The general topics covered in public health studies—all superficially—were vital statistics, environmental sanitation, industrial hygiene, child health, nutrition and food hygiene, and pest control. The approach was based on the work of Max Joseph von Pettenkofer, a nineteenth-century German professor of medical chemistry. Content focused on such matters as the physical and chemical properties of air, water, soil, and food, with little attempt to relate these to social or biological conditions. The textbooks tended to duplicate materials covered in preclinical and clinical courses, especially material dealing with infectious diseases. Epidemiological case studies were notably lacking. Classroom instruction occupied over 50 percent of the time. Field training diminished to the vanishing point, and graduates emerged with no real sense of broad public health issues. Not surprisingly, medical student interest in public health diminished radically.

Meanwhile an experiment in medical education had been launched in the Northeastern Provinces to train a group of physicians specifically for practice in rural areas, where 80 percent of China's nearly one billion people live. Under the program junior- high-school graduates were enrolled and given a three-year program of medical training. The program was subsequently extended to other parts of the country. Graduates were variously known as "physicians" or "physician's assistants."

Meanwhile, medicine and public health education began to go separate ways. The Minister of Health had shown an interest in such an arrangement as early as 1950, and in 1953 the ministry organized a pilot program of specialized public health training. In 1955 the matter was formally concluded, with the announcement of plans to discontinue training of public health physicians and to organize instead separate public health schools for the training of "public health specialists."

医学院的课程是应对学生准备在城市或县医院或研究机构从事临床工作的需求而设置的。但对课程中公共卫生内容的关注很快变得相当敷衍了事。公共卫生研究中涵盖的一般主题（都是肤浅的）是生命统计、环境清洁、工业卫生、儿童健康、营养和食品卫生以及虫害控制。该方法是基于 19 世纪德国医学化学教授马克斯·佩腾可夫的研究。内容集中于空气、水、土壤和食物的物理和化学性质等问题，却很少联系到社会或生物等因素。教科书多重复临床前期和临床、尤其是与传染病相关的内容，但明显缺乏的是流行病学的案例研究。课堂教学占了 50% 以上的时间，现场教学几近消失，毕业生缺乏对广泛的公共卫生问题的真正认识。不出所料，医学生对公共卫生的兴趣急剧下降。

同期，在东北几省开展了一项医学教育实验，目的是培训一群医生以专门为在中国近十亿人口（80% 生活农村地区）的农村地区服务。根据该计划，录取初中毕业生接受为期三年的医学培训。该计划随后扩展到全国其他地区，毕业生被称为"医生"或"医生助理"。

与此同时，临床医学和公共卫生的教育方案开始分道扬镳。卫生部长早在 1950 年就已对此安排表现出兴趣，1953 年卫生部组织实施了公共卫生专业培训的试点计划。1955 年，该项目尘埃落定，宣布停止培训公共卫生医师的计划，取而代之的是组织设立独立的公共卫生学院以培训"公共卫生专业人员"。

Each of the six key medical colleges was to have such a school. One of the six was Sichuan Medical College, which had been organized on the campus of the former missionary-operated West China Union University, and when its public health school was established, I became its acting dean.

Officials of the Ministries of Health and Education formulated the overall framework of a generally four-year curriculum for the new public health schools. It was to cover two to three years of preclinical and clinical instruction, without much practical work, and less than one year for different public health specialties. As the program evolved, it emphasized classroom and laboratory instruction rather than field training at rural sites, where problems existed and required solutions. Graduates of those schools, rather than physicians, were to be the vanguard of new public health leadership.

The new schools accepted high-school graduates for training from the same pool of candidates also being considered for medical, dental, and pharmaceutical training. Although the public health schools were on the same academic level as the schools of medicine, they ranked lower in prestige because the best students were selected for medicine, not public health. Not unexpectedly, science and clinical teachers were quite uninterested in the public health students. Teachers in the public health schools were nearly all trained on short courses of different specialties without practical experience.

THE GREAT LEAP FORWARD AND THE LAUNCHING OF A RURAL HEALTH SYSTEM

In the years that coincided with the Great Leap Forward, there was a surging interest within the CCP in mobilizing the farmers in support of CCP goals and, in this context, in providing support to meet their special needs, including health. Consistent with this political view emanating from the top, medical education was shortened once again to three years after 1958 in most schools. (A few remained under the five-year arrangement.)

在六所重点医学院校中设立公共卫生系，包括在原传教士办的华西协合大学的校园里创办的四川医学院。在成立公共卫生系时，我担任了代理系主任。

卫生部和教育部为新的公共卫生系制定了四年学制的课程框架。它涵盖两到三年的临床前和临床教育，但临床实践很少。还包括不足一年的公共卫生各专业学习。该项目的发展强调了课堂和实验室教育，但忽略了大量急待解决的农村地区问题的现场实习。培训这些非临床医生的公卫系毕业生，是为了造就新公共卫生领导层的后备人才。

这些新的公共卫生学院与临床医学、口腔医学和药学专业一样，生源是通过高考的高中毕业生。虽然公共卫生学院与医学院学术水平相当，但由于最好的生源被选择进入了医学院而非公共卫生学院，因此公共卫生学院声望较低。不出所料，教授科学和临床学科的教师对公共卫生专业的学生缺乏兴趣，而公共卫生学院的教师几乎都只接受过不同专业的短期培训而缺乏实践经验。

"大跃进"和建立农村卫生体系

在"大跃进"时期，党对农民动员的兴趣高涨，宣传动员他们支持党的目标，并满足包括健康在内的特殊需求。教育的价值普遍降低。1958 年后大多数学院的医学教育再次缩短至三年制（仅少数保持五年制教育）。

High-level interest in the needs of the agricultural population was absolutely crucial to the massive expansion of rural health care system that took place beginning in 1958. Without it, this achievement would certainly have never been accomplished so rapidly and perhaps might never have occurred at all. With it, all the power of the central government, and the leverage that power provided, was brought to bear on the task. Given the impetus of the authority and prestige of the party chairman, the buildup proceeded with a degree of speed and deliberation that could hardly have been imagined in the past. In fact, there was so much centralized power that the government could achieve almost anything it set out to do.

While central and provincial health officials had voiced both the desire and the intent to extend modern health care across the country, until the highest authorities intervened, the idea had largely failed to materialize. They had built a few small hospitals in some county seats. Apart from that, however, efforts to date had concentrated on the operation or construction of hospitals and clinics in urban areas in a pattern not unlike the one that I had observed in the Soviet Union some years before.

The agencies that operated these facilities included, besides the Ministry of Health, the health administrations of the provinces and a number of other province-level government organizations, including three municipalities. All were urban-based bureaucracies. They formed the upper-level and urban component of government, as distinct from lower-level and rural component—the counties, sub-counties or communes, and villages or brigades.

Health officials were called to task soon after the Great Leap Forward began. The Ministry of Health came under sharp attack, as Chairman Mao criticized its urban orientation and charged it with being " the ministry of influential people," serving only high officials.

The initial response to the criticism was to dispatch mobile health teams to provide some clinical care to the farmers. Mobile units could go

高层领导对农民需求的关注，对 1958 年开始的大规模壮大农村医疗保健体系至关重要。如果没有这种关注，农村医疗保健体系的建设肯定不会如此迅速完成，或永远也无法完成。正是由于中央政府的权威及其带来的影响，才能胜任这项任务。在党的权威和声望的推动下，农村卫生保健体系以前所未有的速度和审慎的态度开始建立起来。事实上，政府几乎可以完成它计划的任何事情。

尽管中央和省级卫生官员都表达了在全国推广现代医疗保健的愿望和意图，但在最高权威的干预之前，上述想法基本上还没有实现。他们在一些县城建了几所小医院，除此之外，迄今为止的努力都集中在城市医院和诊所的运作或建设上，这种模式与我几年前在苏联观察到的模式并无不同。

运营这些设施的机构除卫生部外，还包括各省的卫生行政部门和其他一些省级政府组织，包括三个直辖市。这些都是地处城市的政府机构，它们构成了政府的上层机构和城市部门，而有别于基层机构和农村部分——县、乡、公社以及村庄或大队。

"大跃进"开始后不久，卫生官员就被派去执行任务。其间卫生部受到了严厉的批评。领导认为其是"城镇老爷卫生部"，仅为高级官员服务。

对该批评的首要整改措施是派遣流动医疗队为农民提供一些临床保健内容。然而，该流动队受到道路条件的限制，所发挥的

only where roads took them, however, and so proved to be of limited use. More importantly, the mobile clinic teams were stunned by the magnitude of need they encountered in rural market towns and villages, especially by the incidence of infectious disease. The authorities thus began to plan some measures of prevention, albeit somewhat hesitantly, as the ideas of some officials about preventive medicine were rather vague.

Before prevention programs could be carried out, however, the rural health system had to evolve. This was to be accomplished through rural administrative organizations and depended on full- scale cooperation from county authorities and input from sub county and commune representatives. County hospitals were already in evidence and county health bureaus were organized or upscaled at this time; however, the most significant development of this period was the development of organizations at the commune level. Ninety percent of communes developed a health facility of some type.

Initially these typically offered either traditional or modern medical care, but not both, and were supported in a variety of ways. The first were cooperative clinics with a traditional practitioner in charge, whose upkeep depended on patient fees. Later subcounty officials and commune committees opened a number of small hospitals and health centers staffed by salaried graduates of secondary medical schools. In time, all three types of facility were combined into commune health centers, in which the patient could obtain either modern or traditional care. Besides providing a relatively large amount of health service, the commune centers trained some village-level health workers in elementary medical work.

EXPANSION FROM COMMUNE TO VILLAGE: THE 1960s

The significant strides made in the control of infectious disease through massive immunization were made possible by the huge aggregate

作用有限。但重要的是，流动医疗队对他们在农村集镇和村庄遇到的巨大需求感到震惊，尤其是震惊传染病的发病率。因此，当局开始计划一些预防措施，但措施有些迟缓，因为一些官员关于预防医学的概念还相当模糊。

然而，在开展疾病预防之前，必须发展农村卫生体系。这将通过农村行政组织来实现，并依托于县当局的全面合作以及县辖区和公社代表的共同努力。县医院已经就绪，此时，县卫生局也已经组建或扩大；然而，这一时期最显著的是公社一级组织的发展。90% 的公社组建了某种形式的卫生机构。

最初，这些公社发展的卫生机构通常提供传统医学和现代医学的医疗照护，但不是两者兼备的方式，并通过多种途径得到支持。第一种是有传统执业医师负责的合作诊所，其运营来源于患者的医疗收费。后来，县辖区官员和公社委员会开设了许多小医院和卫生院，配备了中专医学校的带薪毕业生。随着时间的推移，三种类型的机构全部被合并到公社卫生院，患者可以获得传统医学和现代医学的医疗照护。卫生院除了提供相对大量的健康服务外，还为村级卫生工作者提供初级的医学培训。

20 世纪 60 年代从公社到村的扩展

从 1960 年开始，村级大批卫生工作者致力于集中大规模免疫接种，因此传染病防控工作取得重大进展。这一工作主要依靠

of village-level personnel assembled mainly from 1960 onward. The main component of this aggregate consisted of "barefoot doctors," who, for better or for worse, served as prototypes for many other developing countries as they organized their own rural health services. The barefoot doctors were not, however, the only persons giving immunizations and doing primary health care in Chinese villages in the 1949-1976 period. In immunization work, midwifery, and later, family planning, lay people contributed substantially.

The rural health system that had evolved by the mid-1960s was three-tiered, consisting of the county health bureau at its apex, with commune and village-level facilities below that. The county hospitals had come first, mainly before 1958; the commune health centers next, between 1958 and 1964; and the village clinics at different times between i960 and 1970 or so. Apparently there was a great deal of overlapping in the development of health organizations below the county level, and the whole picture became rather confusing. About all that can be said is that the system developed from the top down, and whatever facilities opened in the communes and villages resulted from decisions of higher authorities.

It is almost impossible to clearly differentiate between the time when village health workers, with little training, and the time when barefoot doctors, with considerably more training, were turned out. About all we know is that barefoot doctors first entered the picture in the early 1960s, and that their number increased greatly during the Cultural Revolution. Some were traditional practitioners or lay health workers who had entered the system as affiliates of commune organizations. Others had been doing practice of traditional medicine or selling herbs in their own villages before becoming barefoot doctors. County hospitals trained some of them, a few for periods of from six months to a year. Commune and subcounty organizations trained others.

The practical training of these barefoot doctors varied from case to case, of course, although presumably the common ground consisted of instruction

赤脚医生，这种模式不管怎样已成为许多发展中国家农村卫生体系发展参照的原型。然而，在 1949—1976 年，并非只有赤脚医生从事中国农村的免疫接种和初级卫生保健工作。在免疫接种方面，助产士和随后的计划生育部门人员以及非专业人员都做出了巨大的贡献。

到 20 世纪 60 年代中期已经发展的农村卫生体系共分三层：最上层是县卫生局，依次为公社和村级机构。最先出现的是县医院，主要集中于 1958 年之前；其次是公社卫生院，集中于 1958 年至 1964 年间；村卫生室则是在 1960 年至 1970 年间陆续出现。县级以下卫生机构的服务和发展明显与上级存在很大的重叠，所以整个情况难以理清。由于整个体系是自上而下发展起来的，所以公社和村庄里的可利用条件和设施，都由上级决定。

很难对"受过很少培训的村卫生工作者的时代"以及"受过较多培训的赤脚医生时代"进行区分。我们所知道的是，赤脚医生最早是在 20 世纪 60 年代初走上历史舞台，后来数量大大增加。其中一些是中医医师，另一些是非专业的卫生工作者，他们来自于公社有关部门。还有一些则是在成为赤脚医生之前，一直在自己的村庄做传统医疗或卖草药。县医院对他们中的一部分人进行了从六个月到一年不等的培训，剩余的人由公社和县辖区组织培训。

当然，这些赤脚医生的实际培训情况因情况而异，但大致的共同内容是一些简单的医疗程序和免疫接种技术。但随后而来的是：许多赤脚医生做的远远超过了这些，他们甚至像普通医生一

in a few simple medical procedures and in techniques of immunization. The time came, nonetheless, when many barefoot doctors were doing considerably more than that, with some doing diagnosis and treatment on the same level as ordinary physicians. Given the variation in their backgrounds and abilities, not to mention those of the persons who trained them, their caliber varied widely. Some were considerably less proficient than others.

Even the most competent, however, had to practice without any planned support from scientific and technical personnel with more advanced training. For there was no suggestion of developing a carefully structured system, such as we had organized at Dingxian, which linked such workers to a hierarchy of more fully trained medical personnel at higher rural levels, or to advanced scientific personnel in the cities. To the contrary, their responsibilities were ill defined, and, lacking systematic supervision, they were free to act most of the time entirely on their own judgment. On a quantitative basis much was achieved in the massive rural health expansion, but later there were indications that the quality of village-level medical care would have to be considerably improved through programs of further training in a post-Mao system.

During the Cultural Revolution universities established branches or teaching points in rural areas. This gave further impetus to rural health development and the system, establishing firm roots in the villages. Also, young teachers were diverted from classroom duty and sent as permanent residents or members of mobile teams to serve the rural areas and to assume some of the responsibility' for training additional barefoot doctors. Health directives issued from the top were channeled through new provincial health administrators who replaced the more experienced personnel.

The push to train barefoot doctors ended about 1972, and perhaps one-third of the total group returned to full-time farming, when funding for the activities became problematical. Rural health continued to develop, although at low standards.

样进行疾病的诊断和治疗。由于专业背景和专业能力差异较大以及他们的培训者本身水平也参差不齐，因此在这些赤脚医生中有些人的熟练程度可能远低于其他人。

然而，即使是最能干的人，他们在实践中也未得到那些受过更高级培训的科技人员的有计划的支持。因为缺乏一个像我们在河北定县组织那样的完备体系，即通过一个分级的体系，把村医与上一级受过更全面培训的医务人员进行对接以及与城市中更高级的科技人员建立联系。与之相反，这些农村医生的责任不明确且缺乏系统的督导，其大部分时间都完全根据自己的经验任意行事。从数量上看，在大规模的农村卫生体系扩展方面取得了很大成就，但后来有实证表明，村一级医疗保健的质量必须通过"后毛泽东时期"培训计划而得到显著提高。

20 世纪 60 年代后期，大学在农村地区建立了分校或教学点，这进一步推动了农村卫生事业发展和体系的完善，使卫生事业逐步扎根于农村。此外，青年教师被调离课堂，被派去常驻或作为流动小组成员为农村地区服务，并承担培训更多赤脚医生的责任。最新指示通过新的省级卫生领导传达下来。

强化对赤脚医生的培训工作约在 1972 年结束。因为该时期赤脚医生的活动资金出现了问题，以至约 1/3 的人回去全职务农。当时农村卫生事业是在一个较低的水平上持续发展。

HEALTH POLICY AND ITS IMPACT: A MID-1970S PERSPECTIVE

Medical and Public Health Education

Meanwhile in the 1960s, medical education in the universities had gone through another cycle of extension and attrition. In 1963 the three-year curriculum established in 1958 was adjusted upward to a full six-year curriculum. The Cultural Revolution, however, led to a reversion to the three-year curriculum once again in 1968, as supporters of the CPP party chairman assented to the idea that even primary school graduates could become medical doctors. In 1972 there was a final upward readjustment once again, echoing popular disillusionment with the Cultural Revolution policies.

The impact of all this on the modern medical field can be assessed when we consider that between 1949 and 1978 almost two generations of medical professionals were produced, while the older generation, trained in accordance with the preliberation six- year curriculum, was moving into retirement age. It was difficult to remain convinced that faculty and students alike, including those students who became teachers after graduation, had not been placed at a disadvantage by these shifting arrangements. Whatever the case, the end result very clearly was great variation in the scope and substance of medical training. Diversity became so great, in fact, that what a physician, physician's assistant, or barefoot doctor trained in this period had or had not studied was an unknown variable.

As for public health education, the pattern of early specialization had continued throughout the period. Theoretically, early specialization had strengthened the discipline. In reality, year after year, premature specialization produced graduates who were ill-prepared, especially because of their lack of clinical training and scientific background. To some teachers, too, they appeared to have failed to gain an adequate understanding of the broader meaning of public health. Students were unable to supplement their deficiencies through self-study. In the final

298

卫生政策及影响：20 世纪 70 年代中期的视角

医学和公共卫生教育

20 世纪 60 年代，大学的医学教育学制经历了另一轮延长和缩短的循环。1958 年建立的三年医学学制于 1963 年调整为完整的六年学制。 1968 年再次恢复为三年学制，因为部分支持者认为即使小学毕业生也可以成为医生。1972 年再次对医学教育学制标准的进行最终调整，反映了民众对 20 世纪 60 年代教育政策的反省。

以上医学教育对现代医学领域的影响可作如下估计：在 1949 年至 1978 年间，大概培养了两代医疗卫生专业人员。而按照建国前的六年学制培训的老一代医务人员已步入退休年龄。很难相信教师和学生，包括毕业后成为教师的学生，没有受到由这些学制改变而带来的不利影响。很明显，最终的结果显示了在医学教育的范围和内容上，差异是很大的。由于医学教育的差异如此之大，事实上在这个时期接受过培训的医生、助理医生或赤脚医生学习或未学习过哪些医学课程，都很难区分。

至于公共卫生教育，在整个时期施行的都是及早专业化的模式。理论上及早专业化是为了强化公共卫生的能力，但在现实中，年复一年的过早专业化却因缺乏临床培训和科学背景而导致培养的毕业生准备不足。某些教师未能充分理解公共卫生的广泛含义，学生也无法通过自学来补充自己的不足，最终他们都被视为用处

analysis they were perceived as health professionals of little use. Perhaps as many as 40 to 50 percent became discouraged and entered other careers. Public health education then became an enigma to those of us who had received a different type of fundamental training.

The Alternative Systems of Medicine

By the mid-1970s, the gains for traditional medicine could be seen in both rural and urban areas. In the countryside, traditional medical practitioners were working together in the same clinics with modern-trained secondary medical school graduates. In the cities, there were, of course, separate traditional medical hospitals, but in some modern hospitals specific areas had been designated in the outpatient departments for traditional medical consultations. Varying numbers of traditional and modern physicians thus often worked side by side under the same roof, although the patients for each type of practice were kept separate. Each system had its own pharmacy, too, but modern physicians were being encouraged to learn how to prescribe traditional drugs.

Separate departments of traditional medicine to be found in the national and provincial health ministries had been authorized to develop traditional medicine on a wide basis. Plans included the organization of special hospitals of traditional medicine in each province and county. Such plans were readily received by the people, who believed in the usefulness of traditional medicine, especially for the treatment of chronic disease.

A MEDICAL SCIENTIST IN THE NEW SOCIETY

As to my personal participation in the Chinese health experience during these years, it had been largely in the capacity of medical educator. Nonetheless, I had also had some opportunity to engage in rural health work in outlying parts of Sichuan Province, and in Yunnan Province, a neighboring province to the south. Initially also I had participated periodically in various conferences and study sessions in other parts of the country.

不大的卫生专业人员，可能有多达 40% 到 50% 的人因气馁而转行。对于我们这些接受过不同类型基础教育的人来说，公共卫生教育成了一个难解之谜。

医学的另一个体系

到 20 世纪 70 年代中期，传统医学在农村和城市都有所发展。在农村，传统医学从业者和受过现代医学教育的中等专科医学校毕业生在同一个诊所一起工作。在城市，传统医学也得到了相同的发展。当然，有独立的传统医院，但在一些现代医院中，门诊指定了特定区域进行传统医学医疗咨询。因此，尽管针对患者的诊疗实践有明确的区分，数量不等的传统医生和现代医生经常在同一屋檐下并肩工作。传统医学和现代医学各有自己的药房，但鼓励现代医学学习如何处方传统医药。

国家和省级卫生机构中单独设立有传统医学管理部门并得到授权以广泛促进传统医学的发展，其实施范围包括在各省、县组建传统医学专科医院。因为传统医学一直以来深入人心，尤其是在治疗慢性病方面，这些政策被群众广泛接受。

新社会的医学科学家

这些年来，我个人主要是作为医学教育工作者参与中国卫生事业。尽管如此，我也有机会在四川和云南的偏远地区从事农村卫生工作。早年，我还定期参加在全国其他地方举行的各种和研讨班。

By the time of liberation in 1949, I had been living in Chongqing for three years and was deeply involved in getting the new medical college at the national university on its feet. This presented endless problems. A fairly strong faculty of medical science was built up in spite of the disastrous inflation. With two teaching hospitals of over 300 beds, the six-year curriculum was carried to completion for the first class of medical students, who graduated in 1952. The CCP meanwhile had accumulated an excellent record in halting the spiraling inflation of the preliberation period.

Graduation of the first class in 1952 provided a moment of personal fulfillment and patriotic pride to many of those involved. In the past most of our medical graduates had come from missionary-run teaching institutions and after completion of their studies had been drawn into the network of modern hospitals and clinics in the cities. Now, however, we had a national university medical college in our own province that we had built entirely with our own resources, and whose graduates were well prepared to work for the benefit of the common people in a newly liberated China. Many would be recruited to work in the provincial health administration or would become professors in different medical specialities.

In 1952 I took eighty students to Yunnan Province on the border of Burma for field training. There we studied malignant malaria and bubonic plague among the minority nationality people at Mangshi, a large market town some distance southwest of Kunming. A surgeon and an obstetrician accompanied us on the trip, which took twenty days by truck, a portion of it by way of the historic Burma Road. Villagers in the area relied on traditional practitioners exclusively, except for a few more affluent peasants who crossed the border into Burma, where they paid a very high price for modern medical attention. Thai people predominated among the three minority nationalities in that sector of Yunnan Province. The area was then under military control by the PL A, but an old tribal government headed by a Tusu chieftain survived.

Mangshi had a small clinic, with a few beds. We rearranged the limited space into consultation rooms and an operating area. Suspicious

到 1949 年中华人民共和国成立时，我已经在重庆生活了三年，并深度参与筹建重庆大学医学院，筹建工作存在很多问题。尽管出现了灾难性的通货膨胀，还是建立了一个拥有强大师资的医学院及两所拥有 300 多张床位的教学医院。第一批医学生完成了六年学习并于 1952 年毕业。与此同时，党成功阻止了在解放前不断恶化的通货膨胀问题。

1952 年首届毕业班中的许多毕业生给我带来了个人成就感和爱国自豪感。过去，我国的医学毕业生大多来自教会开办的教学机构，完成学业后他们被吸引到城市的现代医院和诊所网络中。然而，我们在本省有一所国立大学医学院，完全是用自己的资源建立的，毕业生准备好为新中国的广大人民谋福利。许多人将被招募到省级卫生行政部门工作，或成为各门医学专科的教授。

1952 年，我带了 80 名学生到与缅甸边境接壤的云南省进行现场实习。我们在昆明西南以远的大集镇芒市研究了在少数民族暴发的恶性疟疾和腺鼠疫。一名外科医生和一名产科医生陪同我们坐了 20 天的卡车，经过了历史悠久的滇缅公路。除了少数越过边境进入缅甸的富裕农民能以支付高昂费用获得西方现代医疗照护外，该地区的村民完全依赖当地的传统医生。在云南省的该地区，三个少数民族中以傣族居多。芒市当时仍有一个土司领导的旧部落。

芒市有一个小诊所，只有几张床位，我们把有限的空间重新布置成了诊室和手术区。因为过去少数民族没有得到汉人的友好

at first because they had been badly treated by Chinese in the past, the people came around after a few months of hard work on our part, treating patients with terminal and other conditions and performing preventive work. They began calling on us in a variety of situations.

As a field experience for the students, it was a rewarding interlude, giving substantial insight into health problems among the rural poor and how the application of scientific medical knowledge might elicit improvement. A number of students subsequently became leaders in health organizations serving rural populations.

We reduced the incidence of malaria after mass drug treatment and educated people to use mosquito nets and to open their windows to permit sunlight and ventilation in their houses. We performed surgery, attended cases of difficult childbirth, and treated cardiac failure, all with some success. The people had the habit of depositing their feces around the villages, to be eaten by the pigs. Since they also ate meat raw, a very high percentage of the population was infested with tapeworms. When patients were treated and saw the worms they had been harboring, they were greatly surprised. We then gave some simple lessons about contamination.

We returned home in March 1953 to find that the CCP had taken over all administrative positions, including the deanship of medical schools. For me, this meant that I would be relieved of administrative responsibility but would continue to teach. With the absorption of the Medical College of National Chongqing University by the Sichuan Medical College, my family and I moved to Chengdu, and I quite comfortably started to undertake only public health teaching to medical students. My lectures were well received by the students, and I was to begin my field instruction. The new government was already emphasizing classroom and laboratory' instruction, however, so it became necessary to teach epidemiology without field studies.

In Manchuria, where I had been sent in 1950 to study new patterns in

相待，因此一开始他们持怀疑态度，但经过我们几个月努力治疗晚期病人和其他疾病，并进行预防工作，他们才开始接受我们。他们逐渐在各种情况下和我们进行交流。

作为学生的现场实习，这是一段有益的插曲。学生们深入了解农村贫困人口的健康问题，以及现代医学知识的应用可能会带来怎样的改善。一些学生后来成为服务农村的卫生组织的领导人。

在大规模药物治疗后，疟疾的发病率降低了。我们还教育人们使用蚊帐，打开窗户，让阳光进入室内、保持空气流通等措施。我们在外科手术、处理难产病例和治疗心力衰竭等方面也都取得了一定成功。当地村民有随地粪便并听任猪群食用，加上他们自己有吃生肉的习惯，很多人都感染了绦虫。当患者接受治疗并看到让他们一直承受病痛的绦虫实物时，均大为吃惊，我们则趁机简单讲解了一些有关病原污染的知识。

我们于 1953 年 3 月从缅甸回到重庆，党已经接管了学校所有的行政部门职务，包括医学院院长。对我来说，这意味着我将被免除行政职务，但将继续任教。随着国立重庆大学医学院被四川医学院收并，我和家人搬到了成都，我相当轻松地开始了只承担医学生的公共卫生教学。我的讲座很受学生欢迎，我也开始现场教学。然而，新政府已经在强调课堂和实验室的教育，因此开设了在没有现场实践情况下的流行病学教学。

1950 年，我被派往东北研究医学教育的新模式。在那里，

medical education, I had already seen evidence of trends that seemed to me to somewhat jeopardize the quality of medical education. The stress on classroom lectures, using poorly translated Russian texts, the use of a provisional three-year curriculum, and the passive attitude of students during clinical demonstrations that I had seen all were disappointing. Also disconcerting was the interest in early specialization for public health students evidenced in Beijing at the First National Conference on Health. The neglect of field training was another milestone for me in a journey in the wrong direction.

Then in 1955, I was sent to Beijing to attend the conference of medical educators, at which it was made known that separate public health schools were to be established. A number of persons at the conference were unable to understand the principles underlying the announced curriculum. Participants, however, were not expected to discuss the decision. Whatever our views, a colleague from Shanghai and I were both appointed deans of new schools of public health.

Having made a number of criticisms of the general trends in medical education during the Hundred Flowers Campaign, I was later removed from the deanship and downgraded from second- to fourth-grade professor, with a loss of salary and certain amenities. Thereafter my teaching conformed strictly to official methodology, and my contact with students was more or less restricted to formalities.

Intellectuals had been criticized for preferring the cities and not being willing to help the common people, so between 1958 and 1966 I was twice sent to rural areas to render medical relief. From my own perspective, this was a welcome assignment, for it gave me an opportunity to observe rural conditions firsthand and, as I was still a teacher, to utilize the situation to provide some students with field training. They responded quite well, and we had a good time together.

The 1958 assignment was to provide medical relief in a northern area

我看到了一些在某种程度上危及医学教育质量的隐患。来自课堂授课的压力、使用翻译不佳的俄语文本、临时的三年学制，以及我所看到的学生在临床实习期间的消极态度等都令人失望。同样令人不安的是，在北京举行的第一届全国卫生大会上，人们对公共卫生专业学生的早期专业化产生了兴趣。对我来说，忽视现场实习是另一个重大方向性的错误。

1955 年，我被派往北京参加医学教育工作者会议，会上方知晓将建立独立的公共卫生学系。一些与会者无法理解所公布课程的学理。然而，参会人员也未参与讨论这一决策。不管我们的观点如何，我和上海来的一位同事双双被任命为新公共卫生学系的主任。

在"百花齐放，百家争鸣"运动期间，我对医学教育的总体方向提出了一些批评，后来我被免除系主任职务，从二级教授降为四级教授，降低了工资和福利待遇。此后，我的教学严格遵循官方的教学方法，与学生的接触或多或少局限于形式。

人们批评知识分子更喜欢城市，不愿意帮助农村老百姓，因此在 1958 年至 1966 年期间，我两次被派到农村地区提供医疗援助。从个人角度我非常乐意接受这样的任务，因为它让我有机会亲眼观察农村情况，而且我还仍然是一名教师，我可以利用这种条件给一些学生提供现场实习的机会。学生们对农村现场实习反应很好，我们在一起很开心。

1958 年我的任务是在麻风病和梅毒流行的四川省北部地区

of Sichuan Province where leprosy and syphilis were prevalent. Travel from Chengdu to the destination in the northwestern corner of Jiange County took one day by train. I was accompanied by other teachers from the Medical College and a number of students.

In the principal population center in the county, there was a thirty-bed hospital with an army medical officer in charge. The officer spent his time in the hospital and had no firsthand knowledge of health conditions or problems in the surrounding area. As expected, the local inhabitants depended almost entirely on traditional practitioners for such medical care as they could obtain.

What we saw and experienced in Jiange County made me realize once more just how scientifically unenlightened villagers were and the extent to which superstition and fear still permeated their ideas about disease and its cure. For example, although traditional practitioners had an abundance of theories, neither they nor the army medical officer seemed to have any practical knowledge of diagnostic procedures. So one day I invited a group of eighty or so for a brief talk on the subject. To illustrate the talk, I brought in a few typical patients with leprosy and syphilis into the classroom. Confronted with the patient with leprosy, the traditional practitioners became greatly alarmed. Their anxiety was so great, in fact, that when 1 examined the patient in their presence, many covered their eyes and buried their heads, evidently fearing that they might contract the disease simply by looking at a diseased victim.

That field trip also made me realize how essential it is for anyone in public health to have a good foundation in scientific medicine, both curative and preventive. One day on a visit to Wangcang and Guangyuan Counties nearby to the east, we saw an increasing number of leprosy cases. In one small village, I was introduced to a man who for years had believed he had contracted leprosy. After careful examination, I found that what he actually had was psoriasis, not leprosy. On being informed of this, the man jumped for joy, shouting that he had received his second life. Had the original

提供医疗援助。从成都到剑阁县西北角的目的地，坐火车需要一天时间。同行的还有医学院的其他老师和一些学生。

剑阁县的主要人口居住的中心地带，有一家一名军医负责的拥有 30 张床位的医院。这名军医主要呆在医院，对周围地区的健康状况或卫生问题没有第一手的资料。不出所料，当地居民几乎完全依赖传统行医者提供的医疗服务。

在剑阁县的所见所闻让我再次意识到，村民们在科学上是多么落后，他们关于疾病及其痊愈在观念中仍然渗透着迷信和恐惧。例如，尽管传统行医者有丰富的理论，但他们和军队的医疗官员似乎都不掌握任何有关诊断的实际知识。所以有一天，我邀请了80 人左右的小组就这个问题进行了简短的交谈。为了演示，我把几个典型的麻风病和梅毒患者带入了教室。面对麻风病患者，传统行医者变得异常惊恐。事实上，这些传统行医者极度担心，以至于我当着他们的面对患者进行检查时，许多人都遮住了眼睛且埋下了头，明显是他们担心自己由于仅仅通过目视患者就会感染上这种疾病。

那次现场考察也让我意识到，在公共卫生领域，任何人在治疗和预防上都必须具备良好的科学医学基础。有一天在东部邻近的旺苍县和广元县考察，我们看到了越来越多的麻风病例。在一个小村庄里，让我去看一位多年来一直认为自己得了麻风病的人。仔细检查后，我发现他实际得的是银屑病，不是麻风病。一听到这个消息，这个人高兴地跳了起来，大喊他得到了第二次生命。

diagnostician been more knowledgeable, that patient might have been spared years of suffering. No doubt, concurrently, there were many actual cases of leprosy going undiagnosed and untreated. This reinforced my conviction that it is essential for rural public health workers to be thoroughly familiar with diseases prevalent in the areas in which they work.

By 1960 my status had begun to improve, and gradually restrictions on my activity were relaxed. In time, I was permitted to travel to certain areas, read certain materials, and participate in a number of conferences, all of which had previously been prohibited to me. In 1963, for example, a conference was held in Beijing in an attempt to raise the social standing of the intellectuals and to make for a more comfortable atmosphere, downplaying some of the criticism that "rightists" had received. I was treated as a guest for a few days.

In 1964 several colleagues and I visited rural areas in Anyue and Neijiang Counties, southeast of Chengdu. The Neijiang Regional Health Center was responsible for preventive work in the area, a subject of much interest to us. Disappointed, we found that it was spending most of its resources on laboratory examinations of water and food. Its epidemiological surveys were confined largely to areas in the immediate environs of the city. In the city of Anyue the water supply was quite inadequate, and surface pollution of drinking wells was evident everywhere.

Later I reflected on the importance of systematic organization in rural health care delivery and concluded that intermittent visits by mobile health teams simply cannot do the job. Without systematic organization, the tendency is toward hit-or-miss measures of prevention, while attention is concentrated on institution-based health activities in the urban pattern. Physicians think in terms of the needs of patients in hospitals and clinics, while those of the community as a whole are often neglected.

Another field trip in the same year took me to the Yongxin commune, in Mianyang County, north of Chengdu. A commune health center had not yet been established at that time, but there were clinics in three

试想如果当初诊断的医生更有知识，那个病人会免受多年的痛苦。毫无疑问，同时还有许多实际的麻风病病例没有得到诊断和治疗。这加强了我的信念，即农村公共卫生工作者必须彻底熟悉所工作地区流行的疾病。

到 1960 年，我的处境开始改善，逐渐放宽了对我活动的限制。很快我可以到某些特定地区，阅读指定的材料，参加一些会议，这些以前都是被禁止的。以 1963 年为例，在北京召开了一次会议，我受到了客人般的接待。

1964 年，我和几个同事去了成都东南部的安岳县和内江县的农村。内江的地区保健站负责该地区的预防工作，这是我们非常感兴趣的课题。但失望的是，我们发现它正在将大部分资源用于水和食物的实验室检查。其流行病学调查主要局限于城镇周边地区。而安岳市的供水十分不足，饮用水井的表面污染随处可见。

后来，我思考了系统性的组织在农村卫生保健工作中的重要性，并得出结论，由流动卫生队断断续续地提供服务根本无法完成这项工作。如果没有系统的组织，预防措施往往会是碰运气式的，而注意力仍集中在城市模式、以机构为中心的卫生活动上。医生思考的是医院和诊所里患者的需求，而往往忽略了整个社区的需求。

我在同年的另一次实践考察的地点是成都北部绵阳县的永兴公社。那里当时还没有建立公社卫生院，但在三个集镇都有诊所，

market towns, two practicing modern medicine under the direction of a secondary medical school graduate and the other run by traditional practitioners. One of the modern clinics specialized exclusively in schistosomiasis, and we established ourselves there. Although our diagnostic capabilities were considerably better than those of the young secondary medical school graduates, without any laboratory work, our findings were inconclusive.

After working there for some time, it became quite evident that the quality of health service in the clinics of the area was low. The personnel assigned to antischistosomiasis work engaged in some snail eradication. But neither they nor the clinic personnel had had sufficient training for what they were expected to do.

The poverty prevailing in some villages compounded other problems. This was brought home to us by the case of a woman we encountered in a field. Obviously ill, she was greatly in need of some drugs for which we were expected to charge a negligible fee, but she could not afford even that small sum. Fortunately, a friend helped her out. That incident convinced me that economic improvement of impoverished areas is always a necessary corollary of lasting health improvement.

In 1966 new admissions were suspended. In 1968 they were resumed but this time only for a limited number of junior- and senior-high-school graduates who came on the basis of official recommendation rather than on the basis of a competitive entrance examination as in the past. The institution was moved to the rural areas and classes were conducted mostly by young teachers of peasant or worker origin. Students were given short courses in which political considerations took priority over medical content.

In 1972 classes were reinstituted on the Chengdu campus. Professors and other staff members were called back to work. On my return, the party asked me to do only technical work. Given a choice of several

其中两个由在中等专科医学校毕业生的指导下实践现代医学，另一个则由传统行医者经营。其中之一是专门研究血吸虫病的，我们就在那里也建立了一所现代诊所。尽管我们的诊断能力大大优于年轻的中等专科医学校的毕业生，但由于没有任何实验室工作的支持，我们对疾病仍无法下准确的结论。

在永兴公社工作了一段时间后，可以很明显地发现该地区诊所的卫生服务质量很低。分配去做血吸虫病控制工作的人员主要是从事灭螺工作，但他们和在诊所工作的其他人员都没有接受过完成预期任务的培训。

一些村庄普遍存在的贫困现象使其他问题更为复杂化。在实地遇到的一名妇女的案例让我们体会了实情。这位妇女由于生病而急需药物治疗，我们收取的药费极少，但她仍负担不起，所幸的是一个朋友伸手相助帮了她。这一事件使我确信，在贫困地区要想持久地改善健康状况，必须同时发展经济。

四川医学院 1966 年新生录取工作暂停，1968 年又恢复，但恢复后只接受官方推荐的数量有限的初中和高中毕业生，而非过去通过竞争性入学考试而录取。学校也搬到了农村地区，课堂主要由农民或工人出身的年轻教师授课。学生们上的是短期的课程。

1972 年，成都校区恢复上课，教授们和学校其他工作人员也陆续回来工作。我回来后，组织安排我只做技术性工作。在

alternatives, I finally decided to study the diagnosis and treatment of occupational lung diseases that attacked many farmers working in the mines. This decision was approved by the party.

Between 1972 and 1975 I became the first scientific leader of research on occupational lung diseases. By the end of 1975 my vision became very poor and I tendered my resignation. This was accepted, and I left the college to retire in Beijing. I was in that city when the Gang of Four was overthrown in 1976, paving the way for the emergence of a new national leadership.

几种选择中，我最终决定对在矿山工作的许多农民罹患的职业性肺病的诊断和治疗进行研究，该决定获得了组织的批准。

1972 年至 1975 年间，我成为第一位研究职业性肺部疾病的科学带头人。到 1975 年年底，由于视力变得很差，我提出辞职。组织批准后，我离开医学院在北京退休。1976 年"四人帮"被推翻时我就在北京，这为新的国家领导层出来工作铺平了道路。

译者：冯录召，张婷

Chapter 6

A New Era in Health Development

In 1978 postliberation China entered another phase in its history, and with it my own life passed another turning point. A rightward shift of the political pendulum not long after the death of Party Chairman Mao in 1976 was reflected in the rise to power of a pragmatic reform group, headed by Vice Chairman Deng Xiaoping. In its emphasis on expediency, the reform group adopted a strategy of concerted mobilization for development, launching a campaign of economic modernization whose ambitious targets, if realized, would propel China into the ranks of relatively advanced, industrialized nations by the year 2000. The drive to make modernization a reality has continued unabated over the past decade, carrying socialist China in new directions under strong party leadership.

With science perceived as the key to modernization, advanced scientific and technological training was valued once again, and intellectuals collectively were now treated with respect that had been unknown for decades. After the Cultural Revolution was declared at an end, intellectuals all across the country began returning to their posts. I myself was asked to come out of retirement, and returned, at the request of Sichuan Medical College, to my former position as Director of its Occupational Lung Disease Laboratory.

第6章

卫生事业发展迈入新纪元

　　1978 年，中国发展迈入了新的历史阶段，我的人生也随之迎来另一个转折点。1976 年毛泽东主席逝世后不久，政治形势发生了转变，这反映在以邓小平副主席为代表的务实派走上领导岗位。中央改革领导小组强调务实导向，团结带领全国各界群众，齐心协力谋发展，开启了一场国家经济现代化建设运动；其宏伟战略目标就是力争于 2000 年前把中国建设成为世界上相对先进的工业化国家。20 世纪 80 年代，在党的坚强领导下，现代化建设持续呈现良好势态，社会主义中国正朝着新的方向前进。

　　随着科学被视为现代化建设的关键因素，先进的科学技术培训再次受到重视，被认为是第一生产力；而知识分子也受到了前所未有的尊重。分布在全国各地的知识分子开始重返岗位。应四川医学院的邀请，我被返聘回原来的岗位，继续担任职业性肺病实验室主任。

In the drive to make modernization a reality, policymaking and administrative arrangements assumed utmost importance. With so much concentration of authority in the central government, and in some cases in the provincial government, the formulation of correct policies and their execution through appropriate and effective administrative channels was absolutely critical to the future of the modernization movement. This was true of all constructive efforts, including health improvement.

Somewhat surprisingly, emphasis on modernization had not carried over into medical practice to any significant degree, although science and technology represented one of the "four modernizations" (modernizations in agriculture, industry, science and technology, and defense). Instead, in the decade since emphasis on modernization had begun, traditional medicine had further reinforced its institutional position and in the late 1980s stood on an equal footing with scientific medicine.

Trends in modern medical education were nonetheless consistent with the country's need to build and maintain a scientifically skilled medical community. The institutional structure of higher education in modern medicine had been strengthened, and the general course requirements that had prevailed between 1963 and 1968 had been reinstated. By 1987, a five-year curriculum of advanced study had been standard in most medical colleges for a decade, while a few leading educational institutions offered programs of six or more years.

The same time period passed, however, without reexamination of the patterns of public health education that had been imposed under Soviet influence more than twenty years earlier. Public health education in 1987 therefore continued to be based on the assumption that its work was better left to "specialists" who are not medical doctors and whose training followed a rather narrow channel of interest, rather than to physicians trained in public health. In medical school itself, public health studies are deemed significantly less important than clinical coursework. Because some public health "specialists" become disappointed with their choice

在实施现代化建设的过程中，政策制定和行政管理至关重要。在中央政府集中统筹布置的基础上，结合各地方省政府因地制宜地制定正确的政策，并通过行之有效的行政管理渠道贯彻落实好，对推动现代化建设进程至为关键。这也是适用于所有现代化建设事业的普遍规律，包括卫生事业现代化建设。

尽管科学技术是"四个现代化"（农业现代化、工业现代化、科学技术现代化和国防现代化）之一，但令人有些惊愕的是，在医学实践领域的现代化建设并未受到应有的重视。相反，自全面开启现代化建设以来的十年中，传统医学进一步加强了其建制机构地位，并在 20 世纪 80 年代后期与科学医学处于并驾齐驱之势。

医学教育的现代化进程与国家建立维护一支拥有高水平科学技能素养的医疗人才队伍的现实需求是一致的。期间，现代医学高等教育的体制结构得到了完善与强化，并恢复使用在 1963 年至 1968 年间所制定的教学培养大纲。到 1987 年，五年制高等医学教育在过去十年已成为大多数医学院校的标准模式，少数重点医学院校探索推出了六年制甚或更长学制的培养模式。

然而，过去的同一时期内并未重新审视我国在 20 多年前基于苏联影响下所实施的公共卫生教育模式。因此，直到 1987 年，公共卫生教育仍然基于既往观念在进行：即公共卫生工作最好交给那些有兴趣且接受过培训范围很窄的"专门人员"来做，而不是交给接受过公共卫生规范培训的临床医生做。而且，医学院校本身的公共卫生专业远没有临床医学专业受重视。一些从事公共

and change to other careers while others disappear into large bureaucratic institutions in the cities, public health in rural areas depends largely on the younger, less experienced graduates.

It was, nevertheless, impressive to see the great amount of work that has actually been, and was being, done to improve health in the rural areas, through antiepidemic campaigns, health services for women and children, and other means. In many places the upward turn of the financial situation of farmers under economic modernization had resulted in better living standards and had been accompanied by increased demand for medical and health care. In other areas where, in late 1987, financial conditions were not so good, village household budgets did not permit discretionary spending for health protection or improvement.

With respect to health improvement in the villages, perhaps the most difficult challenge facing the new leadership was the high percentage of untrained physicians and other medical workers serving in rural China—a legacy of efforts at rapid extension in an earlier era. Even those physicians who had received some formal instruction had been disadvantaged by disruptions and dislocations in medical education in the same era. Seemingly, the only solution for this troubling situation was the provision of systematic training programs for health personnel of all types by local authorities.

POSTLIBERATION CHINA: 1976 to 1987

Chairman Mao died in September 1976; Jiang Qing, and her three associates were arrested in October and subsequently exiled. By 1978, however, the issue had quite clearly been resolved in favor of Deng Xiaoping and moderate elements within the party, who by that time had risen to occupy many of the key leadership positions in the party and the government.

卫生工作的"专门人员"也对自己当初的选择感到后悔，他们要么改行从事其他职业，要么遍布在城市各级卫生行政机构中任职。因此，农村地区的公共卫生事业建设则很大程度上依靠一群经验不足的年轻毕业生。

为改善农村地区卫生状况，大量且繁重的工作已经完成或仍在进行，其中包括全民抗疫运动、妇幼保健服务及其他工作，这些工作效果明显，令人称道。在许多地区，随着经济现代化大潮，农民经济状况持续改善，生活水平不断提高，医疗和健康照护需求也随之增加。然而，在 1987 年年底，在一些经济状况不太好的地区，村民家庭收入预算尚难考虑用于健康保护或改善卫生。

在改善农村卫生状况方面，新领导层面临的最大困难可能是在中国农村服务人员系统中，未经培训的医生和其他医务工作者的比例很高，这也是早期快速发展推进的遗留问题。即使是曾接受过规范培训的医生，也因当时医学教育的中断和安排不当而先天不足。因此，解决这一困境的唯一办法是由地方行政管理部门为各类卫生人员提供并使其完成系统的培训计划。

解放后中国：1976 年至 1987 年

1976 年 9 月，毛泽东主席逝世；江青和她的三个同伙在十月被逮捕，随后被逐出政界。到了 1978 年，以邓小平为代表的党内务实派得到普遍认同，已在党和政府中担任着许多关键领导职务。

The pragmatic reform group confronted an array of problems, not the least of which was that, thirty years after liberation, the country had little to show in the way of economic growth. Moreover, its population had increased from 540 million to roughly one billion. This made China the world's most populous nation, creating enormous demand for food, housing, jobs, education, and health care.

The strategy of response involved economic modernization in four areas: agriculture, industry, science and technology, and defense. An emphasis on orderly and pragmatic processes of change, to which intellectuals were expected to contribute as a group, replaced the revolutionary shifts of the previous period and the belief that scientific and technical work could be done by persons without specialized training. Ambitious plans for what were termed the "four modernizations" were widely publicized through mass campaigns to nurture patriotic feeling and encourage youthful enthusiasm.

In time, scientists were afforded some freedom of initiative in research that contributed directly to modernization. A widely her-aided national conference of sciences was convened in Beijing in March 1978, and in the same year Deng Xiaoping declared intellectuals to be members of the working class, after which they were regarded as equal in social status to workers and peasants. The scientific and intellectual community was encouraged to participate in a two-way exchange of information with their counterparts in technologically advanced countries, the flow facilitated by a new "open-door" policy in foreign affairs.

While official interest not unexpectedly focused on the physical sciences, within limits social sciences were strengthened as well. Before 1978, Marxism was considered the only legitimate social science discipline, but in 1979 in the more open-minded environment a Chinese Academy of Social Sciences was established with responsibilities for promoting scientific studies of social phenomena on the basis of worldwide knowledge. Soon afterward, Sichuan Province established its

遵循实事求是原则的改革领导小组面临着一系列问题，其中最重要的是，建国后 30 年，国家在经济增长方面几乎没有取得长足进步。而且，人口已从 5.4 亿增加到约 10 亿。这使得中国成了世界上人口最多的国家，也造成了在粮食、住房、就业、教育和医疗保健方面均存在巨大需求。

发展的应对战略就是全面推进农业、工业、科学技术和国防四个方面的经济现代化。当时强调组织有序、追求实效的改革，希望知识分子群体做出应有的贡献，这扭转了过去由政治主导一切的局面，尤其是抛弃科学技术工作可以由未经专门培训的人员完成的错误观念。通过开展"四个现代化"宏伟战略的广泛深入宣传运动，培养了爱国情怀，激发了青春朝气。

科学家们逐渐被赋予科学创新研究的一定自主权，直接为现代化建设做贡献。1978 年 3 月，在北京召开了极其重要的全国科学大会；同年，邓小平指出，知识分子是工人阶级的一部分，从此以后，知识分子得到广泛尊重，与工人和农民阶级拥有同样的社会地位。得益于对外事务中的全新"开放"政策，科学界和知识界人员被积极鼓励与技术先进国家的同行们进行双向信息交流。

虽然官方聚焦点不出意外地集中在自然科学上，但社会科学也在一定范围内得到了重视。1979 年，在更加开放的环境下成立了中国社会科学院，基于全球知识视野，负责促进开展社会现象的科学研究。不久之后，四川省也建立了自己的社会科学院。

own such academy.

Decisions reached by the Central Committee of the Party in December 1978 set the stage for a series of economic and political reforms whose full realization would produce fundamental change in many aspects of the national life. The implementation of general reform guidelines, however, starting in urban China, commenced at a modest pace, as reform-minded innovators made small headway in persuading old-style administrators to adapt new habits of thinking.1 From 1984, however, after many old Party retainers in provincial and county administrations had been replaced by younger reform-minded functionaries, we began to see some change.

TRENDS IN HEALTH POLICY AND ADMINISTRATION

In health administration, the pattern was more or less the same. Specifically, in the early 1980s a few leading physicians in central research organizations and major industrial territories began to express opinions, take the initiative, and try to influence persons in positions of authority. Technical service organizations and the medical universities received a few benefits from these initiatives. Meanwhile the minister of health had been removed from office and was succeeded by his vice minister.

In general, however, administrators at the provincial level and below were slow to implement reform guidelines as they might apply to medicine and public health. To a number of the older bureaucrats, many of whom were former army medical workers, the suddenness of the ideological turnabout was quite incomprehensible, and they found themselves perhaps unwilling, or perhaps unable, to follow through. Younger men and women appointed as county health bureau directors or superintendents of county hospitals during 1984 and after were more reform-minded.

党中央于 1978 年 12 月做出的决策，为一系列经济和政治改革奠定了基础，而这些改革的全面实现，将使国民生活的诸多方面发生了翻天覆地的变化。具有改革思想的拓荒者努力说服那些思想禁锢守旧的行政人员，要主动适应新思维、接受新理念，但并未取得实质性进展，而从中国城市开始实施的总体改革方针的推进仍然举步维艰。然而，从 1984 年开始，具有改革思想的年轻一代官员逐渐登上历史舞台，我们开始看到一些真正的变化。

卫生政策与行政管理动向

在卫生行政管理方面，模式大致同前。具体来说，在 20 世纪 80 年代初，中央研究机构和主要工业地区的一些有影响力的医生开始发表观点，提出倡议并试图影响相关权力机构的决策者。由此，技术服务性部门和医学高校从这些倡议中获得了一些支持，与此同时，卫生部部长由其副部长接任。

然而，总的来说，省级及以下的卫生行政人员在实施改革方面进展缓慢，因为这些方针政策可能不太适用于医疗和公共卫生。对老一批的卫生行政官员来说，其中很多人是部队医务工作者，思想观念的骤然转变使他们难以理解与适应，他们甚至发现自己可能并不愿意改变，其中或许还有能力不足的问题。自 1984 年开始，一大批年富力强且有改革思想的年轻人，被陆续任命为县卫生局局长或县医院院长。

In 1982, with encouragement from the World Health Organization, the Ministry of Health targeted several county health systems to serve as models and began to look for professional input into these systems. I was approached for advice on rural health personnel and their training.

The changed political climate made possible the convening of a national conference of community medicine in Chengdu in 1984. Most of the delegates at the conference were young, technically trained supporters of the new leadership. Many papers were presented dealing with health conditions in the rural areas. One result was the organization of a National Center of Public Health Administration at Sichuan Medical College. My experience in developing rural health services was again recognized, and I began to advise its staff on field training activities.

Policy Related to Traditional Medicine

Within the central health administration, the creation of a new Bureau of Traditional Medicine in 1984 seemed to signal encouragement to practitioners and supporters of the style of medicine venerated in China over so many centuries. The proliferation of new hospitals, clinics, and schools of traditional medicine seen in the early to mid-1980s reinforced this impression. What the benefits and costs of the policy placing the two systems of medicine on an equal footing might be for future generations remained to be seen; for the present, however, most Chinese seem to want to go along with the equitable treatment.

Accordingly, in just about every area of medical education and practice, agencies and facilities representing both traditional and modern systems may be found. Each system has its own representation in the central government, as well as its own nationally or provincially administered urban clinics, hospitals, and medical schools. At the county level, there are typically also traditional as well as modern medical hospitals, although the major share of funding seems to go to the modern facilities.

1982 年，在世界卫生组织的鼓励倡议下，卫生部选定了几个县卫生系统作为改革样板，并着手为他们寻找专业支撑。与此同时，相关部门向我咨询如何给农村卫生人员做好培训。

1984 年，在成都成功召开了全国社区医学会议。大多数与会代表都是受过专业技术培训的年轻人。会上宣读交流的许多论文内容都是关于农村地区卫生状况的。这次会议的成果之一就是在四川医学院率先成立了国家公共卫生管理中心。我在发展农村卫生服务方面的经验再次得到认可，我也开始就如何开展区域实地培训活动向相关工作人员提供建议和咨询服务。

与传统医学相关的政策

在中央卫生行政部门的管辖下，1984 年新成立了一个传统医学局，这向在中国备受尊崇数个世纪的传统医学的从业者和支持者传递了一种莫大的鼓励。20 世纪 80 年代初至 80 年代中期，新的传统医学医院、诊所和传统医药院校的激增更加强化了这种信号。有关两种医学体系并行发展政策的效益和成本有待后人继续观察与评判；然而，至少在当时看来，大多数中国人是认同两种医学体系并重发展的。

因此，在每一个地区，几乎都有代表传统医学和现代医学这两种截然不同的医学教育与医疗实践、机构和设施。每一种体系在中央政府部门都有自己的代表，以及各自体系下的国家所属或省属的城市诊所、医院和医学院校。即使在县一级，尽管大部分资金似乎用来发展了现代医疗机构，但通常情形下，传统医学医院和现代医学医院仍然同时存在。

As of 1987, organizational conflict has almost entirely disappeared. In the cities modern physicians and scholar-physicians treat patients in some of the same hospitals, and in the countryside secondary medical school graduates and traditional practitioners work side by side, without constraint, treating patients according to their own individual principles without thought of criticism from the other practitioners.

Freedom of choice for the patient can produce interesting results. This was impressed on me in 1979, for example, during a field trip to Deyang County in Sichuan Province. There I visited what was then called a commune health center, where traditional medicine was practiced. It was very busy, full of patients. A dozen "doctors" were prescribing drugs. A few streets away there was a government-run modern health facility. The contrast between the two was startling. The modern facility had only a few patients and its staff had very little to do.

The situation aroused my curiosity. What could explain it? Wherever the two medicines (of which neither is standardized) were available, they were undoubtedly rendering some useful service. So why was the preference so strong? Perhaps only because of long ingrained habit. Perhaps, as I was inclined to think, however, it could be explained in part by shortcomings in the training of modern physicians serving the farmers, which diminished popular confidence in them and made them appear less competent as a group than traditional medical practitioners. Whatever the reason, more training for modern physicians serving in rural areas would be to the advantage of our country.

Policies Relating to Village Health

In the years between 1978 and 1987, a number of economic and social policies had strong effects on the life of the farmers. Apart from the dramatic increase in prosperity in some areas resulting from modernization

自 1987 年起，组织体系的冲突几乎已经完全消失。在城市，现代医师和传统医师可以在同一家医院中诊治病人；在农村，卫生职校的中专毕业生和传统行医者并肩工作，不受制约、完全根据自己的个人经验诊治病人，而无须考虑其他从业人员的评议。

病人在两种医疗机构中自由选择就诊，有可能会产生某些有趣的现象。比如，1979 年，我在四川德阳县的一次实地考察，就给我留下了深刻的印象。在那里，我参观访问了当时被称为"公社卫生院"的一个地方，那里开展的是传统诊疗。现场显得十分忙碌，挤满了病人，十几个"医生"正在为病人开药处方。而在相距几条街之外，有一家由政府管理经营的现代医疗机构。形成鲜明对比的是，那里的病人寥寥无几，医务人员几乎无事可做，这一现象令人吃惊。

这种现象引起了我的好奇。怎么解释呢？无论这两种医疗模式（都没有被标准化）且都可以使用，他们无疑都在提供有价值的服务。那么为什么这种在偏好上的差别会如此强烈呢？也许只是因为长久以来形成的根深蒂固的行为习惯。然而，也许正如我倾向的观点可以一定程度上得到解释，即那些为农民服务的现代医师没有得到足够的培训。由于这些缺陷，削减了人们对现代医师的信心与信任，并使他们这个群体被认为是能力水平似乎不如传统行医者的医师群体。总之，对在农村地区服务的现代医师进行更多的培训总是对国家有利的。

与农村卫生有关的政策

1978 年至 1987 年，一些经济和社会政策对农民的生活产生

reforms, perhaps the most obvious was the reduction in births proceeding from the strictly enforced policy of one child per family.

In 1987, in the counties whose circumstances I am familiar with, contraception is widely practiced, as in other rural areas, although some farmers still want more than one child. Barrier methods, sterilization, and abortion for both married and unmarried women are the most common methods; barrier methods have a 20 percent failure rate, however, and numbers of women become pregnant unintentionally. Chemical preparations are not very well favored. For the married, all surgical operations and treatments of possible complications are free of charge. For the unmarried, there is a charge, assigned in accordance with government regulations.

The benefits of family planning for improved child health are readily evident. With smaller families, household financial circumstances have been upgraded and living conditions improved. All but a very few parents are prepared to spend money to guard their child's health, and they are careful to do so.

The situation reinforces the assertion I had made nearly forty years ago in Chongqing to Dr. Marshall Balfour of the Rockefeller Foundation: public health without birth control may do more harm than good for Chinese farmers. I am now 100 percent in favor of our family planning policy, notwithstanding certain side effects, to whose long-term consequences—both social and emotional—our government is highly sensitive. The government, in fact, has already taken steps to ameliorate such affects.

In one of the model counties of Sichuan Province, Shifang County, which I visited in 1986, now almost all young parents have only one child, and with only one, they take painstaking care of the child's health. Parents pay close attention to immunization, knowing its importance, and reports indicate that 88 percent of the children have been immunized under current control programs. Some parents, on discovering that their child was not given a vaccine when others were, will not rest until they are satisfied that the child was already protected.

了重大影响。除了现代化改革使得一些地区快速繁荣之外，最明显的影响莫过于严格执行计划生育政策。

1987 年，在我熟悉情况的那些县，和其他农村地区一样，虽然有些农民仍想多子生育，但普遍推行节育措施。物理阻断、绝育和人工流产是已婚和未婚妇女最常用的方法。然而，避孕工具仍有 20% 的失败率，许多妇女出现意外怀孕。药物避孕不太受欢迎。对于已婚者，所有的外科手术及其可能并发症的治疗都是免费的。对于未婚者，则根据政府规定收取相应费用。

计划生育政策显著改善了儿童健康状况。随着家庭成员规模的缩小，经济状况与生活条件均得到改善。绝大多数父母都愿意将钱用在孩子的健康保障上，且悉心对待。

这种情况印证了约 40 年前我在重庆对洛克菲勒基金会马歇尔·巴尔弗博士做出的论断：如不实施计划生育，公共卫生政策对中国农民来说可能是利大于弊。我现在百分之百赞成计划生育政策，政府已经采取措施来减少不良影响。

1986 年我考察访问了四川省什邡县，当时几乎所有的年轻父母都只有一个孩子，他们对孩子的健康非常重视。父母都知道免疫接种极为重要，密切关注免疫接种。报告显示，在推行免疫计划政策后，88% 的儿童完成了免疫接种。有一些父母当发现自己的孩子没有接种疫苗、而其他孩子都进行了接种后，他们会感到焦虑不安，直到自己孩子得到了免疫接种后方才满意释怀。

Other directives, including several issued in 1985 by the Ministry of Health, also had important overall and long-term implications. One of these created a new category of physician, the "country doctor," ranking intermediate to the regular medical school graduate and the "barefoot doctor." The "barefoot doctor" who can claim to have passed a formal examination is entitled to the new rank.

Most of those who became country doctors through this new regulation are, in fact, traditional practitioners with a modest overlay of scientific training. The likely inference, then, is that traditional medicine will gain an additional advocacy group, one with more influence and prestige than barefoot doctors or village health workers, and that scientific medicine may be set back farther.

The creation of another category of "doctor" added to an already confusing situation. The term "doctor" had come to have only a very loose meaning. Persons with academic degrees in modern medicine, graduates of secondary medical schools, traditional practitioners, barefoot doctors, and now' country doctors, as well as persons who simply prescribed and sold drugs, were all referred to as "doctors." No criteria have as yet been established to distinguish among these various and, to some extent, overlapping categories, notwithstanding the great variation in their qualifications to practice medicine.

Two other regulations were of interest in terms of their potential for affecting health in rural China, one permitting "barefoot doctors" to engage in private practice, setting their own fees, and the other permitting private entrepreneurs to manufacture and sell drugs for profit. Because "barefoot doctors" in general have had less than optimal training, and because China suffers from a scarcity of published medical reference material, many rural physicians lack a sound understanding of the scientific principles on which the use of certain drugs is based. As private practitioners, how ever, they are legally entitled to prescribe drugs without restriction, under little or no supervision. This can put the patient

其他一些指导方针包括卫生部 1985 年发布的几个文件，也产生了长期深远的影响。其中之一便是官方确认一类新型医生，称为"农村医生"，其介于正规医学院校毕业生和"赤脚医生"之间。而那些确认通过官方正式考试的"赤脚医生"，意味着获得了"农村医生"这一新的职业身份。

事实上，符合这项新规成为"农村医生"中的大多数人，都是传统行医者中仅受过有限的科学培训者。因此，可能推想，传统医学将可能获得更多的拥趸，这些人往往比"赤脚医生"或农村卫生工作者更有影响和声望，如此一来现代医学可能更难普及和深入人心。

而这类"医生"的出现使本已混乱不堪的局面更加雪上加霜。"医生"一词的含义变得模糊不清而且非常宽泛。拥有现代医学教育学位的人、卫生职校的中专毕业生、传统行医者、赤脚医生、现在的农村医生以及那些仅仅处方售药的人，都被称为"医生"。尽管他们的医疗实践资质与岗位胜任力存在很大差异，但仍尚未建立关于他们的任何的区分评判标准，在某种程度上还存在分类重叠、杂乱无序。

另外两项规章对中国农村卫生状况的潜在影响也是值得关注的。其中一项法规允许赤脚医生从事私人执业，提供医疗服务，并可自行制定费用标准；另一项法规则允许私营企业承包生产和销售药品牟利。由于赤脚医生一般都没有接受过正规培训，加上我国缺乏公开出版发表的医学参考资料，许多赤脚医生对某些药物的使用所依据的科学原理缺乏正确的认识。然而，作为私人从

at considerable risk.

Also, the temptation to pursue monetary profit may be irresistible for a few barefoot doctors. This would be difficult for the farmers, who depend on them in health matters and respect their judgment. Rural inhabitants already tell visitors of alleged incidents in which a barefoot doctor has prescribed an injection for only slight illness or has substituted inferior medications for a more costly one.

The private production and sale of medications also had troublesome implications. Until 1985, rural physicians could obtain drugs only at government dispensaries, These dispensaries had been the exclusive agents of all drugs, of which the government was the sole manufacturer. Now, however, physicians may not only prescribe drugs without supervision but also purchase them from any supplier they choose, and any individual who elects to produce drugs may do so. In theory, the quality of drugs purchased from all sources is the same. Private drug manufacturers are subject to official monitoring of standards by a quality-control bureau. The proliferation of small companies makes it increasingly difficult to exercise full control, however, posing the danger that the quality of privately produced pharmaceuticals will fall significantly below that of those manufactured by the government. The current government is still the main drug producer, but its share of the market seems to be declining.

Party and government leaders are not unmindful that problems could develop and in 1986 clearly indicated their commitment to the well-being of farmers and strengthened movement for positive change in their behalf. In that year alone, the Ministry of Health sponsored two major meetings at which delegates focused on rural health concerns and local training issues. Both meetings took place in July of that year in Shandong Province, one a national conference of medical educators held in Qingdao, the other a national rural health conference held in Yantai. Out of the latter movement came the movement to organize a permanent

业者，他们居然有权在几乎不受监督限制的情形下自主地处方开药，而且是合法的，这可能给病人带来相当大的风险。

此外，个别赤脚医生难以抵挡住金钱利益的诱惑。这对在健康问题上依赖并尊重他们的农民来说，无疑会带来灾难。农民已经向参访人员讲述了类似这样的事例，比如有的赤脚医生在诊治过程中"小病大治"，或者用劣质低价药物代替冒充价格昂贵的药品。

药品的私人生产和销售也存在很多问题隐患。1985 年以前，乡村医生只能在政府统一配给药房获得药品，所有药品都是专营的，政府也是唯一的生产方。然而，现在医生不仅可以在没有任何监督下处方开药，甚至还可以自主选择供应商来采购药品，同时任何生产药品的个人都可以随意销售。理论上，从各种渠道购买的药品质量应该是一样的。而且私人药品生产商都接受质量控制监督局的官方监督。然而，小公司的激增使得全过程的质量控制变得越来越困难，这带来的风险就是私人生产的药品质量难以保障，很可能大大低于政府生产的药品质量。当前政府仍然是主要的药品生产方，但其所占市场份额看来正在下降。

党和政府领导人并非没有意识到这些问题及其可能后果，并在 1986 年明确表示，他们致力于保障农民的健康福祉，并加强开展了对农民积极有益的系列活动。仅在那一年，卫生部就主办了两次重要会议，代表们在会上集中讨论了农村卫生问题和地方卫生培训问题。这两次会议都是当年 7 月在山东召开的，一次是在青岛召开的全国医学教育工作者大会，另一次是在烟台召开全

consultative body, the National Rural Health Association. These were highly significant developments and, all in all, it would be difficult to understate the importance they held for discussion and long-term constructive action for rural health.

Meanwhile other forward steps were also being instituted by the national leadership, some with input from international development agencies working in China since the implementation of the open-door policy. The agencies included the United Nations Children's Fund (UNICEF), the World Health Organization (WHO), and the International Bank for Reconstruction and Development (more commonly known as the "World Bank").

Such agencies had an important influence on health policy and administration, although their contribution was usually indirect. For example, when Ministry of Health officials shifted from generally impromptu discussion as a basis for planning and evaluation to scientific methods employing quantitative analysis, foreign technical personnel were consulted for advice as to the best methods for setting up a new statistical bureau in the ministry.

In another example, there is, in our own province, the Shifang model county health program. The World Bank lent support in its establishment and continues to provide some technical assistance; but China runs the project. Shifang County government functionaries and health officials are responsible, and some respected medical and health figures serve as special consultants. I personally, as a professor of community medicine at Sichuan Medical College (now renamed West China University of Medical Sciences), offer suggestions on health training and other matters.

国农村卫生大会。在后一个会议举办期间，还组织建立了一个常设咨询机构——全国农村卫生协会。总而言之，这些都是非常重要的发展进步，而它们对于农村卫生的形势分析和指导制定长期建设措施具有不可或缺的重要意义。

与此同时，国家领导层也在采取其他的积极措施，其中一些得到了自改革开放政策实施以来一直在中国工作的国际发展机构的资金投入支持。这些机构包括联合国儿童基金会、世界卫生组织和国际复兴开发银行（通常被称作世界银行）。

尽管上述机构的贡献通常是间接的，但它们对卫生政策和行政管理均具有重要的影响。例如，当卫生部官员拟对卫生政策计划和评价时的常规及临时性讨论，转为采用定量分析的科学方法，此时就需要向国外技术专家咨询求助。因此他们建议最好就是在卫生部下辖设立一个新的统计局来解决这些问题。

另一个例子是，四川省什邡县被确定为卫生方案示范县。世界银行支持其成立，并陆续提供了一些技术援助；但这个项目由中国自行负责。什邡县政府工作人员和卫生官员具有高度负责感，一些德高望重的医疗卫生人士担任特别顾问。而我个人作为四川医学院（现更名为华西医科大学）的一名社区医学的教授，也对卫生培训等事宜提出建议咨询。

ORGANIZATION OF HEALTH SERVICES

The organization of health services in China today can be described in only broad terms. The system exhibits regional and local diversity and is subject to organizational rearrangements at any given time or place. Even terminology shows no obligation to hold still.

About all that can be said with certainty is that the Ministry of Health, in the central government, is the source of, and final authority on, planning, policy, and budget matters, and all other health agencies are ultimately accountable to it. The Minister of Health is a member of the State Council, or Cabinet.

In the implementation of policy, the Ministry of Health provides technical supervision through a chain of agencies linked together down to the lowest level, the village (see fig. 2) All health agencies, both urban and rural, generally implement central government decisions without modification, although a recent ruling, taking account of the country's great diversity, allows a few provincial governments somewhat more freedom than others. Units at each level select their own staffs, but appointments are subject to approval at the next higher level.

Below the Ministry of Health there are more than twenty province-level governments, including municipalities and autonomous territories, having their own health administrations. Some province-level units are divided into regions having their own health administrations.

All these agencies as well as the hospitals, schools, and clinics they operate are government facilities, staffed by government employees. Together they constitute the urban component of the health system, as distinguished from the rural component. The distinction between the two components is significant and has many implications for sources of funding, personnel, and other matters.

338

卫生服务组织架构

当今中国的卫生服务组织架构只是个一般性术语。整个系统呈现出区域和地方多样性，并在某些特定时空环境下还受到组织架构重组的影响。从具体名称来看，它也不是一成不变的。

可以肯定的是，中央政府的卫生部是制定规划、政策和预算的最高权力机构，所有其他卫生机构最终都要对卫生部负责。卫生部长一般都是国务院成员或内阁成员。

在政策执行过程中，卫生部通过从上到下直至村一级的完整链条的各级卫生行政机构实施技术监督（见图 2）。所有卫生机构，无论是城市还是农村，都常规严格执行中央政府的决策部署，而最近的一项规定则考虑到我国幅员辽阔，各地具体情况不一，中央政府给予少数几个省政府更多的决策自主权。各级卫生机构可以自行选择任用工作人员，但任命需得到上一级的批准。

在卫生部之下，有 20 多个省级政府，包括直辖市和自治区都有各自的卫生行政管理部门。一些省级行政区域又被下设特区并拥有各自的卫生行政管理部门。

所有这些卫生管理部门以及它们主管的医院、学校和诊所都是政府机构，工作人员都属于政府工作人员。这些部门和人员共同构成了有别于农村卫生系统的城市卫生系统。城市与农村卫生系统的区别很大，包括资金来源、人事任用和其他诸多方面均不同。

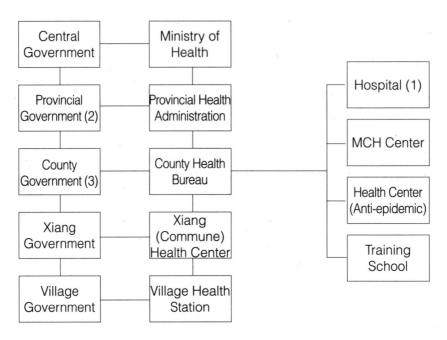

Fig. 2. Organization of Rural Health Services, 1987

The rural component of the health system dovetails with the urban component at the county level of government. County-level governments (the apex of authority in rural China), and the county health bureaus they operate, enjoy considerable autonomy in selecting personnel and carrying out day-to-day operations. They are, nonetheless, ultimately responsible to provincial health administrators, who, in turn, are accountable to the officials of the Ministry of Health.

The organization of health services below the county level varies from place to place. In general terms, however, it can be considered as a three-tiered arrangement consisting of units at the county, xiang, and village levels. (The xiang administration replaces the disbanded communes.) Each of the three administrative tiers has its own responsibilities and functions and operates different facilities. While this arrangement resembles the three-tiered organization at Dingxian in 1930,

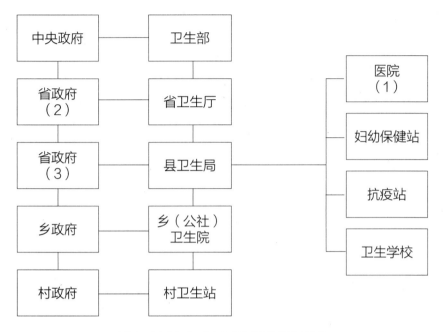

图 2 1978 年农村卫生服务组织结构

卫生系统的农村组成部分与城市组成部分在县一级基本一致。县级政府（中国农村地区的最高行政机构）及其主管的县卫生局在人事安排和日常工作管理方面享有相当大的自主权。然而，他们最终需对省级卫生行政管理部门即卫生厅负责，而卫生厅则需对卫生部负责。

县及以下的卫生服务组织因不同地区而存在差异。但总的来说，它基本可划分为三级结构：即由县、乡、村三级单位组成（乡政府取代了过去的公社）。三个行政管理层级都有各自的职责和功能，并主管着各类机构。虽然这种组织架构类似于 1930 年定县当时的三级组织，包括区、街道和村级单位（安排和承担具体

which encompassed district, subdistrict, and village-level units (and it does entail arrangements for technical supervision), it seems to lack the emphasis on integrated functioning that we considered to be the essence of the Dingxian system.

The general scheme was modified in certain counties, however. Some counties actually have a four-tiered system with an intermediate subcounty level between the county and the xiang level.

The staffs of county-level agencies throughout China are salaried government employees and, like others in that category, are entitled to free health care. In North China—the generally poorer half of the country's traditional heartland, government employment in health generally extends down to the xiang level of health administration, meaning that the staffs of local health facilities at that level have access to free medical care, as do urban government and factory employees. This is seldom the case in South China. Rural health everywhere, however, is supported in various ways, particularly including the provision of subsidies for preventive work.

As to health agencies below the county level, they, too, receive some subsidies, mainly for equipment. By and large, however, the local community provides resources for their establishment and operation; treatment costs are borne by individual patients.

The Urban Component

The Ministry of Health has general responsibility for the health and well-being of the population, although family planning matters are essentially the responsibility of another ministry, with which the Ministry of Health only cooperates. Additionally, the ministry operates various educational, research, and treatment facilities in Beijing and some other cities. These include what are called the "key medical colleges," as well as a number of hospitals, and scientific research institutes.

的技术监督工作），但目前的三级组织架构似乎还缺乏职能统筹和功能协调，而这恰恰是我们所推行的定县模式所拥有的精髓。

虽然在大的框架不变情形下，有些县的三级组织架构进行了调整，比如某些县实际上设置了四级组织架构，即在县和乡之间还增加划分出一个县下辖的区级中间组织机构。

中国各县级卫生系统的工作人员都是领工资的国家公职人员，和其他级别卫生系统的工作人员一样，都享受国家的免费医疗保健。在北方地区——中国传统的中心地区，也有一半的地区较贫穷。政府在卫生系统的工作人事任命直接延伸到乡一级的卫生行政管理部门，这意味着乡级卫生系统的工作人员也可以享受免费医疗保健，这与城市政府和国有工厂职工没有差别。这种情况在南方很少见。各地的农村卫生机构工作人员是以多样化方式得到保障，特别是确保开展预防工作的补贴。

县级以下的卫生机构也可以获得一些补贴，主要集中在设备采购方面。然而，总的来说，地方为卫生机构的建立和运转提供了经费资源；治疗费用则由病人个人承担。

城市部分

虽然计划生育工作基本上是另一个中央部门主管，卫生部只需配合协作，但国民卫生健康事务则由卫生部统管。此外，卫生部还主管着在北京和其他一些城市的直属教育、研究和医疗机构。这些机构中包括俗称的"重点医科院校"，以及一些部属医院和科研机构。

Among others, the research institutions include the monumental Chinese Academy of Medical Sciences (CAMS), with a total working staff of more than 10,000 persons, which was formed by merger with the PUMC and another medical institution.2 The CAMS has yielded a number of high-level research projects against important epidemic diseases, including plague, schistosomiasis, kala azar, and venereal disease. One recent CAMS research project led to a breakthrough in treatment of uterine cancer.

Intent on improving academic standards in higher education, the post-Mao leadership restored the competitive entrance examinations for all prospective university-level students and lengthened the medical school curriculum in regular and key medical colleges to six years or more. In another policy decision, it established departments of community medicine in a number of medical schools.

Quite a few representatives of these new departments attended the National Conference of Community Medicine held in 1984 at Chengdu. Since then a professional journal has been established, and some university departments have launched plans to conduct regular classes for the training of health administrators. As of 1987, however, the scope of activities of the new departments was not yet well defined.

Province-level health administrations also played a key role in urban health care and medical education. A great many of the hospitals and clinics in Chinese cities are administered by provincial and municipal governments, some constructed in the pre-1958 period when much attention was devoted to development of urban facilities and others more recently in the drive for modernization. Some hospitals engage exclusively in scientific medical practice, others practice traditional medicine exclusively, and still others have sections or facilities for either.

这些科研机构中就包括著名的中国医学科学院，其工作人员超过 10000 人，由北京协和医学院和另一家医学研究院合并而成。中国医学科学院完成了一些针对包括鼠疫、血吸虫病、黑热病和性病等重要流行病的高水准科学研究项目，又在子宫癌治疗研究领域取得了突破性进展。

为了更好地提升高等教育的办学质量与学术水平，毛泽东后时代的中央领导层全面恢复了针对所有符合大学就读资质的学生的入学资格考试——高考，并恢复了普通和重点医学院校的学制，并将一些重点医学院校的学制延长至六年或更长。另一项政策就是在一些医学院里建立了社区医学系。

1984 年在成都召开的全国社区医学大会上，有不少参会代表都来自这些新成立的社区医学系。之后不久，社区医学专业期刊创立，而一些医学院校的社区医学系已着手制定常规计划，以用于培训卫生管理人员。然而，直到 1987 年，这些新社区医学系的工作范围尚未得到明确界定。

在城市卫生保健和医学教育方面，省级卫生行政部门也发挥了重要作用。中国城市中的许多医院和诊所是由省、直辖市政府主管的，有些医疗机构是在 1958 年以前建立的，而当时普遍关注城市卫生系统设施发展建设，另一些是在现代化进程中建造的。其中，一些医院专门从事科学医学诊疗，另一些则专门从事传统医学诊疗，还有一些则兼作两者。

Not unexpectedly, while these facilities are all located in the cities, their patients are not exclusively urban. The reputations of the provincial hospitals reach out to the countryside, and in serious cases those villagers who are discontent with the rural medical care and who can afford to come to the city to seek help will often do so. For example, in early 1986, I encountered a well-to-do farmer whose broken fibula had been improperly handled at a xiang health center. When he obtained no relief from treatment by local physicians, he sought help from a highly respected orthopedist at the provincial hospital.

This influx of farmers to urban hospitals is a trend worth noting. Provincial hospitals are already heavily burdened with urban patients, and the influx of villagers imposes an extra load on provincial hospital staff physicians. Because of this patient overload, the staff is hard pressed, and some may be left unsatisfied with their treatment. Moreover, the trips are costly for the farmers who often must wait for several days before being admitted to the hospital and must find, and probably pay for, temporary lodgings somewhere.

Key medical colleges, located in major cities and operated by the central government, arc the most prestigious medical schools devoted to teacher-training responsibilities. Usually, schools of dentistry, pharmacy, and public health are affiliated with each medical college. A traditional medical college in Beijing, administered by the central Ministry of Health, is among the key medical schools.

Provincial authorities operate the other two types of modern medical college—the regular medical colleges and the lower-rated secondary medical schools (which accept junior-high-school graduates for admission), plus some schools of traditional medicine. As of 1987 there were about 100 provincial medical colleges and about 500 secondary medical schools.

不出所料，虽然这些医院都位于城市，但其病人来源却并不仅限于城市居民。省级大医院在农村地区享有很高声誉，尤其病情严重时，那些对农村医疗能力不满意又有经济基础的农民，经常会去城市医院寻医问药。例如，1986 年年初，我遇到过一个富裕的农民，他的腓骨骨折，但乡卫生院对其病情处理不当。经当地医生治疗后其病情并未获得缓解，于是他便到省级医院去寻求一位知名骨科专家的救治。

农村病人涌入城市医院是一个值得重视的倾向。省级医院已经被城市病人压得喘不过气来，加上农村病人的涌入，给医务人员医生带来了超额的工作负荷。由于病人过多，医护人员工作压力巨大，常处于高度紧张状态，而有些病人可能不一定能得到满意的治疗。此外，对于农村病人，出行成本高，而且他们还常常要等上好几天才能办理入院，所以需要找到临时住所并为此付费，这无疑更增加了就医成本。

位于几大主要城市并由中央政府部门直接管辖的重点医学院校是承担师资培训任务的最负盛名的医学院校。通常，每所医学院校都附设有口腔医学、药学和公共卫生学等学系。由卫生部直管的北京中医学院亦是重点医学院校之一。

省级卫生行政部门主管着另外两类现代医学院校——普通高等医学院校和卫生职业学校（招收初中毕业生入学），还包括一些传统医学学校。截至 1987 年，大约有 100 所省属医学院校和 500 所卫生职业学校。

Test scores on the basis of general competitive examinations determine the order in which students can select the medical, dental, pharmaceutical, or public health school of their choice. Because the public health field is not well understood, public health schools are seldom selected first. About one-eighth of the successful medical college candidates are assigned to traditional medical colleges, which under the present administration enjoy almost the same professional standing as modern medical schools. The four-year curriculum in these schools generally consists of an initial two years of scientific study, including courses in pathology and biochemistry, followed by two years of traditional learning.

As to course requirements in public health schools, there is considerable emphasis on laboratory work, entailing examination of air, water, food, and waste products, or animal experimentation. Field training, through which students might profitably be exposed to major health problems in their country and possible solutions, is greatly downplayed. Many graduates are absorbed into provincially administered health research institutions, where examination of various aspects of epidemic, endemic, and occupational disease is conducted. Others join the county-operated antiepidemic stations.

Ranking below the key and provincial medical colleges are the secondary medical schools, which train junior-high-school graduates for service as physicians in rural areas. On the basis of the number of years they had been in operation, and the average class size, by 1987 these schools presumably graduated nearly one million physicians. The schools also train some nurses and a few midwives for rural service.

Clinical training in the secondary medical schools is quite brief; thus, graduates cannot be assumed to be anywhere near as skilled as regular medical college graduates, who in the rural system are concentrated at the county level. Their reputation as a group seems to be declining. They are

入学考试成绩结合志愿填报，决定了学生是被录取到医学系、口腔医学系、药学系或公共卫生学系。由于对公共卫生专业领域了解不多，很少学生会先选择公共卫生学系。大约 1/8 被医学院校成功录取的学生被分配到传统医学院校。按照当时的政策管理规定，这些传统医学院校的学生享有与现代医学院校学生同等的专业地位，其学制一般为四年，前两年学习医学基础课程，包括病理学和生物化学等课程，后两年专修传统医学专业课程。

在公共卫生学系，在必读的课程中非常强调实验室操作训练，主要包括空气、水、食品和废弃物的检测或动物实验。但是通过现场实地培训、学生可以接触到国家的主要卫生健康问题和可能的解决办法并从中获益的培训，已被轻描淡写了。许多毕业生被吸引分配至省级卫生研究机构，那里的工作涉及流行病、地方病和职业病等各方面。其他毕业生则被分配到县级卫生抗疫站。

排在重点医学院校和省属医学院校之后的是卫生职业学校，这类学校是招收初中毕业生并培训他们成为能够胜任农村地区工作的医生。根据这些学校开办时间和招生规模，到 1987 年，大概培养了近 100 万名医生。同时，这些学校还为农村医疗服务系统培养了一些护士和助产士。

卫生职业学校的临床实习相当短暂，因此，不能想当然地认为其毕业生能像医学院校毕业生那样有扎实的技术，后者主要集中在县级医疗卫生机构。而卫生职业学校毕业生在总体上的声誉似乎在下降。即使与许多农村医生或赤脚医生相比，他们业务能

at an apparent disadvantage even compared with many "country doctors" or "barefoot doctors," who may have had little formal training but who have benefited by their considerable practical experience. A 1986 survey reports that among those country doctors evaluated, 75 percent were rated as equally competent or more competent than a physician who had graduated from secondary medical school.

The issue of competency and the need for field training and local training school activity for the benefit of many health personnel was made further evident by statistics published in the mid-1980s by several provincial governments. For its part, for example, the Sichuan provincial government recognizes four grades of "doctor" and two of "medical assistant." Of "doctors" enumerated in the province in 1984, 13.7 percent were college-grade, meaning that they had graduated from a regular or key medical college; 24.8 percent were junior-college-grade, meaning that, on the basis of their experience, they were deemed more qualified than the secondary medical school graduates at the next-lower level; 38.5 percent were secondary-medical-school-grade; and 23 percent had had no formal training whatsoever. Among the medical assistants, 64.28 percent were secondary-medical-school-grade. The remainder, almost one third, had had no formal training of any type.

Zhejiang Province has the highest educational levels in China, but even there many of the "doctors" were totally without formal medical training in 1984. According to official figures for that year, only 19 percent of physicians in the province had graduated from a regular or key medical college; 46 percent had graduated from a secondary medical school. But again more than 33 percent had had no formal medical education.

Meanwhile a survey in the same year from Heilongjiang Province provided further indication of just how critical was the need for additional systematic training. In a sample survey, asked to comment on

力也处于明显的劣势，农村医生或赤脚医生可能没有受过多少正规培训，却拥有丰富的实践经验。1986 年的一项调查报告称，与卫生职业学校毕业的医生相比，接受评定的农村医生中有 75% 被认为具有同等能力或能力更强。

有些省政府在 20 世纪 80 年代中期公布的统计数字进一步证实了上述能力差距问题，为解决这些问题，帮助医疗卫生人员提高专业技能，需要开展有效的临床实训和地方学校培训活动。基于此，四川省政府承认"医生"的四个级别和"医疗助理"的两个级别。在该省 1984 年统计的"医生"中，13.7% 是大学本科毕业级别，这意味着他们毕业于普通或重点医学院校；24.8% 是专科毕业级别，根据其学历经历，这意味着他们比下一地域级别的卫生职业学校毕业生更有资质能力；38.5% 是卫生职业学校毕业级别；23% 迄今没有受过任何正规的培训。在医疗辅助人员中，64.28% 毕业于卫生职业学校，而其余人中的几乎 1/3 没有受过任何形式的正规培训。

浙江省是中国受教育水平最高的省份，但即使在浙江，许多"医生"在 1984 年也完全没有受过正规的医学培训。根据当年的官方数据，该省只有 19% 的医生毕业于普通或重点医学院校；46% 毕业于卫生职业学校。但同样有超过 33% 的医生没有接受过正规的医学教育。

同年，黑龙江省的一项调查进一步表明了在加强系统培训方面需求形势的严峻。在一项抽样调查中，对一组 100 名医生的技

the proficiency of a group of 100 physicians, respondents categorized 22.7 percent as "competent," 51.9 percent as "not competent," and 25.3 percent as "very incompetent."

Because the better-trained and, therefore, presumably more competent physicians prefer to work at the county level and above, such distributions fall particularly hard on the farmers. More than likely, the least qualified physicians are to be found mostly in rural areas.

The Rural Component

The general scheme of rural health services has evolved over the past thirty years. What I know of that system, of course, is based on my familiarity with the situation in my own province and does not necessarily pertain to, or characterize, circumstances in other parts of China.

The County Bureau of Health

The function of the County Bureau of Health is to execute policy designed by higher authorities and approved by local party officials. In this context it engages in both curative and preventive work. Funding comes mainly from the county budget, with small additional increments from the provincial government. The range of total health expenditures probably varies considerably from one county to another and from one part of the country to another. Precise information on this point is not available.

The county health bureau serves as administrative headquarters and provides the most technically advanced level of services available. The service agencies in counties in our province, and in many other Chinese counties, include one or more hospitals (some counties have both a traditional and a modern hospital and sometimes a specialized hospital), a health center, a maternal and child health center, and a training school for continuing health education.

能熟练程度进行了评价，结果 22.7％ 的医生被判定为"称职"，51.9％ 被判定为"不称职"，25.3％ 被判定为"非常不称职"。

由于受过更规范更系统培训而被认为能力更强的医生，更倾向于去县级以上的医疗机构工作。所以这种医生资源的不合理分配对农民就医来说带来了挑战与困难。如此一来，在农村地区服务的医生只能是那些最不合格的医生了。

农村部分

过去30年里，农村卫生服务的总体规划发展有了长足的进步。当然，我对这一系统的了解是基于我对自己所在省份情况的熟悉，不一定能代表或概括中国其他地区的情况。

县卫生局

县卫生局的职能是执行上级行政部门制定的或经当地党委官员批准同意的政策，主要工作就是统筹管理防与治。资金主要来源于县级财政预算，省政府也下拨少部分资金。卫生费用总支出的范围各县以及国家不同地区之间均有差异，但缺乏准确数据资料。

县卫生局作为县级卫生服务的行政管理中心，负责提供现有可及的技术最先进的医疗服务。我所在省的各县以及中国其他许多县的卫生服务机构包括一家或多家医院（有些县既有传统医学医院，也有现代医学医院，有时还有一家专科医院）、一个卫生抗疫站、一家妇幼保健中心和一所进行继续教育的卫生培训学校。

The county hospitals are the apex of the medical care service agencies. They have the most advanced equipment and the most specialized staffs and are supposed to attend to the most seriously ill patients. While physicians trained in secondary medical schools still constitute the majority of staff members, an increasing number of graduates of regular medical colleges are now being appointed to serve with county hospitals.

A county hospital that has the best equipment, specialized manpower, and a dedicated staff may still face many resource deficiencies and technical problems; thus, even the finest county hospital might be unlikely to qualify as a model for rural medical care. The staffs are short-handed. More nurses are needed to relieve families of patient care responsibilities, more nutritionists are needed to attend to special diets, and more architects and engineers specializing in hospital design are needed to focus on such special aspects as water supply and waste disposal. Because many medical personnel have little knowledge of the nature of infection, cleanliness of the surroundings is not a high priority. Even physicians and nurses may fail to assign high priority to cleanliness; for instance, it is by no means unusual to hear that the surgical incision of a hospital patient became infected because the site was not kept unscrupulously clean.

Regardless of what the term "county health center" implies, these facilities generally are intended not for dispensing treatment but for preventive medicine after the Soviet model. Their main responsibilities are communicable disease control, health services in schools and factories, public health education, food hygiene, and collection of vital statistics. Some counties also operate special health centers for endemic disease, such as filariasis.

The maternal and child health centers offer various advisory and oversight services. For example, they provide health care and information on nutrition to pregnant women. After a child is born, they offer regular

县医院是县一级医疗保健服务体系中的最高机构。他们拥有区域内最先进的设备和最专业化的工作人员，理应接收救治当地患病最严重的病人。虽然卫生职业学校培养的医生仍然占医务人员的大多数，但越来越多的普通高等医学院校毕业生被分配到县医院工作。

县级医院拥有最好的医疗设备、专业的人力资源、敬业爱岗的职工，但仍然还会面临很多资源不足和技术方面的问题；因此，即使是最好的县医院也不太可能成为农村医疗保健的典范。在日常诊疗中，医院常常人手不足，常需要更多的护士来减轻由家庭照顾病人的责任，需要更多的营养师制定特殊饮食，需要更多的专门从事医院设计的建筑师和工程师来解决医院供水和医疗废物处理等问题。由于许多医务人员缺乏对感染原由的认知，因此周围环境的清洁及医院感染控制工作并没有受到重视。即使是医生和护士也可能无法确保做到无菌操作；例如，医院病人的手术切口感染的常见原因为手术现场未能保持绝对的清洁。

我们不深究"县卫生抗疫站"一词的来源，它通常都是参照苏联模式建立起来的，是专门从事预防医学而不是用来提供疾病治疗的机构。其主要职责是传染病防控、学校和工厂的卫生服务、公共卫生教育、食品卫生和生命相关统计数据的收集。有些县还建立专门的地方病防控卫生服务中心，如丝虫病。

妇幼保健中心提供各种咨询和监督随访服务。例如，他们会向孕妇提供保健和营养方面的建议。孩子出生后，妇幼保健中心

health examinations, monitor growth, and plan immunizations.

The training schools for health offer continuing education courses for local health personnel. Teachers are drawn from the staff of the county hospital.

Xiang-Level Health Facilities

With county hospitals caring largely for only the most seriously ill patients, the real burden of providing medical relief for a rural population of some 800 million persons falls to the xiang and village-level facilities and personnel. Of the former, there were, in 1981 (according to a report circulated at an international health conference in Singapore in 1981), some 554,000 health centers, averaging fifteen beds each, with a total staff of 935,000. Since then, some consolidation had taken place, with the more accessible and best equipped xiang health centers being upgraded to form so- called key centers, with oversight responsibility for about five smaller health stations in the surrounding areas. Statistics for 1987 are unavailable.

When commune health centers were first organized in the late 1950s, they were financially supported in different ways, ranging from a majority that were completely, or very largely, supported by the commune to a minority organized on some sort of a fee-collecting basis. In recent years, the government has advocated a change-over to a fee-for-service arrangement for all xiang health centers. Xiang-level health authorities are accountable to county officials, but in planning and supervising village-level personnel whom they are responsible for supervising, they have some degree of autonomy.

Xiang health centers provide a wide variety of patient care, treating serious cases of infectious disease and surgical need as well cases of minor illness or injury. They also are concerned with preventive activities, provision of health care for women and children, and family

会定期为其进行健康检查，监测婴幼儿生长发育情况，并完成计划免疫接种。

卫生培训学校则为当地卫生人员提供继续教育课程培训。培训教师都是从县医院的专业技术人员中挑选抽调的。

乡级卫生机构

由于县级医院主要救治照护病情最严重的病人，为约八亿农村人口提供医疗保健的任务实际上都压在了乡和村一级的卫生机构及其工作人员身上。1981 年（根据 1981 年新加坡国际卫生会议上发布的报告），中国大约有 55.4 万个卫生院，平均每个卫生院有 15 张床位，工作人员总数为 93.5 万人。从那以后，政府采取了一些巩固提升措施，更便利、设备更好的乡卫生院升级组成所谓的区域重点卫生院，负责监督指导周围地区约五个较小的卫生院。但还没有 1987 年的统计数据。

20 世纪 50 年代末，当公社卫生院成立之初时，资金来源方式不尽相同，但大多数完全或几乎均由公社支持，少数以集资方式筹建。后来，政府已同意所有乡卫生院实行按医疗服务收费。乡一级的卫生行政部门向县级卫生行政官员负责，但他们在自己负责监督的村子中，对人事的规划和安排具有一定的自主权。

乡卫生院可提供范围很广的医疗照护：如严重的传染病治疗、外科轻症或轻度外伤治疗。同时也开展各种预防工作、为妇女和儿童提供的卫生保健以及承担计划生育工作。乡卫生院的工作人

planning. Typically the staffs included one or more secondary medical school graduates, but in many cases personnel had received only on-the-job training.

Performance of surgery by persons lacking sufficient training is, of course, strictly forbidden. Nevertheless, this seems to occur occasionally when, for one reason or another, physicians overestimate their own capabilities. A rumor circulating in a rural county in 1986, for example, concerned a farmer who experienced bleeding for two weeks following an ineptly performed vasectomy. The farmer was unable to work while recuperating and lost his entire income during that period. Circulation of such stories or rumors could have an adverse affect on the entire birth planning program.

Village Health Stations

The days in prerevolutionary China—when, for example, 220 out of 472 villages in the rural district of Dingxian had no medical facilities of any kind—are gone forever. According to the latest data available to me (from the 1981 conference held in Singapore), China in 1981 had 670,000 village-level health stations, covering 85 percent of all villages. Affiliated with them were 1,348,000 barefoot doctors, 30 percent of whom were women. Additional affiliates included 1.6 million village health workers and about 0.5 million midwives.

Such stations are usually staffed by two or three people, but this number may vary depending on the size of the village. The county government subsidizes the station for its family planning activities and immunization projects. The village provides the treatment rooms and some equipment and medicine. The affiliated barefoot doctors charge fees to the patients for all services including immunizations, which until recently were given free.

The functional distinction between the barefoot doctors and the

员通常包括一至多名卫生职业学校的毕业生，但多数情况下，他们只接受过在职培训。

当然，政府严格禁止未经过充分培训的工作人员施行外科手术。然而，出自某种原因，当医生高估了自己的能力时，这种情况偶尔也可能会发生。例如，1986 年在一个偏远县，一位农民接受了不恰当的输精管结扎术，术后出血长达两周。这位农民在休养期间无法工作，也完全没有了收入。此类故事或谣言的传播可能会对计划生育工作整体产生不利影响。

村卫生所

新中国成立前，以定县农村地区为例，472 个村庄中有 220 个没有任何医疗服务设施，到 20 世纪 80 年代，这样的情形已经一去不复返了。根据我掌握的数据（来自 1981 年新加坡会议），1981 年中国有 67 万个村级卫生所，覆盖了 85% 的村庄。共有 134.8 万名赤脚医生在这些村卫生所工作，其中 30% 是女性。此外，还有 160 万名的村卫生员和约 50 万名的助产士。

此类村卫生所通常配备两到三名医务人员，数量可能因村庄大小而异。县政府为村卫生所的计划生育和计划免疫工作提供补贴。村政府为卫生所提供治疗用房、一些基本仪器设备和药品。赤脚医生可向病人收取包括免疫接种在内的所有服务费用。直到 20 世纪 80 年代末，免疫接种才实行免费提供。

赤脚医生和村卫生员之间的职能区分并不清晰。然而，总的

health workers is somewhat blurred. In general, however, at least in Sichuan Province, the former concentrate more on curative medicine and the latter, on preventive measures. The health workers, who work only part time, earn small fees and engage, for example, in malaria control or health propaganda activities.

Immunization programs were suspended in some places during the Cultural Revolution, except for smallpox immunization, which was continued by popular demand. Since 1978, however, these programs have been resumed, and the Ministry of Health has assigned them a high priority. Volume and coverage have been widely extended, probably exceeding the level of effort at any time in the past. These immunization campaigns, planned by the authorities and carried out by village-level workers, provide one of the major health success stories of the party (CCP) and the government. Life expectancy in China has risen from 40 years of age in 1949 to 68 in 1986, and infant mortality has declined from 200 per 1,000 live births to 34 per 1,000 in the same period. Rising socioeconomic levels contributed to this achievement, but a major share of the credit is attributable to the immunization campaign programs.

In 1987 immunization activities at the local level remained critically important. Unless immunization were administered by people living in the villages, who could follow those who needed vaccination until the work was completed, the level of infectious disease— regardless of whether the government assigns the issue high priority—could not be controlled. Agricultural work demanded that adult members of farming household be at work in their fields, and they could not accommodate their schedules for those of a visiting mobile health team. Instead, the barefoot doctor with fresh vaccine had to seek them out.

The mobilization of village level workers for preventive work has been accompanied by another trend, however, whose long-term implications are far less laudable: the tendency for barefoot doctors,

来说，至少在四川省，前者更关注治疗用药，后者更关注预防措施。村卫生员一般只做兼职工作，赚取少量费用，主要从事疟疾控制或卫生健康宣传等活动。

20 世纪 60 年代，除了天花的免疫接种服务应民众需求继续实行外，一些地方终止了免疫接种计划。但自 1978 年以来，这些接种计划已全面恢复，卫生部也高度重视此事项。免疫接种的数量和人群覆盖面都明显扩大，其效果可能已超过历史上任何一个时期。这些由卫生行政主管部门制定的计划并由村级卫生工作者具体实施的免疫运动，是党和政府在卫生方面的主要成就之一。1986 年，中国人均预期寿命从 1949 年的 40 岁增长到 68 岁，同期婴儿死亡率从 200‰下降到 34‰。当然，社会经济水平的提高是取得这一伟大成就的根本原因，但很大一部分原因要归功于免疫运动计划。

1987 年，在基层的免疫接种工作仍然至关重要。不论政府是否把免疫接种工作放在优先地位，除非免疫接种工作的实施者是生活在农村的卫生工作人员，因为他们可以对需要接种疫苗的人进行追踪直到工作全部完成，否则传染病无法得到有效的控制。农业生产要求农民家庭的成人劳动力在田间劳作，因此在时间上难以配合那些上门接种的流动卫生队。而解决方案是，赤脚医生带着疫苗直接找到他们劳作的田间地头完成接种。

然而，随着动员村级卫生工作人员积极开展预防工作，同时也出现了另一种倾向，即大多只受过急救处理或治疗轻症常见病

most of whom are trained only to administer first aid or treat mild cases of common illnesses, gradually to regard themselves as fully trained physicians capable of practicing medicine.

This poses a frequently serious risk to the farmers. In one case, for example, a barefoot doctor treated a patient with acute abdominal pain by injecting morphine. The patient, who actually had acute appendicitis, suffered a visceral rupture and developed peritonitis. Even physicians with many years of medical education are not always skilled at diagnosis, so the dangers of permitting those with only minimal training to do so are obvious.

THE SHIFANG COUNTY HEALTH SERVICE: A CASE STUDY

It may be useful to share some information and personal impressions gathered in 1984 and 1986 trips to Shifang County, the model county for which I serve as a consultant on rural health training. While general impressions may be valuable, however, China's size and diversity must be constantly borne in mind. Conditions in Shifang are unique to that county and may or may not reflect those in other parts of the country.

Shifang County lies on the northwestern border of the West Sichuan plain, an 863-square-kilometer, kidney-shaped area. Eighty percent of its 384,000 inhabitants live in one or another of nineteen scattered xiang. Its northern sector is hilly and mountainous, and its southern sector is a densely populated, fertile plain, watered by the 2,000-year-old Guanxian Irrigation Works. Rice, wheat, corn, tobacco, and a plant yielding edible oil are among its agricultural products. The area under cultivation averages less than one-sixth acre per person, a plot—if carefully cultivated—just large enough to provide food for one person.

培训的赤脚医生会逐渐自认为自己已经是培训有素、有足够独立行医能力的医生了——此现象的长期影响是负面的。

这种现象给农民病人带来了严重的风险。有一次，一名赤脚医生通过注射吗啡治疗一名患急性腹痛的病人。该病人实际上患有急性阑尾炎，出现内脏破裂并发展为腹膜炎。即使是受过多年医学教育的医生也难免出现误诊，而让这些只受过很少正规培训的赤脚医生来独立完成诊治，带来的潜在危险是显而易见的。

什邡县卫生服务（案例研究）

我在 1984 年和 1986 年两次到什邡县实地调研，什邡县是我担任农村卫生培训顾问的示范县，我在那里收集的资料和信息可能会有所帮助。尽管总体印象可能有价值，但我们必须时刻牢记中国的国土面积和地区的多样性。什邡的实际情况是该县独特的，可能反映全国其他地区的情况，也可能未能反映全国其他地区的情况。

什邡县位于川西平原的西北边缘，面积约 863 平方公里，其地形图似肾脏外形。常住人口 38.4 万这些居民中，80% 分散居住在 19 个乡。北部是多山的丘陵山区地带，南部是人口稠密的肥沃平原，该县农田由有 2000 年历史的都江堰灌溉工程灌溉。主要农产品包括大米、小麦、玉米、烟草和一种可产食用油的植物——油菜。人均可耕种地面积不到六分之一英亩，如果精心耕种的话，人均块地的产粮刚好够一个人吃。

Prosperity is evident in many parts of Shifang County today, in striking contrast to the poverty and isolation of twenty, thirty, or forty years ago. Great changes have occurred since liberation in 1949. Agricultural productivity, measured in monetary terms, made a nearly fivefold gain and industrial productivity, a more than fiftyfold gain in the 1949-1982 period. Primary school enrollment rose from 7,000 in 1949 to 56,000 in three decades. Whereas in 1949 there were no hard surface roads at all, today villages are linked to a network of such roads that cross the county.

Like most other counties, Shifang has a health center that serves as an antiepidemic station. It also has a modern hospital with 160 beds, a traditional hospital with 60 beds, and a special hospital for treatment of skin diseases. A maternal and child health center and a country training school for health are also operated in this model county. There are, of course, also the usual outlying xiang health centers and village health stations.

In the early 1980s about ¥640,000 was expended for health, the equivalent of about 5 percent of the county's annual budget, and representing ¥1.69 per capita. The county hospital received the largest single allocation, ¥140,000, apart from a ¥152,000 sum designated to grants in aid to xiang health centers. The antischistosomiasis program, the antiepidemic health center, and the maternal and child center received smaller sums. Only ¥11,000 was allocated for the county training school for health. Individuals spent an estimated ¥6.00 for drugs.

Declining mortality rates and increasing life expectancy provide telling testimony to recent health improvement. By 1984, according to official county statistics, the crude death rate was 6.84 per 1,000, the infant mortality rate was 27.24 per 1,000 live births, and the natural increase rate was 1.5 percent. Life expectancy was 68.77 years for men and 71.18 for women. These rates compared favorably with those for the

20 世纪 80 年代，什邡县到处呈现一派繁荣景象，这与 20 年、30 年或 40 年前的贫困和封闭的情形形成了鲜明的对比。自 1949 年以来，这里已经发生了翻天覆地的变化。1949 年至 1982 年，农业生产总值增长了近 5 倍，工业生产总值增长了 50 多倍。30 年间，小学入学人数从 1949 年的 7000 人上升到 56000 人。1949 年，县内根本没有坚硬的道路，而到 1980 年，全县公路四通八达，将各个村庄紧密地串通相连。

像其他大多数县一样，什邡有一个卫生中心，其功能如抗疫站；还有一家现代医院，拥有 160 张床位；一家拥有传统医院，拥有 60 张床位；以及一家专门治疗皮肤病的专科医院。这个示范县还开设了妇幼保健中心和县卫生培训学校。当然，还有边远的乡卫生院和村卫生站。

20 世纪 80 年代初，什邡用于卫生方面的支出约为 64 万元，相当于该县年度预算的约 5%，人均约为 1.69 元。县医院获得了最大的一笔拨款是 14 万元，此外，还有 15.2 万元的拨款专门用于建设乡卫生院。血吸虫病防治项目、抗疫卫生站和妇幼保健中心也得到拨款，但金额略少。卫生培训学校只获得拨款 1.1 万元。估计个人用于购买药品的花费为 6 元。

死亡率下降和预期寿命延长有力地证明了该县人们健康水平得到极大地改善。到 1984 年，据该县官方统计，粗死亡率为 6.84‰，婴儿死亡率为 27.24‰，人口自然增长率为 1.5%。男性平均预期寿命为 68.77 岁，女性为 71.18 岁。同年，发达国家的平均粗死亡率

more developed countries of the world, which averaged a crude death rate of 9 per 1,000, an infant mortality rate of 19 per 1,000 live births, and a natural increase rate of 2.0 in the same year.

Cardiovascular disease was the leading cause of death in the county, responsible for 210.0 deaths per 100,000 persons in 1981. In the same year, malignancy, cerebral hemorrhage, and accidents accounted for 63.07, 66.47, and 71.96 deaths per 100,000 persons, respectively. Other major causes of death were chronic respiratory disease, gastrointestinal disease, and tuberculosis.

While rising life expectancy and declining mortality were cause for satisfaction, morbidity data yielded a less positive picture. County statistical records revealed a high incidence of some infectious diseases even while local surveys indicated that many cases of infectious illness went unreported. Hepatitis, for example, is widespread. Tuberculosis is still a serious problem, as is infant diarrhea and dysentery.

For whatever reason, infectious disease rates in rural areas seem to be dramatically higher than those in urban areas. According to a mid-1980s government report, only 2 percent of patients in urban hospitals run by provincial administrators were being treated for infectious disease, as compared with 27 percent in county facilities and 95 percent in xiang-level facilities.

According to a recent estimate, as much as 40 percent of serious infectious disease cases in Sichuan Province are not reported. Regardless of whether this estimate is high, it might reflect an equally high incidence of infectious diseases in other parts of China, which would be of great concern for health authorities. Presumably, the underreporting is attributable to apparent diagnostic failures. Many physicians in rural areas, for example, recognize cases of hepatitis only when they have reached a very advanced stage, by which time family and friends have been exposed to infection.

为 9‰，婴儿死亡率为 19‰，人口自然增长率为 2%，可见，什邡县的这几项人口健康指标与世界发达国家相比是已十分接近。

1981 年的什邡，心血管疾病是主要死亡原因，每 10 万人中有 210 人死亡。同年，恶性肿瘤、脑出血和意外事故分别占每 10 万人中死亡人数的 63.07、66.47 和 71.96。其他主要死亡原因还有慢性呼吸道疾病、胃肠道疾病和结核病。

虽然预期寿命的延长和死亡率的下降令人满意，但发病率数据资料显示的情况却不容乐观。即使当地调查显示许多传染病病例没有报告或漏报，但县官方统计数据显示一些传染病发病率依然很高。例如，肝炎非常普遍。结核病仍然是一个严重的问题，婴儿腹泻和痢疾也是如此。

无论是什么原因，农村地区的传染病发病率似乎远远高于城市地区。根据 20 世纪 80 年代中期的一份政府报告，在省级管理的城市医院救治病人中，只有 2% 的病人是传染性疾病，相比之下，县级医疗机构的这一比例为 27%，而乡级医疗机构的这一比例则高达 95%。

根据估计，四川省有高达 40% 的严重传染病病例未经报告。不管这个估计是否过高，它可能反映了中国其他地区存在同样高的传染病发病率，这一现象应该引起卫生行政管理部门高度重视。据推测，漏报是由于明显的误诊造成的。例如，农村地区的许多患者只有在肝炎已经进展到了非常晚期的阶段才被识别，此时病人的家人和朋友早已经暴露并感染。

Observations in 1984

I made several trips to Shifang County during the mid-1980s to observe health conditions. The first was in 1984, on which occasion I visited several xiang health centers and village health stations.

The health center at Luo Xian was relatively prosperous. Operating on a surplus, it was able to utilize its profits for building repair and the purchase of new equipment. Patients paid to register and were charged for whatever drugs were prescribed, at fees set by government regulation.

A staff of thirty-five attended a caseload of approximately 400 patients each day. Although it included only one regular medical college graduate, the center provided care for all but the most seriously ill patients, who were referred to the county hospital. A number of barefoot doctors were associated with the center on a part-time basis, all of whom had received some training at the county hospital—some for as long as two years. Nonetheless, according to a center spokesperson, as a group they would benefit considerably from further training. Lack of qualified personnel and of necessary equipment, in that order, were the two most serious problems at the center, according to the same spokesperson.

The twenty-nine-member staff of the smaller, fifteen-bed Mian- zhu health center, made up entirely of barefoot doctors, also trained at the county hospital for periods of up to one year. Common illnesses included bronchopneumonia, bronchitis, skin infections, and hepatitis. Eleven active cases of tuberculosis had just been identified. Poisoning from organic phosphorous fertilizer was not unusual. Many older persons suffered from hypertension. One morning I watched several physicians receiving new patients and making diagnoses. They took pulses but not temperatures and, as far as I could see, undertook no physical examination of chest or abdomen. No laboratory tests were ordered.

1984 年的考察

20世纪80年代中期，我几次到什邡县考察其卫生健康状况。第一次是 1984 年，我走访了什邡县几个乡卫生院和村卫生所。

在洛水镇的卫生院经营有方，都能有利润结余，也能够利用其利润进行房屋修缮和购买新设备。病人就诊时需自付挂号费，并按政府规定付费标准支付处方药费。

该卫生院共 35 名工作人员，每天接诊大约 400 名病人。尽管该卫生院只有一名普通高等医学院校毕业生，但除了很严重的病人需要转至县级医院外，均能够满足当地居民的就诊需求。许多赤脚医生也在卫生院兼职，他们都在县医院接受过一些相关培训——有些人员接受培训长达两年。尽管如此，据该卫生院发言人说，赤脚医生将从进一步的培训中获益。该发言人还说，缺乏称职的医疗专业技术人员和必要的医疗救治设备是该卫生院存在的最严重的两个问题。

绵竹乡卫生院规模较小、拥有 15 张床位，其 29 名工作人员全部是赤脚医生，当然他们也在县医院分别接受了最长达一年的培训。收治的常见疾病中包括支气管肺炎、支气管炎、皮肤感染和肝炎。在我去考察的时候，他们刚刚确诊了 11 例活动性结核病病例。有机磷肥料中毒在当地并不罕见。许多老年人患有高血压。一天上午，我观察了几名医生如何为新病人诊治。据我所见，他们只测量了脉搏，但没有测体温，也没有对胸部或腹部进行体格检查及安排实验室检查。

Half a mile from the center there was a village health station, served by two barefoot doctors, one practicing traditional medicine exclusively. Colds, entiritis, dysentery, and chronic bronchitis were treated. The physicians collected fees of which they kept a portion, turning the rest over to village authorities.

At another health station, three barefoot doctors served the villagers, two women and one man. One provided medical care, another provided preventive care, and the third was involved with family planning. While the basic responsibilities were distributed in this fashion, all three medical workers had been trained at the xiang health center and knew how to treat accidents, strained muscles, and other common complaints, as well as how to administer injections. Village health workers assisted the staff, preparing so- called common drugs, performing snail eradication according to traditional formulas, and keeping the vital statistics register.

In the same year I was also able to visit the county training school for health in Renshou County, not far from Chengdu. Closed during the Cultural Revolution, the school had reopened in 1980 with a staff of eighteen and facilities for 180 students. Most of the students, I learned, were barefoot doctors or other types of medical aides. While most of them had been rural health workers since the early 1970s, attending this school was the first opportunity they had thus far had to receive any formal preparation for the work they were doing.

Although the training school had three teachers with scientific backgrounds, the other eight were traditional practitioners, and the primary emphasis seemed to be on the teaching of traditional medicine. Anatomy and physiology, for example, were not taught systematically. Elementary coursework spanned general principles of traditional medicine; Chinese drugs; prescription for treatment; and classical theories regarding internal medicine, surgery, and pediatrics. Advanced coursework focused on traditional medical classics. Some clinical work

370

离绵竹卫生院一公里处有一个村卫生所，由两名赤脚医生负责，其中一名专门从事传统医学诊疗。可治疗感冒、肠炎、痢疾和慢性支气管炎。医生可收取诊疗费用，其中部分归己所有，余额上交村政府。

在另一个村卫生站，有三名赤脚医生照护村民，其中两名女性，一名男性。一名从事医疗救治，另一名提供预防保健，第三名负责计划生育工作。虽然进行了分工和明晰基本职责，但他们都在乡卫生院接受过培训，知道如何处理意外伤害、肌肉拉伤和其他常见疾病，以及如何注射打针。村卫生员协助三名赤脚医生开展工作，如准备所谓的常用药物，按传统方法消灭钉螺，并进行死亡统计登记等。

同年，我还参观考察了离成都不远的仁寿县的县卫生培训学校。该校在 20 世纪 60 年代关闭，1980 年重新恢复，有 18 名教职员工和 180 名学生。据我所知，大多数学生都是赤脚医生或其他类型的医疗辅助人员。虽然他们中的大多数人自 20 世纪 70 年代初以来一直是农村卫生工作者，但进入这所学校进修学习，是他们迄今为止第一次有机会为他们正在从事的工作而接受正式培训。

虽然该培训学校有三名具有科学医学背景的教师，但另外八名则是传统医学从业者，主要培训重点似乎是教授传统医学，没有被系统地教授如解剖学和生理学等。基础教学课程包括传统医学一般原理、中药学、方剂学以及关于内科、外科和儿科的古典

in the local county clinics followed the classroom studies. Students enrolled for anywhere from three months to two years.

Walking around the school, which had four classrooms, I saw only a few teaching aides: some models of human embryos, a few types of pathological specimen, some anatomical drawings, and a few books and journals. One student showed me his textbook, which was one used in secondary medical schools.

Observations in 1986

In April 1986 I returned to Shifang County to observe its primary health care conditions, and the visit provided some interesting comparisons. In the interim, implementation of the new economic policies had infused the farmers and their wives with enthusiasm for creating lucrative activities. Some had banded together to operate small enterprises, such as a cement factory. Other ventures were coal mining, marketing handicrafts, or leasing small tractors for transport. Wives were raising chickens, ducks, and pigs to gain more cash income. Through these endeavors, per capita income had increased from ¥350 to ¥503, a marked rise in household income. As the number of children had been reduced, discretionary funds were used to add to or build new farm houses or to purchase bicycles, fashionable clothing, or more expensive foods. While a general climate of prosperity prevailed, a healthy young farmer seeking a license to sell ice cream or a group of older men whiling away daytime hours playing cards suggested the existence of pockets of underemployment in parts of the county.

One of the most remarkable consequences of social and economic policy was the reduced size of the family, which, in turn, had resulted in increased care for the sick, particularly the precious one child. It was evident that our success in family planning in the rural areas was making a critical contribution to overall reconstruction. In fact, the lowered maternal mortality rate of 1 per 1,000 live births and the infant mortality

理论。高级课程则专注于传统医学经典著作的讲解分析。课堂学习结束之后，学生在当地县区诊所进行一些临床实习。学生培训时间从三个月到两年不等。

在参观考察过程中，我看到学校共有四间教室，只看到了少数教学工具：一些人类胚胎模型，几样病理标本，一些解剖图谱，几本书籍期刊。一个学生给我看了他的课本，是卫生职业学校用书。

1986 年的考察

1986 年 4 月，我再次回到什邡县考察其初级卫生保健状况。这次考察让我发现了一些有趣的对照。在此期间，新经济政策的实施为农村家庭注入了致富的满腔热情。有些人联合起来经营小企业，如水泥厂。也有些人尝试开小煤窑、制作销售手工艺品或租赁小型拖拉机从事运输。妇女们则养鸡、养鸭和养猪，以获得更多的现金收入。通过辛勤努力，人均收入从 350 元增加到 503 元，家庭收入有了明显增加。随着子女数量的减少，积累的可自由支配的资金被用来增加或建造新的农舍，购买自行车、时髦的服装或更昂贵的食品。虽然气氛浓厚，但还可看到努力谋取冰激凌销售许可证的年轻力壮农民或一群白天打牌消磨时间的老人，这些还是反映出该县部分地区存在劳动力未被充分利用的现象。

社会和经济政策最显著的成果之一是随着家庭规模缩小，反过来又刺激了医疗保健需求的增加，尤其是对独生子女而言。显然，农村地区计划生育的成功为全面推动四个现代化建设做出了重要贡献。事实上，产妇死亡率明显降低，每 1000 名活产婴儿

of 27.2 per 1,000 live births was directly attributable to the family planning program.

On our visit, we made an on-the-spot investigation of the condition of medicine, antiepidemic activities, health services for women and children, and family planning at the county, xiang, and village levels. We also visited some farmer's homes to learn something about their living standards, culture, and medical and health conditions. Our general impression was that health work was being carried out broadly and deeply. The achievements were highly impressive, and there had been a noticeable improvement in the physical well-being, spirit, and outlook of the local population.

Antiepidemic work was formulated in principle on a nationwide basis by the Ministry of Health, supervised by the county-level health (antiepidemic) center and organized and implemented by xiang and village-level personnel. In Shifang County results were highly impressive, although the funds provided by the county health bureau for these activities were insufficient. Other less serious problems also remained to be solved, but in general the success of the program could be credited with contributing significantly to a decrease in morbidity from infectious disease in the county. Vaccines against measles, epidemic meningitis, tuberculosis, rabies, diphtheria, tetanus, and leptospirosis were in use.

A cold-chain arrangement to ensure adequate refrigeration for vaccines over the distribution network now covers the entire county, donated by UNICEF. That equipment strikes me as the most useful contribution of a foreign agency in the health field, far more so than such equipment as high-power microscopes and rotating slide projectors, which few persons know how to operate.

The public was responding positively to prevention efforts. In 1984, for example, of the target number of cases vaccinated in the county

有 1 名产妇死亡；婴儿死亡率也显著降低，每 1000 名活产婴儿中有 27.2 名婴儿死亡，这些都直接归功于计划生育政策。

在我们的考察中，我们实地调研了县、乡、村三级的医疗条件、抗疫活动、妇幼保健服务、计划生育等情况。我们还参观了一些农民的家，了解他们的生活水平、文化、医疗和卫生状况。总体印象是，卫生工作正在广泛深入开展。取得的这些成就给人留下了深刻印象，当地居民的身体健康状况、精神面貌和眼界视野都有了显著的提升。

抗疫工作条例由卫生部基于全国范围的原则制定，由县级卫生（抗疫）服务中心监督，乡、村两级卫生工作人员具体负责组织实施。在什邡县，尽管县卫生局为抗疫活动提供的资金不足，但取得的效果令人印象深刻。虽然还有一些其他相对次要的问题也有待解决，但总的来说，抗疫工作取得的成就是毋庸置疑的，该县传染病发病率的大幅下降即归功于此。抗麻疹、流行性脑膜炎、结核病、狂犬病、白喉、破伤风和钩端螺旋体病的疫苗大规模接种使用。

在联合国儿童基金会捐助下，一个确保疫苗得到充分冷藏保存的冷链系统已分配覆盖至整个县。在我看来，比起很少有人知道如何操作的高倍显微镜和旋转幻灯机等设备，这种冷链设备是外国机构对我国卫生领域最切实有用的捐赠贡献。

公众对预防工作反应积极，密切配合。例如，在 1984 年什

measles immunization campaign, 99.5 percent were actually done; in the BCG campaign 92.7 percent were done; and in the whooping cough and poliomyelitis immunization campaigns 93.6 percent and 97.4 percent, respectively, were achieved.

In each xiang center one or two persons were assigned to work on disease prevention, planning immunizations, and the operation of the cold chain. On the thirteenth day of each month vaccines were sent to the center from the county health (antiepidemic) center. The staff members immediately summoned the barefoot doctors and assigned work to them. A refrigerator was used to store the vaccines, which could be kept for only one week. The barefoot doctors were told to take the vaccines to the village stations and to complete their work by within two days.

After accepting an assignment, the barefoot doctor takes the vaccines in a cold storage packet and goes directly to the village. The women's leader in the village has meanwhile announced the impending immunization program at the school. Parents take the children to the barefoot doctor's home, who may visit from house to house. The cold chain generally seems to be working effectively; however, villagers report that a few barefoot doctors carry the vaccines around with them without too much regard for its safety. This should be discouraged, because when the vaccine is not kept sufficiently cold, the 100 percent acceptance rate becomes meaningless.

Financing the arrangements can be a problem as costs sometimes exceed the sum provided by the county health bureau by 100 percent. In vaccinating children, there is generally no problem in carrying out the work or collecting money to cover the cost, except for those parents who occasionally balk in the winter, fearing that children may catch cold by rolling up their sleeves or removing their clothing. Not infrequently, however, workers encounter resistance from adults, who may be too busy in the fields, or may regard vaccinations as necessary only for children.

邡县开展麻疹免疫接种工作的目标人群中，99.5% 实际完成了接种；在卡介苗接种中，完成了应接种人群的 92.7%；百日咳和脊髓灰质炎的免疫接种率，也分别达到 93.6% 和 97.4%。

在每个乡卫生院，均有一或两个人被分配制定从事疾病预防、计划免疫接种和冷链保障方面的工作。每个月的第 13 天，疫苗从县卫生（抗疫）服务中心运送到卫生院。乡卫生院工作人员立即召集赤脚医生，并给他们分配工作任务。用冰箱储存疫苗且只能保存一周。赤脚医生将疫苗带回到村卫生所，并须按工作要求在两天内完成全部接种工作。

接受工作任务后，赤脚医生们把疫苗装在冷藏包里，直接带回村子。与此同时，村里的妇女主任通知学校即将实施免疫接种工作。父母带着孩子去赤脚医生的家，或由赤脚医生挨家挨户上门接种。总的来说，冷链系统是有效的。然而，有些村民们报告说，有些赤脚医生带着疫苗到处跑，不太注意疫苗的安全保存。这种行为应加以防范，因为当疫苗没有被冷藏在适当温度时，即使完成 100% 的接种率也毫无意义。

保障免疫接种的筹资可能是个问题，因为实际费用有时会100% 超过县卫生局提供的资金总额。一般来说，给儿童接种疫苗通常都很顺利，包括收取一定费用来保障开销也是没有问题的。除了那些偶尔在冬天犹豫不决、担心孩子卷起袖子或脱衣服可能会感冒的父母，他们可能会以此为由不给孩子接种。然而，接种工作人员还是经常会遇到来自成年人的阻力，原因可能是成年人

Some villagers also may be less interested in vaccinations for themselves or their children now that they must pay for something once provided free of charge.

The new regulations on private practice raise further concern that the issue of vaccination will receive less attention, since providing immunizations is not very lucrative for the physician. Most of the ¥0.1 fee has to be turned back in to the authorities, with the physician keeping only ¥0.03.

Apart from immunization work, considerable success had been achieved in the county in preventing and treating schistosomiasis since an antibilharzia station had been founded. The plan was to eradicate the disease by the end of the year. It was said, too, that malaria would be eradicated the following year. Morbidity from tuberculosis stood at 640 per 100,000 however, and morbidity from hepatitis was also relatively high. Infant diarrhea was a serious concern.

After familiarizing ourselves with the spectrum of disease and efforts to prevent it, we proceeded to study the available medical work in the county, the focal point of which was the well- equipped, well-staffed Shifang County People's Hospital. The equipment of the hospital was adequate and reliable, its staff was of good quality, and a variety of medical specialties were represented. Modern medicine was practiced there, but the county also operated a traditional hospital and a skin disease hospital, which were not included in our visit.

We also visited the training school for health, another county- level organization, which offered a two-year training program. Most of the teachers are staff physicians from the county hospital, soundly grounded in theory and with extensive practical experience. One of several problems confronting school officials, however, is that workloads of the physicians who also serve as teachers are heavy, often preventing them from conducting their classes as scheduled.

在地里的劳作太忙或认为只有儿童才有必要接种疫苗。还有一些村民也可能对给他们自己或孩子接种疫苗不太感兴趣，尤其是在过去都是免费接种转而需要付费的时候。

对医生来说，其实提供免疫接种本就不太赚钱，而且关于私人行医执业的新规定更减少了该群体对疫苗接种问题的关注。因为按照规定，0.1 元的接种费用必须大部分上缴，接种医生只保留 0.03 元。

除免疫接种工作外，自血吸虫病防治站建立以来，该县在预防和治疗血吸虫病方面取得了相当大的成功。该县甚至计划在当年年底前彻底消除这种疾病。据说，该县还将在下一年消除疟疾。然而，结核病的发病率仍然高达每 100000 人中有 640 人，肝炎的发病率也相当高。此外，婴儿腹泻同样是一个严重的问题。

在熟悉了该县的疾病谱和为预防这些疾病做出的努力后，我们开始进一步研究考察该县现有的医疗工作，关注的重点是设备齐全、人员充足的什邡县人民医院。该医院的设备充足可靠，医疗人员素质良好，各医学专业均有学科带头人，在那里实践着现代医学，但该县也同时运营了一家传统医院和一家皮肤病医院，但它们都不在我们的此次实地走访计划中。

我们还参观考察了卫生培训学校，这是另一个县级卫生机构，提供为期两年的培训。大多数教师都是县医院的在职医生，理论基础扎实，实践经验丰富。然而，学校也面临不少问题，其中之一是，兼任教师的医生本身临床工作量就很大，经常会因临床医疗救治工作而妨碍他们按计划进行授课。

At the maternal and child health center we spoke to two secondary medical school graduates who headed the staff. They were supported by other physicians who had studied at the county training school for health and other staff aides. Most of the ¥100,000 income that the center earned in 1985 came from fees for pre- and postnatal care, but the county government also provided a subsidy for outreach activities in women's health care.

Theoretically, the xiang health centers took care of patients less critically ill than those sent to the county hospital but more seriously ill than those seen at the village health stations. In part because of decreases in morbidity from infectious disease, some xiang health centers received fewer patients than in the past and, accordingly, were experiencing some financial difficulties. In Shifang County people now have bicycles, and villages even usually have tractors. Thus it has become quite easy in recent years to transport people to the county hospitals.

Whether a given center was in difficulty or not depended on many circumstances, including the location of the center, the convenience of transportation, the numbers of residents in the community, whether they specialized in certain kinds of cases, the skill and reputation of the physicians on the staff, the number of retired staff members, and the relationship between the center and the village government. Only one or two health centers we visited had a regular medical college graduate on the staff.

The tasks of the health centers are more or less the same. They maintain fixed hours and a fixed timetable for work and have four main responsibilities: management of antibilharzia programs, other preventive activities, provision of medical care for women and infants, and family planning. Their laboratories are equipped for routine tests only. For women of childbearing age, the centers are responsible for providing contraceptive information and performing abortions. Unless they are deemed inadequately equipped, they perform first-trimester abortions,

在妇幼保健中心走访时，我们采访了两位毕业于卫生职业学校的中心领导。他们手下还有已在县卫生培训学校完成学习的其他医生和其他辅助人员。该中心在 1985 年赚取的 10 万元收入，大部分来自孕期产前和产后护理保健费用，但县政府也为妇女保健方面的外展服务提供补贴。

理论上说，乡卫生院照护的病人没有送到县医院救治的病人危重，但又比村卫生站的病人病情严重。部分原因是由于传染病发病率的下降，一些乡卫生院收治的病人比过去少，因此也遇到了一些财政困难。在什邡县，人们有自行车，有的村还常有拖拉机。因此，他们可以很方便地把病人直接送到县医院救治。

一家卫生院是否陷入困境取决于许多因素，包括卫生院的地理位置、交通的便利程度、附近社区居民的数量、本院是否擅长某些疾病的诊治、医务人员的技能和声誉、退休医务工作人员的数量以及卫生院与各村政府的关系等。我们去考察过的所有卫生院中，只有一两个有普通医学院校毕业生。

各卫生院的工作任务大致相同。他们有固定的工作时间和固定的工作时间安排表，有四项主要职责：血吸虫病防治管理、其他预防活动、为妇女和婴儿提供医疗保健和计划生育。卫生院实验室只配备了常规检验仪器设备。对于育龄女性，这些乡卫生院负责向她们提供避孕知识和实施人工流产。除非缺乏设备，卫生院会对三个月内的早孕施行流产，但对妊娠中期者则送到县医院。

but second-trimester patients are sent to the county hospital. The centers also perform sterilization procedures on request. In Shifang County, tubal ligations are becoming a popular method of female sterilization.

A new and recent challenge for those in Shifang has been the decision to provide retirement income for aging staff, reflecting the new retirement policies adopted at the county level since 1984. The difficulty arises from the way this is being done. The retired physician is retained at 75 percent of the former salary, while another person, usually a family member, friend, or acquaintance and not necessarily trained for the work, is added to the staff. For this reason, in some cases retired members may outnumber other members of the staff, imposing a heavy financial strain on the facility, while the new distribution of the workload may increase the burden of some staff members.

Barefoot doctors and country doctors affiliated with xiang health centers and village health stations are doing very well. Typically they continue to farm but do medical practice on the side, serving perhaps twenty or persons in their own locales, or possibly, by dint of good reputation, drawing additional patients from other areas. The typical fee is ¥0.7 for a diagnosis and ¥0.5 for an injection. They may prescribe either modern drugs or Chinese herbs, for many physicians use both systems of medicine. The patient pays not for the prescription as such but for the cost of the drug, plus a surcharge for the physician of 15 percent on standard drugs and 25 percent on Chinese herbs.

Under current regulations, barefoot doctors in many areas of the country are earning quite a good income. In Shifang County at least ¥100, and at most ¥200 to ¥300 per year, exclusive of income from field harvest and trade sidelines. In the Shanghai metropolitan area, it is reported that those with the best reputations may earn as much as would a professor of internal medicine in a medical college.

这些卫生院也会应病人要求施行绝育手术。在什邡县，输卵管结扎是女性绝育的常用方法。

什邡面临的一个新挑战是决定为老龄职工提供退休金，这反映了自 1984 年以来县级所采取的新的退休政策。然而，政策执行过程中出现了困难。退休医生仍然领取原工资的 75%，而另一个人，通常是家庭成员、朋友或熟人且从未受过正规工作培训，却被有意地也安排到了这些退休人员的队伍中。因此，在某些机构可能出现了退休人员数量超过在职医务工作人员的情形，给医疗机构带来沉重的财政压力，而退休留下的工作岗位任务被重新分配，可能会增加在职工作人员的工作负担。

乡卫生院和村卫生站的赤脚医生和农村医生都十分称职。在通常情形下，他们一边务农，一边行医，为大约 20 人或者在其所在区域附近村民提供卫生照护。如果积累了良好的声誉，也可从其他地区吸引更多的病人前来就医。一般都是诊断费 0.7 元，注射费 0.5 元。他们可能会开现代药品或中药，因为许多医生同时使用两种医学体系。病人支付的不是处方费，而是药品费用，外加支付医生 15% 的标准药品附加费和 25% 的中药附加费。

根据政策规定，全国农村许多地区的赤脚医生收入颇丰。在什邡县，每年至少 100 元，最多 200～300 元，还不包括农业耕作收益和副业收入。据报道，在上海大都市区，声望最好的赤脚医生可能挣得和医学院内科教授一样多。

While most patients seem to be able to afford the expense of treatment, poorer farmers may seek credit or delay treatment, especially at times when seasonal income fluctuations have temporarily reduced family resources. Another alternative is to ask for treatment in accordance with the resources that are available; for example, the patient may ask for treatment worth ¥1. Our impression is that physicians will generally extend credit, although a rare few have been known to refuse.

The quality of physician care in rural areas is contingent on not only the physicians competency but also the utility of medications dispensed. Thus we were interested in visiting the government- run Shifang Medicine and Pharmacy Company. The company conducts a large business, selling about ¥2.4 to ¥2.5 million worth of products yearly, mainly to hospitals. In maintaining a supply of almost any product on the market, the government agency has some advantage over the more than two dozen private enterprises in the county that now also sell modern drugs, whose stocks are smaller and where a customer may find items temporarily out of stock or not carried at all. By the same token, the products are much cheaper in the private stores. In Chinese herbs, there is a very active free-market trade, with hospitals among the buyers as well as physicians in private practice.

The shortage in rural areas of physicians with a high degree of technical competency was hardly remarkable. Chinese physicians are no different from their counterparts around the world. They prefer to work in the cities, in comfortable surroundings, with the potential of professional and monetary reward. In China, regular medical college graduates have until recently generally been easily able to find positions in any one of hundreds of urban hospitals, clinics, and research facilities. With the turnout of medical schools increasing, some graduates have joined county facilities in recent years; but perceived hardships still limit willingness to work at the xiang level. If at least some medical school graduates could be persuaded to serve the village population in xiang centers, the

虽然大多数病人似乎能够负担得起治疗费用，但较贫穷的农民可能会寻求赊账或推迟治疗，尤其是在季节性收入波动暂时造成家庭财力减少时更是如此。另一种选择则是根据现有资金支付能力选择相应的治疗；例如，病人可要求施行价值 1 元的治疗。我们的印象是，除极少例外，医生通常都会允许病人赊账。

农村地区医生医疗质量不仅取决于医生的能力，还取决于他们对所分配派送的药品的使用水平。因此，我们饶有兴致地参观了县政府经营的什邡医药公司。该公司经营着大量的业务，每年销售经营价值约 240 万 ~ 250 万元的产品，主要销售给医院。在维持向市场上供应几乎所有产品的能力方面，政府运营的医药公司比该县大约 20 多家也销售现代药品的私营企业有明显优势，这些私人企业的库存较少，客户可能会发现商品暂时缺货或根本没有库存。不过私人药品商店的产品也便宜很多。在中草药领域，当地自由市场交易非常活跃，买家中有医院，也有私人执业的医生。

农村地区缺少具有技术能力强的医生的现象不足为奇。中国医生与世界各地的医生没有什么不同，他们都更喜欢在城市工作，城市有更舒适的环境，有发挥职业潜力平台，可以获取优厚的报酬。在中国，普通高等医学院毕业生通常都很容易在成千上百家城市医院、诊所和研究机构中找到工作职位。随着医学院的激增，一些毕业生开始进入县级医疗机构；但是基层的艰苦仍然降低了他们前往乡一级卫生机构工作的意愿。如果至少能说服一部分医学院毕业生去乡卫生院工作，真正为农民服务，那么传染病的早

possibility of early diagnosis and treatment of infectious disease cases would be greatly enhanced. With good public health training, these graduates might even begin to think in terms of practicing community medicine.

WESTERN MEDICAL EDUCATION SEEN THROUGH THE "OPEN-DOOR"

As I had long since come to realize, this issue of the quality of personnel—the largest area of vulnerability in our rural health service—could not be solved without rendering our regular medical school graduates more community-minded. This is the reason for the intensification of my interest in medical education and for eagerness of my response when the Ministry of Health, acting in accord with the "open-door" policy, made it possible for me to go abroad to study patterns of medical education in Canada and the United States in 1979.

My views had begun to be of some interest to the authorities, and in early 1979 I had been called to Beijing to attend an official seminar on medical education and public health education. Then, in the fall of the same year, the Ministry of Health delegated me to travel to North America to study the medical school curricula in Canada and the United States with respect to how they could be adapted for use in our own country. On my return, I prepared a report with some recommendations to the Ministry of Health. The next year, on another study trip, I visited the Institute of Rural Reconstruction established in the Philippines in 1967 by James Y. C. Yen, my long-time friend from Dingxian days who had founded and directed the Mass Education Movement in prerevolutionary China.

On the 1979 trip to North America, the first stop, in Canada, entailed visits to the Medical School of the University of Toronto, in Toronto, Ontario and the McMaster University Medical School in Hamilton, Ontario. My brother, a university teacher, met me at the airport after a

期诊断和治疗的可能性将会大大提高。接受了良好的公共卫生培训，这些毕业生甚至可能开始考虑从事社区医学。

从"对外开放"中看西方医学教育

我早就意识到，如果不使我们的普通高等医学院校毕业生更具社区意识和基层思想，农村卫生服务中最薄弱的领域也就是人员素质问题将无法解决。这就是为什么我对医学教育的兴趣越来越浓厚，这也是当卫生部响应执行"对外开放"政策时，我为什么如此急切地在 1979 年出国考察研究加拿大和美国医学教育模式。

我的观点开始引起主管部门的一些兴趣，1979 年年初，我应邀到北京参加了一个关于医学教育和公共卫生教育的官方研讨会。同年秋天，卫生部委派我前往北美，研究考察加拿大和美国的医学院课程，研究其如何更好地适用于我们自己的国家。访问归国后，我随即向卫生部递交了一份带有建议的调研报告。次年，在另一次考察中，我参观了 1967 年晏阳初在菲律宾建立的农村建设研究院，晏阳初是我在河北定县时的老朋友，他创立和发起了平民教育运动。

1979 年北美之旅的第一站是加拿大，我参观了安大略省多伦多市的多伦多大学医学院和安大略省汉密尔顿市的麦克马斯特大学医学院。我的弟弟是一名大学教师，他到机场迎接了我，与以往穿越太平洋的旅程相比，那次旅行非常短暂。1946 年，乘飞机

journey that, compared with previous Pacific crossings, had been very brief. In 1946 it had taken three days by air to reach the Western coast of North America; this time it had taken fewer than twenty hours.

While favorably impressed by the Medical School at the University of Toronto, especially by its research in immunology and biomedical engineering, I found the visit to the Medical School of McMaster University more rewarding because of its innovative approach to teaching. There was a great deal of creative thinking behind the planned program. For example, emphasis on self study, using available resources, was begun at admission. Students and teachers worked in close relationship. Public service, rather than personal reward, was stressed. All in all, it seemed a good model for China.

In the United States, I was eager to see what developments had taken place in the twenty-five years since relations between our two countries had ended. At Harvard University, I visited the Schools of Public Health and Medicine. The faculty had increased enormously, and its interests seemed to revolve less around challenging the students than in generating papers on subjects of high academic interest. Many research topics, as far as I saw, had no connection with major health problems. An encouraging sign at the medical school was the development of a new department of family medicine, with a relatively generalized focus. As to efforts to instill any interest in public health in the students, however, I was not aware of much.

With one exception, other schools I visited seemed to have changed greatly in size but to have changed their teaching methods, educational objectives, and field training activities very little. There was no evidence that the teaching of preventive medicine and public health was respected in the medical schools; possibly the separation of teaching of clinical medicine and public health contributed to this situation. Instruction seemed to be less generally characterized by intellectual stimulation than by reliance on audiovisual aids. It was gratifying to note at Cornell

到达北美西海岸需要三天时间；这一次用了不到 20 个小时。

虽然多伦多大学医学院给我留下了良好的印象，尤其是在免疫学和生物医学工程方面的研究，但我发现参观麦克马斯特大学医学院更有帮助。因为它采用了创新的教学方法，在既定的教学大纲中包含了大量的创造性思维。例如，在入学时就开始强调利用现有资源自学钻研。学生和老师关系融洽，形成了良好的氛围，他们一起工作学习。学校更强调的是为公共服务，而不是个人报酬。总而言之，对于中国来说，这似乎是一个好的学习榜样。

在美国，我急切地想知道自从两国断交后的 25 年里发生了什么变化。在哈佛大学，我参观了公共卫生学院和医学院。学校的教师人数大幅增加，他们的兴趣似乎不是围绕着学生将面临挑战的那些问题，而是更侧重于在撰写发表高水平的学术主题论文。据我所知，许多研究课题与主要的卫生问题关联不大。一个令人鼓舞的迹象是，医学院把对一般医学问题比较关注的"家庭医学"作为一个新的学科给予支持与发展。然而，我却未发现他们做出努力以引起学生对公共卫生专业的兴趣。

除一所外，我参观的其他学校几乎都在规模上有了很大的变化，但在教学方法、教育目标和现场培训方面却几乎没有变化。没有证据表明预防医学和公共卫生的教学在医学院受到重视；这也许是由临床医学和公共卫生教学的脱节所造成的。课堂教学似乎缺乏思维开发而是大量地依赖视听辅助设备。然而，令人惊喜的是，康奈尔大学医学院要求学生进行现场实地调查。

University Medical School, however, that the students were being asked to do field surveys.

The exceptional school was the Medical School of the University of Missouri in Kansas City, which, under a pilot program, was accepting high-school students for admission and in its coursework was emphasizing a population-based approach to medical studies. The director, E. Grey Dimond, M.D., a cardiologist, impressed me as a talented administrator.

In the light of this trip, I felt that the United States was not doing much through its medical education system to imbue its students with a sense of public service and a responsibility to think beyond individual casework and specialized research. I regret that in the medical schools I visited I did not see departments of public health as strong as that of the PUMC in the era of leadership by John B. Grant half a century ago. The schools of public health that I visited in the eastern part of the United States had become research institutions where technology and publication of technical papers generally dictated educational direction.

唯一例外的学校就是在堪萨斯城的密苏里大学医学院，根据一项试点计划中，该校接受高中生入学，并在课程教学中对医学生特别强调以人群为基础的医学研究方法。印象中，部门主任是格雷·戴蒙德博士，他是一名心脏病专家，更是一个颇有才华的管理者。

从这次访问来看，我觉得，美国没有通过其医学教育系统向学生不断灌输公共服务意识，没有培养学生超越个人临床工作和专业研究工作以外的责任担当。感到遗憾的是，在我所访问的医学院中，我居然没有看到哪个公共卫生系能像半个世纪前兰安生领导时代的北京协和医学院公共卫生系那样强大。我在美国东部访问的公共卫生学校都已经成了研究性机构，在那里技术探讨和技术论文的发表成为主旋律，而这些也通常影响着教育的方向。

译者：马礼兵，张婷

Part 3

Sharing Insights

Medicine in Rural China
A Personal Account

交流见识

Chapter 7

Reflections on the Health Experience

All told, my life and work as a modern physician and medical educator span well over fifty years, during which time my primary consideration has focused on community medicine and public health. Even after that long interval, I have no final answer to the question that has absorbed me persistently: "How best can we introduce scientific medicine into an untutored population and make it take root there for the benefit of the common people?"

The course of my life has, nevertheless, yielded a number of insights that I believe should be shared with other persons in medical education, community medicine, and public health around the world. Those working in developing countries may find the Chinese experience in organizing rural health care to be particularly relevant.

A DEVELOPING NATION AND ITS HEALTH CARE SYSTEM

Before sharing those insights, however, it might be well to point out certain assumptions that underlie my thinking about health care delivery in developing countries and, for that matter, health care in any society, for those beliefs shape the specific judgments at which I have arrived.

第 7 章

关于卫生工作经验的
几点反思

总而言之，作为一名现代医生和医学教育工作者，我在过去50余年的职业生涯中首要考虑的问题是类群医学。然而经年累月，我仍无法最终回答一个一直困扰我的问题："如何才能最好地将科学医学引入一个未受过正规教育的人群，使其在那里扎根，造福一方老百姓？"

尽管有困惑，我这一生还是悟得了诸多见解，我认为这些见解应该与世界各地从事医学教育、社区医学和公共卫生工作的人们分享。那些在发展中国家工作的人也许会发现，中国在组织农村卫生保健方面的经验很有意义。

一个发展中的国家及其卫生保健系统

然而，在分享这些见解之前，最好先提出某些假设。这些假设是我对发展中国家卫生保健服务提供思考的基础，就这一点而言，任何社会的卫生保健都是如此，因为这些信念塑造了我得出

The first of these is the conviction that the strength of any nation lies in its common people, and that the best possible health care, therefore, should be available to the population as a whole, not just to a privileged few. I have the deepest respect for the common people of my own country—most of whom are village-dwelling farmers—and see them as the bedrock of our nation. Their agricultural capacity and their fortitude in adversity contribute greatly to national stability.

The belief that the common people are the bedrock of the nation, anchored in ancient Chinese teaching, has been revitalized and given new meaning under CCP rule. The philosophy of hard work and equality has already yielded better lives for the people. Since liberation in 1949, economic well-being has increased, educational opportunity has expanded, and for many, living conditions have improved. Combined with greatly improved health care and the curtailment of population growth, these developments have brought a remarkable decline in mortality and increase in life expectancy.

The common people, I suspect, are the wellspring of national vitality in many other countries besides China, especially those whose economies are also based on agriculture and whose populations consist predominantly of village-dwelling farmers. Some developing countries, as well as some highly developed nations, however, may fail to see a correlation between the national interest and the well-being of the grass-roots population. Promoting public health in such societies may be an especially difficult task.

A second belief that is fundamental in my personal thinking about health care is that medicine based on scientific principles is inherently superior to any system that lacks that foundation. This statement in no way is intended to denigrate the traditional medicine of my own country or that of any other. Indigenous Chinese medicine, for instance, has provided medical relief to countless millions of persons over the ages,

怎样的具体判断。

首先，我坚信，任何一个国家的力量来自于人民，因此，最好的卫生保健应该提供给全体国民，而不仅是少数特权阶层。我对自己国家的老百姓，特别是广大农民，怀有最深切的敬意，并将他们视为我们国家的基石。农民的农业生产能力和在逆境中的坚强斗志为国家的稳定做出了巨大贡献。

在中国共产党的领导下，植根于传统文化中的"民为贵，社稷次之，君为轻"的理念得到了复兴，并被赋予了新的含义。努力工作和人人平等的理念已经改善了人民的生活。1949 年以来，人们经济状况好转，受教育机会扩大，许多人生活条件得以改善。加之医疗保健水平大幅提升，人口增长减缓，使得中国人口死亡率显著下降，预期寿命增加。

我推测，在中国以外的很多国家，特别是那些经济上也以农业为主，人口主要由农村居民组成的国家，老百姓是其民族生命力的源泉。然而，一些发展中国家和一些高度发达的国家可能看不到国家利益与其基层民众福祉之间的关联性。在这些国家，促进公共卫生工作可能困难重重。

我对卫生保健工作的个人思考中，第二个基本信念是：基于科学原理的医学，在本质上是优于任何缺乏科学原理支持的医学体系的。这种说法绝不是有意诋毁我自己国家或其他任何国家的传统医学。例如，土生土长的中医药为千百万不同年龄的人提供

withstanding the test of time, and offering sustained evidence that many of its remedies indeed have some degree of efficacy. The same is apt to be true, to varying degrees, of the indigenous medicines of other countries.

Nevertheless, in my view, because it is formulated and systematized in accordance with verifiable general laws, scientific medicine enjoys an unsurpassable margin of superiority over any competing system of medicine. In the substance of traditional Chinese medicine, for example, there is nothing comparable to the scientifically informed explanations of anatomy, physiology, and pathogenesis that are basic to modern medicine.

In methodology and application as well, the differences are no less significant. The criteria of diagnosis, rationale for treatment, methods of physical and laboratory examination, and analysis of laboratory results found in modern medicine simply have no counterpart in our traditional system. As to application, the vantage ground is clear. Concern with health protection and improvement is all but self-defeating without attention to preventive measures, which can have a crucial impact on health levels. For evidence, one has only to consider the contribution of China's mass-immunization campaigns to the dramatic decrease in mortality in our country since 1949. Yet, whereas scientific medicine assigns some importance to preventive measures, traditional medicine in practice neglects them almost entirely.

In passing, it must be recognized, of course, that scientific medicine, too, has limitations. In any event, regardless of what treatment is used, a patient's successful recovery may at times be attributed as much to nature's intervention as to the ministrations of the physician. We have no way of knowing all that is involved in the natural course of development of an illness. Getting the public to understand the complexity of cause-and-effect relationships is a problem in medicine, as elsewhere.

了医疗救助，它经受住了时间的考验，提供了经久不衰的证据，其中许多中医疗法被证实确有疗效。其他国家的本土药物在不同程度上亦有类似情况。

然而，我认为，现代医学是遵循可证实的普遍规律，并进行了确切阐述和系统化的学科，因此，它比其他任何相提并论的医学体系都享有不可逾越的优势。例如，在中国传统医学的基本内容中，就找不到任何能与现代医学基础中对解剖学、生理学和病理学的科学解释相媲美的东西。

在方法学和应用方面，两者差异也同样显著。现代医学的诊断标准、治疗原理、物理和实验室检验方法以及实验室结果分析等在传统医学体系中根本找不到相对应的描述。在实际应用方面，现代医学的优势显而易见。如果不重视预防，那么即便关注健康保护与服务改善措施，结果只是弄巧成拙，有可能还对人群健康水平产生重要影响。现代医学重视预防，例如，中国开展的大规模疫苗接种运动就对全国 1949 年以来人口死亡率急剧下降做出了贡献。而且，科学医学重视预防，传统医学在实践中几乎完全忽视了预防。

当然，必须承认科学医学也有其局限性。在任何情况下，无论采用何种治疗方法，病人的成功康复有时既归功于医生的照护，也要归功于大自然的干预。我们无法知晓疾病在自然发展过程中的方方面面。让公众了解这些因果关系的复杂性在医学界和其他领域都是个难题。然而，尽管现代医学有其局限性，我仍然相信，

Notwithstanding the limitations of scientific medicine, however, I remain convinced that its application to our national health problems is more in the interest of the people than undue support and expansion of our traditional system.

For those who hope for growing confidence in scientific medicine and its broadened application for the public benefit in any country where traditional medicine has deep roots, time and effort are required in order to achieve organizational change. Meanwhile it is up to us to help to promote scientific understanding throughout the general population and to advocate qualitative improvement in modem medical training.

Like my commitment to the welfare of the common people and my conviction of the relative superiority of scientific medicine, the third and final premise of my medical philosophy derives from the experiences of childhood and youth. Since a young age I have taken it for granted that no worthwhile national goal can be achieved without attention to education. This is no less true in medicine and public health than in any other realm. Anyone interested in seeing the further application of scientific medical knowledge in any country, developing or otherwise, cannot escape responsibility as an educator.

This responsibility assumes special importance with respect to the villagers and nomadic peoples of developing countries. Given the educational levels of modern, industrialized societies, it can fairly safely be assumed that the majority of their populations have at least a fundamental store of scientific knowledge. By extension, therefore, we can further assume that they have been at least minimally exposed to the idea that infectious disease is caused by microorganisms that enter, grow, and multiply in the body, and that many diseases are transmitted by contagion.

In developing countries, however, we can make no such assumption. As is widely recognized, their populations are generally partially or

与不适当地支持和扩大传统医药体系相比，将现代医学应用于解决我国的健康问题，更符合人民的利益。

在传统医学根深蒂固的国家，那些希望增强民众对现代医学的信心并扩大其应用以造福公众的人，需要时间和努力来实现组织变革。与此同时，我们有责任帮助普通民众加强对现代医学的理解，并主张现代医学培训要在质上有所提升。

正如我对老百姓健康福祉的承诺和我对现代医学相对优越性的笃信一样，我的医学哲学思想形成的第三个，也是最后一个依据来源于我童年和青年时期的经历。从很小时候起，我就理所当然地认为，如果不重视教育，任何有价值的国家目标都不可能实现。这一点在医学和公共卫生领域是千真万确的，在其他领域亦是如此。任何有兴趣目睹现代医学知识在各国，无论是发展中国家还是其他国家，得到进一步应用的人都不能逃避作为一名教育工作者的责任。

这种责任对于发展中国家的村民和游牧民族来说尤为重要。鉴于现代工业化社会的教育水平较高，可以相当有把握地假定，其大多数人口至少拥有基本的科学知识储备。因此，我们可以进一步假设，他们至少略有耳闻，知道传染病是由微生物进入人体，并在人体内生长和繁殖引起的，而且许多疾病都是通过传染而蔓延开来的。

然而，在发展中国家，我们不能做出这样的假设。众所周知，

wholly uninformed about basic scientific matters. Many villagers around the world have no idea how infection is contracted or disease transmitted. In fact, illness is often attributed to the work of malevolent spirits. As long as this notion prevails among villagers, we cannot expect them to be concerned about maintaining personal cleanliness or taking aseptic precautions in their daily lives. They will simply adhere to their old ways.

Thus, regardless of the immense challenges that confront health professionals in Third World countries in trying to treat the sick, it is important, at least initially, that they spare some time for health education efforts. Pressures from other directions must be balanced by the need to develop a scientifically informed population made up of men, women, and children who have at least some elementary understanding of scientific principles. Otherwise we can anticipate that efforts to protect and improve health through the application of scientific medicine will have only a short-term and superficial impact.

This was the rationale for the progressive action that several other PUMC students and I took in establishing the Binying Weekly, the newspaper health supplement that we wrote and published as medical students in Beijing. Our aim was to make the educated newspaper readers of the city better informed in health matters and to encourage them to press the warlord regimes for improved health care. Medical students today have no less a responsibility to educate the public, and their teachers, in turn, should encourage them along these lines. The education of the public in health matters is one avenue through which community-oriented physicians can discharge their professional obligations.

THE PROCESS OF RURAL HEALTH DEVELOPMENT: LESSONS FROM CHINA

Making modern medical care accessible to the entire population

发展中国家的人们通常对基本的科学问题都是全然或部分地不知情。世界各地的许多村民不知道感染是如何发生或疾病是如何传播的。事实上，疾病常常被归咎于恶毒神灵的作用。只要这种观念在村民中盛行，我们就不能指望他们在日常生活中注意保持个人清洁或采取无菌预防措施。他们只会坚持用老办法。

因此，尽管第三世界国家的卫生专业人员在试图治疗病人方面面临着巨大挑战，但他们应该至少先抽出一些时间开展健康教育工作，这一点至关重要。必须向民众传播科学知识，使男人、女人和孩子们对科学原理至少有一些基本的理解，以平衡来自其他方面的压力，特别是迷信和某些特殊疗法。否则，我们可以预见，通过应用现代医学来保护和改善民众健康的努力只能产生短期和表面的影响。

这就是我和其他几个北京协和医学院学生开展的一项进步行动，即创办《丙寅周刊》的原因。《丙寅周刊》是我们医学生在北京撰写和出版的新闻副刊，旨在使这个城市受过教育的报纸读者更好地了解健康问题，并鼓励他们向军阀政权施压，要求改善卫生保健服务。今天的医学院学生同样有责任教育公众，他们的老师也应鼓励他们这样做。对公众开展健康教育是服务社区的医生履行其职责的一个重要途径。

农村卫生发展进程：来自中国的经验

使发展中国家的全体人民都能获得，并且广泛接受和使用现

of a developing country, and fostering its acceptance and use, cannot be accomplished overnight. The process requires time and patience. It implies fundamental change in the way people think and behave as well as the education and training of scientific personnel, and the organization of a health system, in which those persons can function effectively.

Six somewhat overlapping stages seem to be involved in the process. First, an appropriate relationship must be worked out with whatever indigenous medical system exists. Next, it is necessary to identify and educate a vanguard of young medical scientists and to imbue them with idealism and enthusiasm to undertake a difficult pioneering venture. Prepared for the task, the new leaders must produce, through trial and error, a model of health care suited to the needs and resources of that particular society. Foreign models are usually unsuitable, at least in part. The government must lend strong support, preferably before, and certainly after, the model has been developed, so that modern medical care can be made accessible in all parts of the country within the framework of an integrated, nationwide system of health care. Besides facilitating the countrywide establishment of the health network, the government must provide initial and continuing education for technical and support personnel at all levels. Finally, refinement and improvement of the system must be fostered through an ongoing two-way exchange of ideas, knowledge, and experience with other countries engaged in comparable efforts.

Scientific medicine was first introduced into our society over an urban bridgehead from the West well over a century ago. Thus China has already moved through many of these stages. Perhaps it is not too early to gain from our experience, enabling us to enlarge on the promising results for better health and long life that we have already achieved. There may be lessons also for other predominantly agricultural countries, whose young leaders are just now confronting issues and challenges that our leadership faced on the eve of our liberation, now nearly 40 years ago.

代医疗服务，不可能一蹴而就。这个过程需要时间和耐心。这意味着要从根本上改变人们的思维和行为方式，对科学领域从业人员进行教育和培训，并建立一个有效运作的卫生系统，让所有人受益。

这个过程可能涉及六个有些重叠的发展阶段。第一，必须与本土医疗体系建立适当的关系。第二，有必要发现和培养一批年轻的医学科学家，并给他们灌输理想主义思想和热情，使他们进行艰难的创业。第三，新产生的领导者必须通过反复试验，建立一种适合该特定社会需求和资源的医疗保健模式，为完成创业任务打基础。第四，国外的模式通常不合适， 至少在一定程度上不适用。政府必须提供强有力的支持，最好是在新模式形成之前，当然在模式创立之后亦应如此，以便在全国综合性医疗保健系统的框架内使各地都能获得现代医疗服务。第五，除了促进全国医疗保健网络的建立，政府还必须为各级技术和支持人员提供基础和继续教育培训。第六，应该与其他开展类似建设项目的国家开展经常性的思想、知识和经验的双向交流，来促进该系统的完善和改进。

一个多世纪前，科学医学第一次从西方以城市作为桥头堡引入我们的社会。之后，中国历经了多次医学模式发展阶段。也许我们应更早地从过去的经历中总结经验，以便进一步详述在健康改善和寿命延长方面取得的预期成果。其他以农业为主的国家也可借鉴这些经验，因为他们国家年轻的领导人现在正面临着中国领导人在建国初期所面对的类似问题和挑战。

Dealing with Traditional Medicine

In rural China, traditional medicine remains very powerful. Traditional hospitals and clinics are crowded with patients, traditional practitioners are prospering, and the farmers generally use more herbs than standardized pharmaceuticals. Traditional medicine, along with scientific medicine, receives strong support from the central government, and many high officials seem to be persuaded that traditional medicine offers benefits possibly not found in a scientific medical system.

One might well ask how this could be possible. Scientific medicine had been introduced into China more than a century earlier and had quickly obtained a firm footing in urban areas. Moreover, intellectual and reformist currents that swept our country in the 1920s had vaulted science and scientific thinking to a pinnacle of approbation among influential intellectuals of the day, who saw its potential for bettering human life as almost boundless.

A century, in terms of our country's long and complex past, is a relatively brief time span, however, and for the answer one has to reach much more deeply into the ages. Chinese as a people have a strong sense of history. We cherish our ancient cultural heritage and value traditional medicine as a component of that heritage. Moreover, many, if not most, of us have full confidence in the time-tested measures of medical relief that traditional medicine affords. In rural areas, this confidence may be especially engrained, associated as it was for centuries with the endorsement of respected imperial scholars.

The power of traditional medicine in the contemporary scene is, in part, explicable in these terms. Probably still more important however, is the lingering effect of the century after century during which its scholar-physician practitioners ranked in the highest strata of society and enjoyed the confidence and support of the imperial rulers. The social and political

与传统医学打交道

在中国农村，传统医学仍然非常强大。传统医院和诊所挤满了病人，传统行医者生意兴隆。相对标准化药品，农民更普遍使用草药。传统医学和现代医学一样，都得到了中央政府的大力支持，许多高级官员似乎已被说服，认为传统医学提供的益处可能在科学医疗体系中找不到。

人们会问，这怎么可能？现代医学早在一个多世纪之前就传进了中国，并迅速在城市地区站稳了脚跟。此外，20 世纪 20 年代，知识分子和改革派潮流席卷中国，使科学和科学思想在当时有影响力的知识分子圈中的认可度达到了顶峰，他们认为，科学和科学思想改善人类生活的潜力几乎是无限的。

然而，就我国漫长而复杂的历史而言，一个世纪是相对短暂的时间跨度，要找到答案，必须更深入了解各个时代。作为一个民族，中国人有着强烈的历史感。我们珍视自己古老的文化遗产，并将传统医药视为这一遗产的组成部分。此外，我们中的许多人对传统医学提供的久经考验的医疗救助措施充满了信心。在农村地区，这种信心可能特别根深蒂固，因为几个世纪以来，它一直得到受人尊敬的皇家和士大夫的认可。

传统医学在当代社会的影响力在一定程度上也可以这样来解释。然而，还有一点可能更为重要，那就是由士大夫认可的医师身处最高社会阶层，享有皇家统治者的信任与支持，这种影响历

influence of traditional practitioners in urban China today mirrors that historical position.

Ironically, the outspoken minority of modern physicians who, in the early twentieth century, campaigned to have traditional medicine legally abolished suceeded only in increasing its public support. The failure of their strategy reflected a blindness to important cultural realities. Unlike modern medicine, traditional medicine had been developed in Chinese soil by Chinese physicians, who shared a philosophical and intellectual background with the highest officials. Among a people who revered their millennia-old civilization and culture and respected the wisdom of classical scholars, that was more than sufficient to ensure its survival. Had modern medicine advocates steered a more moderate course, traditional medicine would very likely be far less powerful than it is today, and the circumstances would have been more conducive to the diffusion of scientific medicine in our society.

Those who had tried to ban traditional medicine had miscalculated both the political resources of the urban-based scholars and the depth of public attachment to traditional medicine. More explicitly stated, perhaps, the idea was unrealistic. Advocates of abolition entirely ignored the attitudes and circumstances of the villagers, who formed the majority of the population. The peasants by and large lacked access to any other kind of medicine, but, tradition-bound as they were, they were unlikely to have tried it even if they had had access.

Although modern medical care is widely available in rural China today, attempts to prevent the general population from using traditional medicine would be as ill-advised in the late 1980s as they were then, especially in areas where well-trained modern physicians are rare. Traditional medicine is much more acceptable to Chinese of all walks of life than is scientific medicine because it is more closely linked to our thinking and philosophy of life. People believe in it, and when they are

代相传，挥之不去。在当今的中国城市地区，传统行医者群体具有的社会和政治影响力反映了其曾经的历史地位。

具有讽刺意味的是，在 20 世纪早期，少数直言不讳的现代医生曾发起运动，要求合法地废除传统医学。其结果是非但没有成功，反而增加了公众对传统医学的支持度。他们战略的失败反映了他们对重要文化现实的视而不见。与现代医学不同，传统医学是由中国医生在中国土地上发展起来的，他们与统治阶级有着共同的哲学思想和知识背景。在一个尊重千年文明和文化，尊重古典学者的智慧的民族中，这足以确保传统医学的生存。如果现代医学的倡导者采取一种更为温和的方式，传统医学的影响力很可能远不如今天强大，其环境也将会更有利于科学的医学在社会中得到传播。

那些试图取缔传统医学的人错误地估计了身处城市中的学者的政治资源和公众对传统医学的依赖程度。更明确地说，这个想法可能不现实。主张废除传统医学的人完全忽视了占人口大多数的农民的态度和处境。农民基本上得不到除中药外的其他任何药品，但是，即使他们有机会得到任何其它的药品，由于受传统束缚，他们也不大可能去尝试。

尽管现代医疗照护已在中国农村地区普及，但在 20 世纪 80 年代后期，仍有人试图阻止普通民众使用传统医药，这个做法与 20 世纪初时的尝试一样不明智，尤其是在缺乏训练有素的现代医生的地区。传统医学比现代医学更容易为各行各业的中国人所接

ill, many, if not most, people want to consult a traditional practitioner, not a modern physician. In our country, modern medicine will supplant traditional medicine only gradually and slowly, possibly only among distant generations, and then only as a result of careful scientific education and demonstration of its efficacy.

The confrontation between scientific and indigenous medicine in our country, then, has perhaps been especially instructive. As we saw in the chapters on preliberation China, the introduction of science, including scientific medicine, into a largely uneducated population is never an easy matter, especially when its indigenous medicine is widely endorsed and culturally valued. In any modernizing society, social and intellectual, as well as technical, difficulties always exist. A scientific mentality must be encouraged in the general population. Where there is strong political support for traditional medicine, as in our country, the problem becomes even more complicated. Tolerance toward traditional medicine may be the wisest choice. Meanwhile efforts should be made to apply scientific methods to the study of any medications or procedures used by indigenous medicine that seem to be useful.

Notwithstanding previous problems, in China today relations between the two systems of medicine are cordial; practitioners respect each other. Thoughtful minds on both sides recognize that to the extent that it interferes with health care delivery, it is a waste of time to dwell on differences. The important point is to develop a health care system that works as a united force to improve the health and prolong the lives of the people.

While it is pointless to dwell on differences, it may not be very realistic to think in terms of "integration." Perhaps in some countries it might be possible to integrate scientific medicine and the indigenous medical system with beneficial effect. In our case, in fact, some highly placed party and government officials have advocated that idea.

受，因为它与我们的思想和人生哲学更密切相关。人们相信中医，当他们生病时，许多人想要咨询的是传统医生，而不是现代医生。在我国，现代医学取代传统医学的步伐只能是渐进和缓慢的，也许只有遥远的未来，通过认真的科学教育和其功效被证明后，才能实现吧。

因此，我国现代医学和本土医学之间的对抗可能特别具有启发意义。将科学（包括科学医学）引入一个大部分没有受过教育的人口中绝非易事，尤其是在其本土医学得到广泛认可且文化上普遍认同的情况下。在任何一个现代化社会中，无论是社会、知识还是技术方面的困难总是存在的。必须在普通民众中鼓励科学精神。在传统医学在政治上得到强有力的支持之处，犹如中国，该问题更具其复杂性。对传统医学的宽容可能是最明智的选择。与此同时，应该努力将科学方法应用于本土医学中那些似乎有利用价值的药物或疗法研究中。

尽管存在上述问题，但在今天的中国，两种医学体系之间的关系是友好的，医生之间相互尊重。双方经过深思熟虑，都认识到，在某种程度上，纠结于中西医的差异会干扰医疗服务的提供，本质上就是浪费时间。重要的是要建立一个医疗保健系统，团结一心来改善人们的健康状况和延长寿命。

虽然纠结于差异毫无意义，但从"整合"的角度来思考问题可能也不现实。也许在一些国家，将现代医学和本土医学体系整合起来并产生有益的效果是可能的。事实上，在中国，一些政府

Seemingly, they are convinced that, in such a synthesis, traditional medicine would play a significant role, given its time-tested theories, abundant clinical experience, and attraction as a subject of study by Western medical specialists. Recently, however, other officials have expressed a less sanguine point of view, cautioning that in an integrated discipline, traditional medicine might actually be absorbed and disappear.

Personally, I am compelled to ask myself what "integration" might mean when so little common ground is shared. Modern medicine had its beginnings in Europe after the Renaissance in the work of such great men as Andreas Vesalius in the sixteenth century, whose work—based on a precise record of observed facts, rather than opinion and speculation—laid the groundwork for scientific anatomical observation.

Traditional medicine is by no means entirely unscientific; it is partly the result of a large amount of experience, just as is modern medicine. But it has no such foundation in scientific observation. Common ground is also lacking in such other areas as methods of examination, consideration of side effects, and attention to prevention. For all these reasons, there will always be areas where physicians on one side or the other will have difficulty understanding each other.

We can see the consequences of the lack of shared ground in the dilemma in which some of our traditional medical students apparently find themselves. Their course of study is challenging. Nowadays they are required to study scientific subjects, including anatomy and physiology. Beginning with the third year, they work under the guidance of an experienced practitioner, learning case by case, through clinical experience, examining patients, and seeing the effects of the drugs they use. Familiarizing themselves with the immense number of Chinese drugs during this period is a formidable challenge in itself. The student must also, of course, become informed about the underlying theories of traditional treatment; traditional medical texts are by no means easy to read. The meaning of passages containing an admixture of description of empirical observations and metaphysical theory may be quite obscure.

的高级官员已经提出了这个想法。他们似乎确信，通过这样的综合举措，传统医学可以发挥重要作用，因为其理论久经考验，临床经验丰富，还吸引着西方医学专家去深入研究。然而，最近有些官员表达了一种不太乐观的观点，他们警告说，在一个综合学科里，传统医学实际上可能被吸收，甚至消失。

就我个人而言，我不得不问自己，在几乎没有共同基础的情况下，"整合"可能意味着什么。现代医学起源于文艺复兴之后的欧洲，基于 16 世纪安德列·维萨里等伟人的工作成果，他们精确记录了所观察到的事实，而不是个人观点和推测，这为科学的解剖学观察奠定了基础。

传统医学并非完全不科学；它的部分内容像现代医学一样，汇集了大量的经验。但它没有基于科学的观察。在检查方法、副作用的考虑和注重预防等领域也缺乏共同点。因此，现代医学和传统医学的医生总会在一些问题上难以理解对方。

我们可以看到缺乏共同点的后果，那就是一些传统医学生发现自己陷入了困境。他们的学习过程充满挑战。他们被要求学习现代科学课，包括解剖学和生理学。从第三年开始，他们要在一位经验丰富的医生的指导下工作，通过积累临床经验逐案学习，检查病人，并观察他们的用药效果。在这段时间里，要熟悉并了解大量的中药本身就是个艰巨的挑战。当然，学生还必须了解传统治疗的基本理论。传统医学的书籍并不容易读懂：文字段落中混合了经验观察与形而上学理论的描述，其含义可能非常难懂。

All this is challenging enough. Additionally, however, students must somehow correlate the traditional theories with scientific observations and explanations to which they have been exposed during their first two years of study. This can lead to problems in understanding the reason for the diagnosis and treatment prescribed.

Under such circumstances, interesting young people in both traditional and modern medicine concurrently can be very difficult. The teacher trying to make traditional and modem medicine compatible, either in theoretical discussion or in practical work, faces a real challenge. I personally have taken short courses in traditional medicine, and because of my background in modern medicine— which, needless to say, is quite different from that of a traditional practioner, the more I studied it, the more confused I became.

At present it is difficult to predict the outcome of our educational program and activities designed to promote integration. It does, however, seem quite apparent that neither political authority nor popular response alone can bring it about. Possibly for many years to come the two types of practitioner will be working on their own basis, side by side, each receiving government support. Meanwhile, whatever else may be said, our solution to the coexistence of two medicines is uniquely Chinese and has produced a uniquely Chinese health system.

Before leaving the subject of traditional medicine, it might be noted that Chinese research institutes have given high priority to research on drugs, which is not surprising given the historic tendency in our country to regard the dispensation of drugs as the essence of medicine as a discipline. Priority research areas include cancer, retinal disease, and fertility, with the focus on finding drugs that have never been known to the outside world and that would produce an effect not obtainable in scientific medicine. A global breakthrough in medical research would be a source of great national pride to our country, as to any other country.

所有这些都极具挑战性。然而，除此之外，学生必须设法将传统理论与他们在头两年学习期间所接触到的科学观察和解释进行关联。这可能会导致学生在理解所描述诊断和治疗的原因时出现问题。

在这种情况下，对传统医学和现代医学都同时感兴趣的年轻人就很为难了。无论在理论研讨还是在实际工作中，那些具有试图将传统医学和现代医学兼容起来的想法的老师就确实面临着挑战了。我个人曾参加过传统医学的短期课程，我有现代医学教育背景，这与传统医生的专业背景大不相同，因此，我越学习，就越感到困惑。

目前，很难预测我们的医学教育和实践在推动整合方面可能会得到的结果。然而，显而易见的是，不管是政府当局还是来自群众的反应，都无法实现这一目标。可能在未来若干年里，这两种类型的医学从业者将在各自原有基础上并肩工作，分别接受政府的支持。同时，不管怎么说，我们对两种医学共存的解决方案是中国独有的，并且已形成了一个独特的中国卫生体系。

在离开传统医学的话题前，也许应该指出，中国的研究机构高度重视药物研究，这并不奇怪，因为我国历史上倾向于将配药视为医学学科的精华。研究的优先领域包括癌症、视网膜疾病和生育能力，重点是寻找不为外界所知的药物，这些药物能产生在科学医学中无法获得的效果。在医学研究中取得全球性突破，是我国和其他国家伟大民族自豪感的源泉。

Developing Pioneer Leadership

The introduction of scientific medicine into societies undergoing modernization requires dedicated pioneer leadership and at least a handful of gifted teachers to bring it along. On the basis of my experience, in fact, I would say that the nurturing of innovative and idealistic leadership in the first generation of newly trained modern medical scientists is crucial to future public health development in any country. In this context, the inspiration of a few good teachers to even a minority of students can make a critical difference, especially if those teachers are concerned with broad issues affecting health rather than with specific clinical interests.

Consider, for example, John B. Grant, the physician who was for many years the Rockefeller Foundation representative in the Far East and concurrently the head of the Department of Health at the Peking Union Medical College (PUMC), which I attended. To me and many of my classmates, Grant was a crucially important source of direction. Most PUMC students tended to regard public health courses as the least welcome elements in the curriculum. Grant accepted that view as a challenge and went on to develop an innovative public health program involving intensive field study that caught the imaginations of many participants. His success lay in confronting students with the scope of health problems in the general population and relating this to the capacity of scientific medicine to alleviate them.

Under Grant, students who might otherwise have entered private practice became interested in the diffusion of modern medicine for a common good. I, for example, at Grant's recommendation, became health director for the Mass Education Movement (MEM) at Dingxian in the 1930s. In subsequently pioneering the organization of our country's first systematic rural health care organization in that county, I was never unaware of Grant's influence on my thinking.

416

培养先锋领导力

将现代医学引入正在经历现代化的社会，需要有献身精神的先锋领导人和至少一小群有天赋的教师来推动。事实上，根据我的经验，我认为对于第一代新培训的现代医学科学家来说，培养他们具有创新精神和满怀理想主义的领导能力，对任何国家未来的公共卫生发展来说都至关重要。在这种情况下，少数优秀教师对学生的启发，即便是少数几个学生，也能产生重大影响，特别是如果这些教师关注的是影响健康的广泛内容，而不是具体的、在临床上的兴趣。

例如，兰安生医生多年来一直担任洛克菲勒基金会远东地区代表，同时兼任北京协和医学院公共卫生系主任。对我和我的许多同学来说，兰安生是指导我们发展方向的至关重要的人。当时大多数北京协和医学院的学生通常都会认为公共卫生课是课程中最不受欢迎的科目。兰安生承认，有这种想法的确是个挑战，继而他开发了一个创新性的、涉及深入现场调查研究的公共卫生项目，激发了众多参与者的想象力。他的成功在于首先让学生直面普通大众的健康问题，然后告诉大家科学医学有能力缓解这些问题。

在兰安生的帮助下，那些本来可以进入私人诊所的学生为了一个共同的目标，开始对现代医学的普及工作产生了兴趣。例如，在兰安生的推荐下，我在 20 世纪 30 年代成为定县平民教育运动卫生部主任。后来，我在该县率先建立了我国第一个系统化的农村卫生保健组织。那时，我从未忘记兰安生对我思想的影响。

He convinced me that insight and experience gained in field training is as important a component of public health studies as is substantive knowledge acquired in the classroom, if not more important. I quickly came to see, too, that knowledge, however gained, is to be valued not for its content, but for its applicability to the problems at hand. The rewards of pursuing knowledge for its own sake must be left to others.

This exposure later brought me to realize the merit of the PUMC decision to use English as the language of instruction, rather than Chinese, as was done at a number of missionary medical schools. I am convinced that the use of English as the teaching vehicle greatly enhanced the value of our education. Taught in Chinese, we would have acquired the substantive knowledge necessary to practice modern medicine as well as the clinical skills. Our scientific training would have been complete. We would, however, have been left with no real sense of the intellectual and philosophical underpinnings of Western medicine, nor would Grant or other teachers really have exercised much influence on our personal spiritual and moral perceptions. This humanistic side of our education was important; for the education of a modern medical student should involve far more than the mere transfer of substantive knowledge of clinical skills. Medicine is an art, as well as a science.

Admittedly, there was a negative side to this issue. The use of English presented difficulties on both sides, and more than one potentially excellent candidate was excluded from the PUMC program because of the language barrier.

By singling out one teacher and that teacher's influence, I mean in no way to diminish the general overall value of the education we received at the PUMC and the contribution of the institution as a whole on my thinking. That was of crucial importance in our development as pioneering national leaders in health. Many of our medical professors were outstanding specialists in one clinical field or another, and our training under their guidance was invaluable.

兰安生使我确信，在现场培训中获得的洞察力和经验，与在课堂上获得的实质性知识同样重要，甚至可能是更重要的。我很快意识到，无论获得了多少知识，其价值不在其内容，而在于它是否能解决手头的问题。而那些为了知识本身而追求知识所得到的回报，还是留给别人吧。

与兰安生这次接触后，我意识到北京协和医学院决定使用英语作为教学语言的优势，而不像某些教会办的医学院那样使用中文教学。我确信，使用英语作为教学工具极大地提高了我们教育的价值。用中文授课，我们可以获得现代医学实践所必需的基本知识以及临床技能，我们的科学培训也就此完成了。然而，我们对西方医学的知识支柱和哲学基础并没有真正了解，兰安生或其他老师也不会真正对学生个人的精神和道德观念产生很大影响。这些人文教育是很重要的。对现代医学学生的教育应该远远超过仅仅传授其临床技能的基本知识。医学是一门科学，也是一门艺术。

诚然，这个问题也有消极的一面。使用英语教学给双方都带来了困难，不止一个潜在的优秀候选生由于语言障碍而被排除在北京协和医学院之外。

以上我着力说明了一名老师及其影响力，绝无意贬低我们在北京协和医学院所受教育的总体价值，以及学校整体对我思想的塑造。北京协和医学院的教育对我们成长为国家卫生领域具有开拓精神的领导者来说是至关重要的。我们的许多医学教授都是某个临床领域的杰出专家，我们能在他们的指导下接受培训非常宝贵。

The insistence on high standards of medical excellence benefited not only the PUMC students themselves but also other Chinese medical schools whose more modest institutional administrations struggled to emulate the model. As a result, over a period of several decades the poor standards of many struggling missionary, Japanese, and government-run Chinese medical schools gradually improved to a marked degree.

Fulfillment of the Rockefeller Foundation goal of providing medical leadership for China had begun as soon as the first students left the walled campus in Beijing to pursue their careers. The PUMC produced just over 300 graduates in twenty-five years, but the influence of those few' was far out of proportion to their number, and a majority of graduates figured importantly in public health, medical education, and medical administration in our country over the next half-century and beyond.

Over the years the reputation of the PUMC came to be based largely on its contributions to scientific research and clinical medical education, its input to national development not going much beyond significant accomplishment in these spheres. As to the contribution made by the few faculty members who interested students in tackling the ordinary and immense medical problems of the general population, and who imbued them with high ideals and a spirit of resourcefulness in so doing, little was said. In the long run, however, the role of the PUMC in educating public health leaders may have been in every sense as important to China, if not more so, than its role in developing clinical specialists, research scientists, and professors of medicine.

Fifty years ago ignorance and superstition shaped the lives of the Chinese peasantry, just as it does the lives of rural inhabitants of many developing countries today. Educational opportunity was lacking for most urban inhabitants as well, and the population of the cities, if somewhat better educated, was no less superstition- ridden. Until this

坚持高标准的医学英才教育不仅有益于北京协和医学院的学生，还惠及其他中国医学院校。这些院校的管理较为温和，一直努力效仿协和这种模式。其结果是，在过去几十年里，许多由教会、日本人和中国政府创办的医学院经过不懈奋斗，教学水平都得到显著提升。

从第一批协和毕业生离开北京院墙围筑的校园、开启他们的职业生涯起，洛克菲勒基金会为中国提供医学领导力的目标就开始实现了。25 年间，北京协和医学院共培养了 300 多名毕业生，但这些毕业生的影响力远远超过他们的人数，而且大多数毕业生在未来半个世纪里，为我国公共卫生、医学教育和医疗管理事业做出了重要贡献。

多年来，北京协和医学院的声誉主要基于它对科学研究和临床医学教育的贡献，而对国家发展的贡献从协和在这些领域所取得的重大成就却未超出前述的贡献。至于少数教职员工有兴趣辅导学生研究解决老百姓的一般性和重大医疗问题，并激发出学生崇高的理想和智谋来为民服务的，这些师德典范，很少有人提及。然而，从长远来看，北京协和医学院在为中国培养公共卫生领导人方面的作用，可能与其在培养临床专家、研究科学家和医学教授方面的作用同等重要，甚至更为重要。

50 年前，无知和迷信成了中国农民生活的底色，正如当今许多发展中国家农民的生活一样。大多数城市居民同样缺乏受教育机会，而城市人口，即便受到更好的教育，也同样受迷信困扰。

medieval mentality was replaced with some understanding of science, and until most Chinese more fully appreciated the need for cleanliness and sanitation, not much progress could be expected in diffusing modern medicine throughout the society.

The fact that a minority of PUMC recognized popular ignorance of scientific principles as an obstacle to health improvement and tried to provide a remedy and proceeded to concern themselves with the medical realities in rural areas is, I believe, part of the special legacy of the PUMC to our country. Unless there had been at least a few graduates prepared to undertake public health work in rural China, under difficult conditions—and willing to sacrifice their own personal and monetary gain and to persist, despite the often frustratingly slow pace of change—rural health services would have improved far less rapidly. Social change in every society requires leaders with creative ideas and high ideals.

Notwithstanding the significant contribution of the PUMC to China, a few aspects of its policy, even for that time, seem to have been less than closely attuned to the needs of the country. For example, the PUMC gave meticulous attention to the advanced technical training of a few nurses. In itself, this was a valuable undertaking. What China really needed at that time, however, was also an army of practical nurses who could do bedside work, train other practical nurses, and imbue in the patients some practices that could enable them to improve their standards of cleanliness and comfort.

An elite institution can be an effective educational tool, as the PUMC clearly showed. It provided its students with many advantages, including, most conspicuously, but not exclusively, a fundamental appreciation of science and the scientific method, and a solid grounding in the disciplines concerned with sickness and health. It set an admirable level of technical standards.

直到这种中世纪思维方式被一些科学知识所取代、且大多数中国人更充分地认识到清洁和卫生的必要性时，现代医学在全社会中的传播才有望取得进展。

北京协和医学院中的少数人已认识到，公众对科学原则的无知是健康改善的障碍，并试图找到补救方法。他们继而开始关注农村地区的医疗现实。我认为，这是北京协和医学院给我国留下的一份特殊遗产。除非有一些毕业生愿意在困难条件下去中国农村从事公共卫生工作，并且愿意牺牲自己的个人利益和经济利益，在农村卫生变革步伐往往令人沮丧又缓慢的情况下仍坚持下去，否则，农村卫生服务的改善速度将远远不会很快。每个社会的社会变革都需要具有创造性思维和崇高理想的领导者。

尽管北京协和医学院对中国做出了重大贡献，但其一些政策，即使在当时，看来也没有与中国的需要密切配合。例如，北京协和医学院高度关注对为数不多的护士进行高级技术培训。就培训本身而言，很有价值。但是，当时中国真正需要的是一支实用的护士队伍，她们可以做临床工作，对其他从事实际操作的护士进行培训，并指导病人一些实用操作以提高其洁净标准和舒适度。

一个精英机构可以成为一个有效的教育工具，北京协和医学院即是。为学生提供了许多优势资源，其中最明显但不是唯一的优势，是对科学和科学方法的根本认同，以及在疾病和健康相关学科方面打下的坚实基础。它将技术标准设定在了一个令人钦佩的水平。

The real problems with an approach that emphasized technical excellence to such a degree, however, is that it risks the deprivation of any developing country of the very kind of physicians it most needs, dedicated innovators and idealists willing to roll up their shirt sleeves and work at the grass-roots level, attacking problems in the soil where they exist.

Had its students lived under conditions that were more in keeping with those of the surrounding population, rather than on a level with those of the elite group in a highly industrialized Western country, perhaps a larger number of graduates would have been prepared to serve their country. As it was, some graduates, accustomed to the lifestyle they had enjoyed as students, left China for the West. Of those who remained, very few were willing to live under uncomfortable conditions among the rural peasants.

Another observation based on the PUMC experience that might be useful to an institution of its type in a developing country today concerns the role of indigenous leadership in institutional policymaking. Although China in the 1920s had its own modern-educated class, input from the Chinese side into PUMC decisions was seldom encouraged. In developing countries today, where educated and experienced leadership is apt to be in short supply, it may be particularly important that country nationals be given an opportunity to participate in policymaking along with the foreign advisors. This will not only provide experience for some people but will also facilitate integration of the institution with the society at large.

Whatever the value of an elite educational institution in a developing country may be, it should not be perceived as the sole source of competent leadership, cither for the organization of health care or for any other modernization goal. Able leaders are to be found everywhere, not just in a small pool of exceptionally gifted students, or of students who have particular social origins, a special language capability, or a certain level of formal education.

然而，如此强调技术卓越带来的现实问题是，它可能使任何发展中国家失去它最需要的那些医生，那些敬业的创新者和理想主义者，他们愿意卷起袖子在基层工作，解决基层那些源自泥土的实际问题。

如果北京协和医学院学生的生活条件与周围人群相当，而不是与高度工业化西方国家的精英群体看齐，也许会有更多的毕业生愿意为自己的国家服务。事实上，由于一些毕业生已习惯了学生时代的生活方式，离开中国去了西方。留下来的学生中，很少有人愿意在农村那种不舒服的条件下生活，与农民打交道。

另一项基于北京协和医学院的观察体验可能对今天发展中国家的这类医学教育机构有用，是关于本土领导人在机构决策中的作用。尽管中国在 20 世纪 20 年代拥有自己的现代教育阶层，但中国方面很少鼓励他们参与北京协和医学院的决策。在当今发展中国家，受过正规教育且经验丰富的领导人往往供不应求，让本国国民有机会与外国顾问一起参与决策，这一点特别重要。这不仅为一些人提供了经验，还将促进该机构与整个社会的融合。

无论发展中国家精英教育机构的价值如何，它都不应成为挑选能干领导者的唯一来源，不管他是领导卫生保健组织还是为实现其他现代化目标服务。有能力的领导者无处不在，不应局限在一小群天赋出众，或者有特殊社会出身、特殊语言能力或受过一定程度正规教育的学生群中。

I remember once at Dingxian expressing concern to Andrija Stampar, the public health leader from Yugoslavia who was visiting our site, as to where I would find competent people to work with me in the districtwide health system we were establishing. "What?" Stampar asked. "You have 400,000 people here, and no leaders?"

His question was appropriate. It may be that too often we think in terms of stereotypes and have fixed conceptions of leadership, blinding us to its existence when we find it other than where we expect it.

Competitive examinations for university entrance, for example, or rigid academic standards often serve a useful purpose; at times, however, they may deprive a society of the talent it sorely needs. Bright, energetic, and able young people, regardless of their personal or educational circumstances, have something to contribute to pioneer leadership in health development. In addition, we may have to uncover their innate capacities by the simple process of giving them a chance to show what they can do, weeding out the less competent through trial and error. There should be more than one fixed path to leadership.

Directing Change Through Experimentation

In the late nineteenth and early twentieth centuries, China theoretically accepted the Western pattern of private medical practice as appropriate for its own use only to realize that, whereas this health system might suit the needs and resources of a modern, industrialized society, it was not compatible with Chinese conditions. In the midtwentieth century China once again turned to a foreign model, emulating Soviet patterns in medical and public health education and in institutional organization for research. An alternative in both cases would have been to work out our own models, or to modify the borrowed ones, in accordance with social and economic conditions specific for our country.

在定县，记得有一次，我向来访的南斯拉夫公共卫生领导人安准加·斯坦帕尔表达了自己的担忧，主要忧虑是到哪里去找有能力的人与我一起完善正在建设中的全区卫生系统。"什么？"斯坦帕尔问道，"你们这里有 40 万人，却没找到领导人？"

他问得很好。这可能是因为我们经常用陈规定式来思考问题，对领导力形成了固定概念。当我们发现某个事物的存在并非我们所期望时，就对它视而不见。

例如，大学入学的竞争性考试或者严格的学术规范常常能起到积极作用；然而，考试和规范有时会让社会失去它急需的人才。聪明、精力充沛、能干的年轻人，无论他们的个人或教育背景如何，都有可能在卫生发展领域起到先锋领导的作用。此外，我们可能得给他们一个展示自己能力的机会，通过一个简单流程来发现他们的天赋，并通过反复试验来淘汰能力较差的人。走上卓越领导力的道路应该不仅是已固定的那一条。

通过实验来指导变革

在 19 世纪末 20 世纪初，中国在理论上承认，西方的私人医疗实践模式适用中国。结果发现，尽管这种医疗体系可能适合现代工业化社会的需要和资源，但它不符合中国国情。20 世纪中叶，中国再次转向外国模式，在医疗和公共卫生教育以及研究机构组织方面仿效苏联模式。除了这两种情况，还有一种选择，就是根据我国特定的社会和经济条件修改完善借鉴来的模式，制定中国自己的模式。

Cost was a major factor in the inappropriateness of the Western system of medical practice for China. Outside support had been required to establish and maintain its urban-centered hospitals and clinics, and, to any thinking person, it was clear that should that external support ever be withdrawn, the system was likely to collapse. Moreover, its philosophical basis engendered wasteful competition among individual physicians rather than a collective response to the overwhelming medical problems of a modernizing country.

More importantly, Western medical practice served only a privileged minority of urban Chinese, largely ignoring the needs for medical attention among the millions upon millions of peasants in the countryside, who constituted the vast majority of the population. In many rural districts there were no medical facilities of any kind; in some there were even no traditional practitioners. After 1928 the Guomindang party somewhat succeeded in organizing urban health administrations and establishing a number of urban hospitals and clinics; however, rural needs were generally neglected. By and large, the villagers remained deadlocked in the grip of poverty, disease, and ignorance of a feudal era.

There were, during the 1920s and 1930s, however, a few privately assisted groups working in areas of rural China, experimenting with various innovative measures to enhance the lives of the peasants. The Mass Education Movement (MEM) based at Dingxian—with which I served as health director for more than seven years—was one of these. As we have seen in chapter 3, it was this organization that provided me with the opportunity I had been seeking since medical school, namely, to experiment with a health system to reach the peasants.

Working with the MEM offered several advantages that may not always be available to developing country health personnel framing programs in their own countries. First, at the MEM we were not trying to

西方医疗实践体系不适合中国国情的一个主要因素是成本问题。建立和维持以城市为中心的医院和诊所是需要有外援支持的。对任何有思想的人来说，很明显，如果外部支持被撤销，这个系统很可能会崩溃。此外，西方医疗实践体系的哲学基础导致个体医生之间进行浪费性竞争，而不是用集体合作的方式去应对现代化国家中压倒性的医疗问题。

更重要的是，西方的医疗实践只服务于中国城市中的少数特权阶层，基本上忽视了农村数百万农民的医疗需求，而这些农民占中国人口的绝大多数。在许多农村地区，没有任何形式的医疗设施；有些地区甚至没有传统的医生。1928 年以后，国民党成功地组建了一些城市卫生管理机构，建设了一些城市医院和诊所；但是，农村的医疗需求被普遍忽视了。总的来说，村民们仍然陷于贫困、疾病和封建时代的无知之中。

然而，在 20 世纪 20 年代和 30 年代，一些私人援助的团体在中国农村地区试验了各种创新措施以改善农民的生活。以定县为基地的平民教育运动就是其中之一，我在那里担任了 7 年多的卫生部门主任。正如我们在第三章中看到的，正是这个组织为我提供了从上医学院以来就一直在寻找的机会，通过试验建设了一个惠及农民的卫生保健系统。

与平民教育运动的共事让我获得了一些好的经验。但这些经验对于发展中国家的卫生人员制定本国方案来说未必总是有用。首先，在平民教育运动中，我们并没有试图孤立地处理各社区中

deal with the health problems of the community in isolation. Rather, we were part of a closely correlated four-point program of socioeconomic change. Education, agricultural techniques, farm credit, and civic training were simultaneously receiving close attention; for even at that early time the MEM leadership had already recognized that the roots of rural problems are interwoven and that coordinated programs for socioeconomic improvement need to be developed. The quality of preventive medicine and of available treatment is just one of the influences affecting the health of a population.

Another advantage I enjoyed as health director was that I had a great deal of autonomy and was able to work systematically and without undue haste. The MEM was a privately organized group, and as such could offer its administrative staff greater leverage for experimentation than a government agency can usually afford, as private groups are accountable to the public or the government only in the broadest sense. In testing some rather unusual ideas through trial and error, therefore, I was relative unhampered by external constraints or by any pressure to come up with a quick answer. This was important, for a model must be tested as it is devised. Components may not work and will need to be adjusted before the model is adapted by administrators in other parts of the country.

Freedom to experiment and time to formulate viable solutions had permitted us to develop a system that received global recognition for its resourceful solutions to knotty problems. Since then, some of our ideas have been disseminated around the world and after some fifty years may no longer seem quite so innovative. At that time and place, however—Dingxian China in the 1930s, we broke ground in many respects. Of our basic working ideas, four were particularly noteworthy.

First, we based our approach to health care on local needs and conditions. Rather than coming in with any preconceived ideas, we

的卫生问题。相反，我们是一个紧密相关的社会经济变革的四大教育计划（教育、农业技术、农业信贷和公民培训）中的一部分。教育、农业技术、农业信贷和公民培训同时受到密切关注；平民教育运动的领袖在早期就认识到，农村问题的根源是相互交织的，需要制定协调一致的社会经济改善方案。预防医学和现有医疗治疗服务的质量只是影响人群健康水平的因素之一。

作为卫生部主任，我还享有另一个优势，就是我有很大的自主权，能够系统地工作，而无须操之过急。平民教育运动是一个私营组织团体，其行政管理人员对开展的试验通常拥有比政府机构更大的掌控权，因为私营团体只对公众或最广义上的政府负责。因此，在通过反复试验来测试一些独特想法时，相对而言，我没有受到外部限制或要求我快速响应的压力。这一点很重要，因为模型必须在其设计时进行测试。如果测试时某组件无法工作，那就需要在该模型被国内其他地区的行政采用之前进行调整。

可以自由地进行实验和有了足够时间制定可行的解决方案，这些条件使我们开发出了一个系统，该系统因其针对棘手问题提供丰富的解决方案而获得了全球认可。从那时起，我们的一些想法就在世界各地传播开来，大约50年后，这些想法看起来可能不再那么有创意了。然而，在那个特定的历史时期的特定地区，——20世纪30年代的中国定县，我们的确在许多方面取得了突破。在我们的基本工作思想中，有四点值得特别注意。

第一，我们开展卫生保健工作的方法是基于当地的需求和条

conducted our own statistical surveys as a basis for planning and consulted with local community leaders to obtain their ideas of the major problems in the district. The notion of taking surveys as part of a planning procedure was virtually nonexistent in our country at that time.

Second, we devised a system that was locally affordable, diminishing the economic barrier that previously had rendered modern medical care inaccessible to most villagers. We did this by basing plans on the collective use of the very small funds available in the village, amounting to less than U.S. $0.10 per capita annually.

Third, we constructed a bridge over which modern medicine as practiced in China's larger cities was carried to the rural areas. Student doctors and nurses from the leading urban hospitals of China came to the Dingxian field training site, where they saw and treated rural patients who heretofore had relied solely on untrained village practitioners.

Fourth, and last, we insisted on community responsibility for the operation and continued effectiveness of the system. In our physicians, nurses, and health workers, as well as among the villagers themselves, we tried to foster habits of cooperation for good community health, such as the early reporting of infectious diseases and the encouragement of a sanitary environment. Beyond this, we made local community organizations responsible for the ethical and responsible conduct of local health workers.

Building the infrastructure

All these attributes of the Dingxian model were noteworthy. As its originator, however, I believe that its most critical attribute was its emphasis on systematic procedures and careful regulation of technical responsibility at each level. I am a strong believer in effective organization,

件。我们没有提出任何先入为主的想法，而是自己开展统计调查，以此作为规划的基础，还与当地社区领袖协商，了解他们对该社区主要问题的看法。在当时的中国，将健康调查纳入卫生规划程序的观点是绝无仅有的，甚至可以说几乎不存在。

第二，我们设计了一个当地负担得起的系统，减少了之前大多数村民获取现代医疗服务的经济负担，这一点我们是通过集体使用村里每年人均不到 0.10 美元的小额资金来实现的。

第三，我们搭建了一座桥梁，将中国大城市的现代医学带到了农村地区。来自中国主要城市医院的见习医生和护士来到定县现场培训基地，在那里他们看到了农村的病人并为他们诊治，这些病人以前只能依靠未经培训的农村行医者。

第四，也是最后一点，我们坚持"社会应对卫生保健系统的运作和持续有效性承担责任"这一理念。在我们的医生、护士和卫生工作者以及村民中，我们努力培养大家的合作习惯，共建良好社区卫生，例如，及早报告传染病，鼓励大家保持环境卫生等。除此之外，我们请当地的社区组织负责管理本地卫生工作者在伦理和责任心等方面的问题。

建设基本卫生体系

定县模式的所有属性都值得仔细研究。然而，作为该模式的创始人，我认为，它最关键的属性是强调系统性流程以及对各个级别的技术责任开展细致监管。我坚信富有效率的组织的重要

and it is this aspect of the Dingxian model that I hope health workers from other countries will find of particular interest. We might have offered modern medical care of sorts to the villagers under several different circumstances, but the high quality of care to which they gained access was possible only because systematic organization was fundamental to our approach.

At Dingxian, health care was rendered through a three-tiered system of village, subdistrict, and district units. Different responsibilities were assigned to each type of unit, in accordance with the different degrees of training of the senior staff at each level. The marked difference in the technical competency of those in charge at each level ensured control of quality.

The system allowed not only for effective collaboration of all levels but also for careful supervision up and down the line. No one was expected or permitted to undertake tasks beyond one's technical capability, and staff at each level respected the superior knowledge and skill of those of higher grade.

From what I have seen in Shifang County in the mid-1980s, I could imagine that some barefoot doctors today have come to regard themselves as more competent than the secondary medical school graduates in charge of the xiang health clinics. This is an unfortunate situation and places the patient in an awkward position. At Dingxian, however, we had been able to circumvent this difficulty through a policy of graduated responsibility based on marked differences in the degree of technical training among personnel at each level.

Our system at Dingxian was built from the bottom upward. By this I mean that we used the least trained workers in the villages, better trained persons at the intermediate level, and the best trained at the county level. We trained our own village-based workers, giving them only simple instruction in health fundamentals, first aid, and techniques of

性，并希望这一属性也能引起其他国家卫生工作者的注意。我们本可以为村民提供不同情况下的各种现代医疗照护，但将系统性组织作为我们方法的基础，可能是让村民获得高质量照护的唯一原因。

定县的卫生保健服务通过村－乡－区（县）三级卫生保健网提供。各级医疗机构的职责根据其高级职员的受训程度而分别制定。各级负责人技术能力的显著差异确保了整个网络对质量的控制。

该卫生保健网保证了各级间的有效协作以及上级对下级的细致监督。该系统不要求也不允许任何职员承担超出其技术能力的任务，各级工作人员都需尊重其上级人员的卓越知识和技能。

联想到 20 世纪 80 年代中期我在什邡县观察到的情况，我可以想到今天有些赤脚医生已经开始认为自己比从中等卫生职业学校（中专）毕业并负责乡卫生室的医生更能干。此情况是很不幸的，也令患者处于尴尬的境地。而在定县，根据各级人员在技术上的受训程度不同而制定不同的分级责任，这一政策能有效规避前面提到的问题。

我们的卫生保健体系是自下而上建立起来的。我的意思是，我们把受过培训最少的工作人员放在村一级，受过较好培训的人员放在乡一级，而县级人员则安排那些受过最好培训的人员。我们培训自己的村保健员，只简单指导他们有关卫生的基础知识、

immunization, and impressing on them the necessity of referring patients to the subdistrict unit for early diagnosis of serious illness or for further treatment. Each subdistrict unit was supervised by a graduate physician, who managed a junior staff, while I headed the district unit, whose senior staff were the most technically competent people in the system.

Dingxian was built from the bottom upward also in the sense that we based our approach on what our surveys and our informants identified as the major health needs of the community, rather than coming in with any prefixed idea of how our system would operate. I am convinced that this is the logical starting point. After all, if many people believe or want something, there is considerable social force behind that collective opinion, and in trying to respond to the need, you will get cooperation. When you start at the top and work downward, as the missionaries tried to do in our country, you often find yourself dealing with relatively few individuals and relatively rare conditions while neglecting the chronic problems of the community at large.

In a three-tiered modern health care system such as we had at Dingxian, the technical training of the key people at the middle level must be unarguably superior to that of the health workers in the villages. Otherwise, one of two circumstances will develop, neither one of which is conducive to the spread of scientific medicine. Villagers may either fall back on traditional practitioners or they will rely on barefoot doctors who may not be sufficiently trained or supervised to provide quality care. Villagers will either develop confidence in modern-trained sources of relief or rely on the village health workers to do more than they have been properly trained to do, and the quality of care will suffer.

To anyone attempting to establish a rural health system in a developing country, I would recommend, on the basis of our experience, recruiting for local leaders in the existing community organizations and preparing them to do the elementary tasks that are most needed in that

急救和免疫技术，并嘱咐他们需将病人转诊到区保健所开展重症早期诊断或进行进一步的治疗。每个区保健所由一名大学毕业的医生负责监督指导，其手下还有一名初级员工。当我负责县保健院时，该院的高级专家是整个保健网中技术能力最强的队伍。

定县也是自下而上建立起来的，因为我们的方法是基于调研和知情人士确定的社区主要健康需求开展建设，而不是根据我们对系统运作的预设模式进行建设的。我相信这是合乎逻辑的起点。毕竟，如果有很多人相信或想要某样东西，这种集体意见背后必有庞大的社会力量，在努力应对解决需求时，定会开展合作。而当你像传教士在中国所做的那样，从上层开始向下工作时，你会发现自己处理的是相对较少的个体和相对罕见的情况，却忽视了社区大部分人群存在的长期问题。

在我们定县这样的三级现代卫生保健系统中，中级医疗机构的骨干人员接受的技术培训必须要优于村级的卫生人员。否则，就会出现以下两种情况，其中任何一个情况都不利于现代医学的传播。村民们可能会掉头继续依赖传统医学医生，也可能会依靠没有经过充分培训或监督的赤脚医生来寻求高质量的卫生保健。他们要么对经过现代医学培训的人员产生信心，要么对村卫生人员产生依赖，要求其进行超出其受训能力的工作，这样，卫生保健服务质量就会受到影响。

如有人拟在发展中国家尝试建立农村卫生系统，根据我们的经验，我建议在现有社区组织中招募当地领导人，并准备其使之

community. These needs will vary from place to place, particularly in an immense and diversified country such as ours. In one area, for example, potable water may be a priority issue and in another area, the control of malaria. The safest way to determine those needs is by consulting local leaders and by conducting preliminary surveys. Needs should be identified on where they actually emerge, not out of textbooks.

Health workers who live in the villages are essential to the maintenance of quality care, but if their training is minimal, their services should be limited to immunization and first aid work. Learning to use a few instruments is a rather simple matter; however, disciplined scientific thinking comes much harder, and this is why diagnostic responsibilities should be reserved to those with sound scientific knowledge and more advanced clinical training. To make such persons available to seriously ill village patients obviously requires that the intermediate and higher levels of the infrastructure be organized as soon as possible after the village health workers have been selected and trained.

No matter how suitable a model for rural health services may seem through experimentation, no one will gain much unless the government is active in extending it. Our experience under Guo- mindang officialdom taught us that. Party officials had recommended in 1934 that the Dingxian model be adopted throughout China, but there had been little follow-up, not so much because of the outbreak of war in 1937 as because of lack of genuine commitment on the part of the goverment to addressing rural needs.

Even for a decade after liberation in 1949, little was done in rural health other than construction of a few county hospitals and clinics and the dispatch of mobile units to distant areas. Once CCP Chairman Mao Zedong became disillusioned with urban intellectuals, however, and criticized the Ministry of Health as the "ministry for influential people," rural health development accelerated rapidly. Without his strong backing, it is most unlikely that the massive and abrupt expansion of

有能力执行一些该社区急需解决的简单任务。各地的需求会因地而异，尤其是在我们这样一个幅员辽阔且多元化的国家。例如，一个地区的优先事项可能是饮用水问题，而另一个地区的优先事项则可能是疟疾控制问题。最安全的方法是通过咨询当地管理者并开展初步调查来确定需求。应根据当地实际出现的问题来确定需求，而不是从教科书找答案。

居住在村庄的卫生人员是保证优质卫生保健的根本，但如果他们接受的培训很少，其工作应仅限于免疫接种和急救。学会使用一些工具是一件相当简单的事情；然而，要获得训练有素的科学思维却困难得多，这就是为什么诊断责任应该留给那些具有良好科学知识并受过更加高阶临床培训的人员。显然，若要让村里的重病患者能够接触到这些专业人员，就需要在选拔和培训村卫生人员后尽快组织建设中级和高级的相关体系。

无论定县实验显示出农村卫生模式有多么合适，如果政府不积极推广，谁也不会受益。国民党执政期间所经历的历史就告诉我们了这一点。国民党政府官员曾在 1934 年就曾提出建议，要在全中国推广定县模式，但后续几乎没有任何行动。这并不只是因为 1937 年爆发了抗日战争，而是因为当时的国民党政府没有真正致力于解决农村问题。

即使在 1949 年建国后的前十年，中国的农村卫生也没有太多发展，只是建设了几家县级医院和诊所，以及派遣医疗队到偏远地区开展巡诊活动。但是，当毛泽东主席对城市知识分子感到失

rural health care service and the recruitment of the required personnel that this entailed would have occurred. Rural health development in other countries today probably also demands strong input from the central government.

The buildup of the county health system of three levels in rural China was both directly and indirectly based on preliberation experience. Authorities drew heavily on the Dingxian model. They did, however, differentiate from it at points where they evidently thought that adherence was inessential or impossible. For example, lower priorities were assigned to development of adjunct training programs and attention to quality control through integration and careful gradation of responsibility.

The remarkable achievement realized from the expansion of the infrastructure in our country was the astonishing amount of prevention work that was done within the villages and by persons who lived right in the villages. This, again, reinforces the importance of the lowest level of the three-tiered system. By 1959, in many areas of the country, plague, smallpox, kala azar, typhus, and relapsing fever had all been brought under control. Environmental sanitation improved as a result of mass health campaigns to promote cleanliness and eradicate insects. In the 1960s, malaria and schistosomiasis were great reduced. Later attacks were launched on smallpox, measles, diphtheria, whooping cough, typhoid, and poliomyelitis.

The point that warrants emphasis is that the work was done right in the villages. In my view, there is no hope of controlling infectious diseases without such a contingent of health workers who do actually live in the village, regardless of how high a priority central authorities assign that aim. Effective immunization cannot be accomplished merely by sending in mobile teams. Farmers often cannot comply with their schedules and are neither able nor willing to bring their children to mobile stations in sufficient numbers. One may elicit a 50 to 60 percent response at most, but not the 90 percent necessary for effective control.

望并批评卫生部是"老爷卫生部"之后，农村卫生得以迅速发展。如果没有毛主席的坚强后盾，根本不会有中国农村卫生保健服务突然的大规模发展，也不会出现后来的大规模卫生人员招聘。今天，其他国家的农村卫生发展可能也需要中央政府的大力投入支持。

中国农村三级县级卫生保健网的建立直接或间接地基于建国前的经验。政府主要借鉴定县模式开展系统建设，但在他们认为不必要或不可能沿用定县模式的地方则出现了不同的做法。例如，相关培训项目的开发以及通过综合且细致的分级责任制开展质量控制等事项并未受到重视。

通过卫生体系规模的扩大，我国取得了显著的成就，在各村由村民开展了大量预防工作。这也再次强调了三级保健网中最基层工作的重要性。到 1959 年，鼠疫、天花、黑热病、斑疹伤寒和回归热等疾病在中国许多地区已经得到控制。通过开展群众卫生运动，改善了环境卫生并消灭了部分害虫。20 世纪 60 年代，疟疾和血吸虫病已经大大减少。后来又针对天花、麻疹、白喉、百日咳、伤寒和脊髓灰质炎开展了专门防治工作。

值得强调的是，我们在村里开展了正确的工作。在我看来，不管中央政府有多重视，如果没有这样一支居住在村里的卫生人员队伍，传染病就不可能得到控制。如果仅仅依靠派遣巡回医疗队，根本无法实现有效的免疫接种。农民往往无法遵守时间安排，他们不能也不愿按要求、如数地将孩子们带到移动免疫接种点。其响应率最多也只会有 50% ～ 60%，不可能达到能实现有效控制的 90%。

Providing Trained Personnel

In the fifth step of building a nationwide health care system, personnel must be developed to staff the expanding infrastructure. Ideally, the infrastructure develops only as swiftly as personnel can be trained to meet requirements. In reality, of course, this is seldom possible, and compromises may have to be made.

Rapid extension often means the lowering of personnel standards and the inadequacy of facilities. There can be no guarantee of quality in service or teaching. Qualified personnel cannot be properly recruited and trained in a short time, and any system built on unqualified personnel may defeat the purpose of rendering good care to the general population. A government is generally aware of the disadvantages associated with rapid expansion, but usually for political reasons, large-scale extension with inadequate personnel, equipment, and financial support is carried out at the expense of quality. The only remedy thereafter is to improve the quality of personnel by local training.

Such firsthand opportunities as I have had to observe rural medical care corroborate my belief in the importance of field training and the local training school for health for personnel in our country. In Shifang County I have personally seen a number of instances where an unfortunate situation might have been avoided if the physician in attendance had received better training. There was, for example, a patient with shoulder pain whose shoulder was dislocated by the examining barefoot doctor. Another patient with a fracture paid for a costly x-ray that was essentially worthless because it had been taken by an untrained medical assistant who did not know how to use the equipment properly.

Even in relatively routine situations, it would be helpful if barefoot doctors had more training, and consequently more confidence in their own competency. For example, a barefoot doctor, unsure of what is

提供训练有素的人员

建立全国卫生体系的第五步是必须培养卫生专业人员，充实到不断扩大的卫生体系中工作。在理想情况下，卫生体系的发展速度应与所需人员的培养速度相当。当然，在现实中，这几乎不可能，且可能不得不作出妥协。

卫生体系的快速发展往往意味着工作人员招募标准的降低以及卫生机构的缺乏，且可能无法保证医疗卫生或教学的质量。短期内往往不可能招募到合格的工作人员并进行适当的培训，但任何建立在不合格人员基础上的系统，都不可能达到为大众提供合格健康照护的目的。政府普遍意识到快速发展的弊端，但通常出于政治原因，在人员、设备和资金不足的情况下，以牺牲质量为代价进行大规模扩张。此后唯一的补救办法是在当地为工作人员提供培训以提高其业务能力。

通过我对农村医疗保健发展的亲自观察，确证了我的信念，即现场培训和当地培训学校对我国卫生工作人员非常重要。在什邡县，我亲眼目睹了许多不幸的发生，如果在场的医生接受了更好的培训，就可以避免类似悲剧。例如，有一位患者肩痛，是因为他的肩膀在赤脚医生检查时被弄脱臼了。另一位骨折患者支付了昂贵的费用进行 X 射线拍片，钱却白花了，因为给他做 X 光检查的人员是一名未经培训且不懂得如何正确使用 X 光机的医疗辅助人员。

如果赤脚医生能接受更多培训，那他们对自己的能力会更有信心，那样即使在相对常规的情况下，也会带来很多帮助。例如，

causing the cough and fever of a small child, and without anyone with more advanced training to turn too, as a precaution may prescribe penicillin when, in fact, the simple suggestion of bedrest and plenty of fluids would have served just as well. In such a situation, the mother of the precious "one child" will almost certainly spend her money for the expensive, but needless, prescription.

The difficulty of doing this well in China is very great, however, in part because the county training schools for health schools must deal with people whose educational backgrounds are so extremely limited. What we greatly need, therefore, is some pioneer effort to show the sizable positive impact that a really effective county training school program can have on rural health.

Benefiting from Foreign Contact

In the sixth and final phase, responsible health leaders must take deliberate steps to constantly refine and improve the health care system, relying not only on their own ideas but also on fresh inspiration from outside. If the doors are left open to foreign contact, health administrators, medical educators, physicians, nurses, and other health professionals from other parts of the world can be a rich source of innovative ideas in a two-way flow that benefits both sides.

Free exchange of ideas and knowledge, as I learned as a child, leads to mutual understanding and appreciation. This is a principle of human life equally applicable to relationships between individuals, groups of persons, and great nations. China has appreciated this principle over most of its long history. Classical scholars knew the importance of stimulation and encouragement from others, and the Han, Tang, and Ming emperors, to varying degrees, fostered links with other peoples and cultures.

当赤脚医生诊治一个咳嗽和发烧的儿童患者却不能确定病因时，在没有更加专业的人员可以提供帮助时，预防起见，他可能会开出青霉素进行治疗。而事实上，这种情况可能经过简单的卧床休息和多喝水就能起到同样的作用。那这样，这位宝贝"独生子女"的母亲就会白白把钱花在昂贵但没必要的处方上。

但是，在中国要做好这件事的难度很大，部分原因是县级的卫生培训学校接收的都是受教育程度极低的学生。因此，我们极为需要做一些开拓性的工作，确保县级培训学校项目真正有效，并对农村卫生产生积极可观的影响。

在国际交往中获益

第六步也是最后一步，负责卫生的领导必须深思熟虑，不断完善和改进卫生保健系统，不仅要依靠国内人员的想法，还要从国际上获取新鲜灵感。如果打开国门进行对外交往，来自世界其他地区的卫生管理人员、医学教育工作者、医生、护士和其他卫生专业人员可以和国内人员开展双向交流，互惠互利，碰撞出丰富的创新性想法。

就像我小时候学到的那样，自由的思想和知识交流会带来相互理解和欣赏。这是人类生活的一条原则，同样适用于个人、群体和大国之间的关系。中国历史悠久，大部分时间都奉行这一原则。传统学者深知他人启发和鼓励的重要性，汉代、唐代和明代的皇帝在不同程度上都加强了与其他民族和文化的联系。

In the modern world, domestically derived ideas and perceptions alone are insufficient to ensure the safety and security of a way of life, much less of progress and modernization in any field, including medicine. Our country's fate under the Qing dynasty testified to this all too clearly. Even the relatively short moratorium on international contact during the 1960s and early 1970s cost our country very dearly. I hope that we Chinese will never again return to a state of intellectual isolation under the guise of self-reliance.

With our present shortage of teachers, the programs of scholarly exchange with the outside world can probably do more good than any other attempt to upgrade the efficiency of our health system. What forms these programs should take is a matter that must be constantly evaluated, in China as in any other country.

It may or may not be appropriate for public health graduate students from the Western democracies to restrict their interest to a relatively narrow range of advanced theoretical topics. It is clearly inappropriate, however, for those from developing countries to do so. Their graduate education should equip them for attacking the commonplace health problems of the Third World, whose remedies lie in such areas as improved sanitation, nutrition, maternal and child health care, and communicable disease control.

A number of cooperative agreements between Western and Chinese institutions were signed in the first flush of newly reestablished relations with the United States; however, there have been fewer as the fever subsided. In general, their full potential has not been realized because of difficulties at various levels of implementation. A fairly well established consensus in the mid-1980s seemed to hold that with limited resources on both sides, the focus should be on an exchange of individual scholars.

Two points in this context deserve some attention. First, when foreign scholars come to a developing country to study or teach in its

在现代世界，仅凭国内衍生的思想和观念不足以确保生活方式的安全，更不用说保障包括医学在内的各领域的进步和现代化。我们国家在清代的命运，已经清楚地证明了这一点。20 世纪 60 年代至 70 年代初期，我国短暂地停止了对外交往活动，即使时间相对较短，仍使国家付出了沉重的代价。我希望我们中国人永远不要再回到以自力更生为名的智识隔离状态。

鉴于目前我们缺乏师资，要提高我们卫生系统的效率，开展国际学术交流可能较其他项目活动都要有效。开展国际学术交流的形式，在中国和在其他国家一样，都需要不断进行评估。

西方国家的公共卫生研究生将学习领域限制在相对狭窄的高级理论研究，这可能合适，也可能不合适。但是，若发展中国家的公共卫生研究生这么做，显然是不合适的。研究生教育应该是使他们有能力去解决第三世界国家常见的卫生问题，包括环境卫生改善、营养、母婴保健和传染病控制等。

在中美恢复建交初期，中国和西方国家签署了大量机构间合作协议；然而，随着热度的退却，后续签署的协议就变少了。总体来说，鉴于后续各级落实困难，合作协议的潜力并没有得到充分发挥。在 20 世纪 80 年代中期，双方达成了一个较为明确的共识，即鉴于双方资源有限，合作重点应放在个别学者交流上。

在这方面有两点值得关注。首先，当外国学者来到发展中国家在其卫生系统内开展研究或教学工作时，在大多数情况下，他

health system, the value of their contribution in most instances has some proportion to the length of their stay. Even a brief visit may be quite beneficial to scholars for their own purposes. Yet, unless a scholar is prepared to remain for five years or longer, it is very difficult to surmount cultural barriers or to gain an in-depth perception of the problem under study; thus, the visiting scholar will be disappointed in not being able to contribute as fully as hoped. The foreign missionaries who came to China to study and teach before liberation in 1949 seemed to have appreciated the difficulty as many chose to spend their entire working lives in our country.

Second, when developing country medical students do graduate work abroad, the value of their experience to their country depends greatly on the topic on which they spend their research time. Too often such students are guided into areas of narrow research interest in highly technical areas. What the Third World needs is not so much people with greatly advanced specialized scientific medical knowledge, but medical and health professionals trained to respond to chronic, common problems, especially the common health problems in their own countries. Emphasis on advanced technology and specialized research in medical education and practice may serve the industrialized countries well—although even there it is evident that accelerating costs are an unwanted side effect. For students from developing countries, however, it is indisputably inappropriate.

ISSUES FOR THE FUTURE

Where do we go from here? The people of my country, of whom more than 80 percent are farmers, represent more than one-fifth of the total population of the world. That figure lends global significance to both our past experience in rural health development and the future direction of our health endeavors. What happens in China will have crucial

们的贡献价值与其逗留的时间长短有一定比例关系。对学者们来说，即使是短暂的访问也可能使他们受益匪浅。然而，除非他们准备留任五年或以上，否则很难跨越文化障碍或深入了解所研究的问题；所以，访问学者将不能按预期做出充分的贡献而感到失望。1949 年解放前来中国从事研究和教学的外国传教士可能已经意识到其中的困难，所以有许多人选择将他们的全部工作生涯都放在中国。

其次，当发展中国家的医学生赴国外进行研究生学习时，他们的学习经历对其祖国的价值有多少在很大程度上取决于其花费时间研究的课题。在很多情况下，这些学生会被指导去研究狭窄的高技术领域。第三世界国家更需要的并不是那么多的拥有高端专业现代医学知识的人，而是经过培训后可以应对长期存在的常见问题的医疗卫生专业人员，特别是可以应对他们本国常见的卫生问题的人。重视医学教育和医疗实践中的先进技术和专业研究可能会很好地服务工业化国家——尽管在那里，增加的成本也显然是不需要的副作用。然而，对发展中国家的学生来说，这无疑是不合适的。

思考未来的问题

今后我们应当往哪里去？我国的人口占世界总人口的 1/5 以上，其中逾 80% 是农民。这个数字意味着中国过去在农村卫生发展方面的经验以及未来卫生工作的方向都具有全球意义。中国

implications on the level of "health for all in the year 2000."

In retrospect, we see that in China the expansion of the rural health infrastructure since 1958 has brought conspicuous, tangible benefits to our farmers. The increase in access to modern medical care in the countryside is, in fact, nothing short of remarkable. Every county in China, no matter how remote, now offers some form of scientific medical care to its inhabitants. County facilities not only exist but are being used extensively. Xiang centers, employing both modern and traditional methods, are treating a great volume of patients. The familiarity of attending physicians with the personal situations and problems of their neighbors and friends enhances the quality of the physician-patient relationship. Meanwhile, in the villages, barefoot doctors and village health workers, notwithstanding their need for further training and closer supervision, are rendering a very important service, essentially doing primary health care and preventive work.

Medical care, of course, is just one of the influences on health; the total health experience in China is a combination of external circumstances together with improved curative and preventive care that resulted in the striking health improvements since liberation in 1949. Educational and health improvements played a significant role; no one as yet has made a scientific examination of the probable correlation between higher family income and improved nutrition. Yet, it is fairly safe to assume that parents are spending some of their added income on better food for the children. Education has contributed to improved habits of cleanliness among the farmers, helping to reduce the prevalence of diarrhea and trachoma, often associated with poor personal hygiene. It has also made the peasants more conscious of the potential for infection and more interested in maintaining a sanitary environment.

The most critical determinant of development in health, as in all other realms of the national life, however, has been the centralization of political authority in the CCP and the government. The countrywide extension

发生的事情将对"2000 年人人享有健康照护"战略目标的实现产生重要影响。

回顾过去，我们看到，1958 年以来中国农村卫生体系的扩大和发展给农民带来了显著且实实在在的好处。事实上，农村增加了获得现代医疗的机会是非常了不起的。中国的每一个县，无论多么偏远，现在都为其居民提供了某种形式的科学医疗照护。县级医疗机构不仅存在，而且正在广泛发挥作用。乡镇卫生中心利用现代和传统医学方法治疗了大量患者。主治医生对邻居和朋友的个人情况以及问题的熟悉程度改善了医患关系的质量。与此同时，在村子里，赤脚医生和村卫生人员虽然仍需要接受进一步培训和密切督导，但他们提供的初级卫生保健和疾病预防工作却非常重要。

当然，医疗保健只是对健康的影响之一；中国全部的卫生经验集合了外部环境以及强化的防治结合措施，并自 1949 年以来，大大改善了中国人民的健康状况。教育和卫生水平的提高发挥了重要作用；目前，还没有人对增加的家庭收入与营养改善之间可能存在的相关性开展过科学研究。然而，我们有充分的理由推测，家长将部分增加的收入用于为孩子提供更好的食物。教育帮助农民养成了清洁的习惯，而那些与个人不良卫生习惯相关的疾病，如腹泻和沙眼的患病率也随之降低。教育还使农民更加意识到潜在的感染风险，并更加注意保持环境卫生。

然而，就像与国民生活的所有其他领域一样，卫生发展最关

of the rural health infrastructure could never have been accomplished at so swift a pace and might never have been accomplished except in the distance future, had it not been for the strong backing of the Communist party and its then party chairman.

Absolute authority provided other advantages for improving the national health situation as well. For example, the government can encourage top students to attend medical school and can distribute them among the various medical training institutions in the manner most advantageous to the country. Also, after their graduation, it could send them to work where they were needed, rather than where they necessarily preferred to work, although there was some leverage for individual choice within the system.

Given what we have already been able to do, perhaps no other country has a better opportunity than China now enjoys to refine and elaborate a really outstanding health service from which other nations may draw inspiration. If quality and quantity arc kept in balance, continuous penetration of scientific medical knowledge and skill into the everyday lives of our millions of villagers is all but guaranteed. It is a chance that we do not want to waste.

All in all, we have made a promising effort. Our level of health has been significantly improved, and we have an infrastructure in place, fully staffed. I believe that the next step is enlarging the promise by raising the quality of service. This raises several important issues, including the need for further training of local health personnel.

In any scheme to improve training, provincial authorities should, in my view, accept responsibility for improving the skills of county- level health personnel, who should be sent to provincial hospitals and clinics for this purpose. A selected few county health workers might even be enrolled in key medical schools or sent abroad for advanced study if that were deemed necessary.

键的决定因素是党和政府的集中领导。如果没有党的正确领导和大力支持，就不可能如此快速地完成全国农村卫生系统的建设，甚至可能永远不会成功。

就提高国民健康状况而言，政府强有力的管理有很多优势。例如，政府可以鼓励优秀学生就读医学院，并能以对国家最有利的方式将其分配到各种医学培训机构。也可在其毕业后，将他们输送到需要的工作岗位上。当然，安排工作时系统内也会考虑个人的选择。

鉴于我们已经能做到的和已经取得的成果，也许现在没有其他国家比中国拥有更好的机会来完善并提供真正出色的健康照护了，而其他国家也可以从中受到启发。如果能保持质量和数量的平衡，那几乎可以肯定，科学的医学知识和技能将不断渗透到我们数以百万计的村民的日常生活中。这个机会我们不想浪费。

总而言之，我们非常有盼头。我国民众的健康水平得到了明显改善，我们的卫生体系到位，人员配备齐全。我相信下一步的任务是提高服务质量。这就提出了几个重要问题，包括需要对地方卫生人员开展进一步培训。

我认为，在所有培训计划中，各省级政府都应对县级卫生人员技能的提高负责，安排县级卫生人员到省级医院和诊所进修。如有必要，可以选派少数县级卫生人员到重点医学院或者去国外深造。

My strong conviction, however, is that the most of the retraining of rural health workers should be done right in the rural areas, as the responsibility of county and xiang authorities. If country doctors, secondary medical school graduates, or rural nurses are sent to the city for training, they will be apt to seek means to avoid returning to the countryside. Conversely, the diversion of urban personnel to rural areas for service would serve no useful purpose either, since—unused to village conditions and uninterested in rural problems—they would soon become restless. In any event, there are plenty of candidates for remedial training already in the ranks of local rural health personnel.

Time and effort need not be spent on the construction of new educational facilities, as existing hospitals, maternal and child health centers, antiepidemic stations, and training schools can serve the purpose quite adequately. What is required of the existing training schools is that they maintain academically rigorous standards. Also, a program to bring more uniformity in the length and substance of training, at least in schools within each province, would go a long way toward ironing out some of the unevenness that now exists in the training of rural health personnel. Relatively uniform standards for the selection of students would also be helpful in this context.

Training schools should be given a modicum of suitable equip-merit, which need not be elaborate. This might include a tape recorder, a microscope, a centrifuge, a refrigerator, an incubator, and scales. A model training school in one selected county, appropriately equipped and staffed by dedicated teachers comfortable in a rural assignment, might draw favorable attention from other county authorities.

Implicit in these ideas is the underlying idea that secondary medical school graduates and country doctors should be given an opportunity to learn more about what they are already doing, and not that the scope of their responsibilities should be expanded. For example, the country doctors and village health workers are already doing effective

但是,我坚信农村卫生人员的大部分再培训项目应该在农村地区开展,这是县和乡政府的责任。如果把农村医生、中等卫生职业学校毕业生、农村护士送到城市培训,就容易出现他们想方设法避免返乡的情况。反之,如果将城市卫生人员派到农村去服务也无济于事,因为他们不习惯农村的条件,对农村问题也不感兴趣,很快他们就会变得焦躁不安。无论如何,地方农村卫生人员队伍中已有许多人需要进行再次培训。

目前并不需要花时间和精力去建设新的教育设施,因为现有的医院、妇幼保健中心、抗疫站、培训学校就足以开展各项培训教育工作。应要求现有的培训学校保持严格的学术标准。此外,应制定规划统一培训时长和内容,至少要保证各省内部的学校统一,这样将对消除目前农村卫生人员培训项目中存在的不平衡现象大有裨益。同样,相对统一的招生标准也会有所帮助。

应给培训学校配备少许合适的设备,这不需要详细说明。这些设备可以包括录音机、显微镜、离心机、冰箱、培养箱和秤等。对于选定县区的示范培训学校,应配备适当设施以及适合农村教学任务且认真敬业的教师,这样可吸引其他县政府进行学习。

这些建议的基本出发点是:应该给中等卫生职业学校毕业生和农村医生一个机会,让他们更多了解自己在做的事,而不是扩大他们的职责范围。例如,农村医生和村卫生人员已经在开展有效的预防接种工作。然而,如果疫苗接种工作人员能更多地了解

immunization work. Yet it would be helpful to the program if those administering the vaccines understood more about why they produce immunity, what side effects may result, how long the immunity lasts, and why only a certain number of immunizations are given. Or, as another example, more emphasis should be given in the training programs to symptoms of communicable disease, especially infectious disease, which may be more widespread in rural areas than we realize.

The continuing education programs for local health personnel that are most urgently needed, then, are those that will further qualify physicians and village health workers to carry out preventive programs, to treat common ailments without producing harmful side affects, and to identify cases of communicable disease at an early stage so that the patients can be hospitalized immediately and the spread of infection to others prevented.

As long as workers in this category are performing relatively limited functions, simple first aid work, and vaccination, they are fulfilling an important service in many cases. When they are permitted to engage in curative practice, however, prescribing any drugs for any patient, the stage is set for problems.

For instance, with little or no training, a country doctor, failing to understand the source of the problem, may all too easily administer morphine to relieve the acute abdominal pain of a patient suffering from appendicitis, with the result that the patient eventually suffers a ruptured appendix. Rather than trying to organize graduate training for practitioners of that type, it seems more appropriate to limit the scope of their activities and leave the skilled work to others with appropriate training.

More difficult to solve are economic issues, the question of how country doctors might be appropriately remunerated, and how state medicine might eventually be brought to the xiang level and below. The solution of the former question in terms of letting country doctors engage

疫苗为什么会产生免疫力、可能导致什么副作用、免疫力持续多长时间以及为什么只进行一定数量的免疫接种，这将对免疫工作大有帮助。应更加重视传染病症状培训项目，特别那些在农村地区更有可能普遍流行传染病。

因此，目前地方卫生人员最迫切需要的继续教育项目，应该是能进一步提高医生以及村卫生人员执业资格，开展预防性的项目，治疗常见疾病且不会造成有损害的不良反应，并在传染病早期阶段及时识别患者，以便患者可以立即住院并防止感染传播给他人。

只要这类工作人员履行相对有限的职责，实施简单的急救和疫苗接种工作，在许多情况下，他们都在提供重要的照护。然而，如果允许他们参与治疗工作，如可以为任何患者开具任何药物时，问题就出现了。

例如，一名没有经过专业培训或者经过很少培训的农村医生，在无法判断病因的情况下，可能很容易给阑尾炎患者服用吗啡来缓解急性腹痛，结果导致患者阑尾穿孔。所以，与其尝试为这类从业者安排学位培训，还不如限制他们的执业范围，并将专业工作留给接受过适当培训的人。

更难解决的是经济问题，包括如何适当地向农村医生支付报酬，以及国家药物如何最终输送到乡级及以下地区。关于前一个问题的解决办法，前面我已经提到过，如果是让农村医生进行私

in private practice is fraught with many difficulties, already cited. These questions need to be further studied.

Another matter of great consequence in our health future lies in the area of prevention. In my view, there is a very urgent need to tighten up supervision by the xiang-level authorities of the immunization work being done in the villages, so as to ensure quality control.

The village is the place where immunization work has been done and should be done. Nevertheless, village-level personnel seldom fully understand the scientific principles inherent in the immunization procedure. Therefore, they can make serious mistakes that undermine the value of the entire prevention campaign. They may, for example, fail to appreciate the importance of age as a criterion for immunization and immunize members of the wrong age group, or they may not understand the importance of proper vaccine storage. UNICEF has made a major contribution to child health in the Third World with its development and distribution of equipment to maintain vaccine at proper temperatures while it is in transit to the villages. So that full advantage is taken of that concept, however, xiang-level personnel who know so much more about the scientific fundamentals of a vaccination program absolutely must work in close cooperation with the village personnel. Unless the vaccination efforts are continuous, their long-term value will be lost.

Improved education of public health specialists is another issue that needs further study in our country. As noted earlier, public health education as modeled after the Soviet system currently emphasizes topical discussion, for example, of physical elements in the human environment, and performance of laboratory experiments rather than the application of scientific knowledge to common health problems. In my view, a shift away from the theoretical toward the more practical side of the public health field, particularly if field training were more widely used, would be of greater benefit to the country and would perhaps attract a higher quality student to the public health field.

人执业，则困难重重。这些问题都需要进一步研究。

在未来的卫生工作中，另一个重要的方面在预防领域。我认为，目前极为紧迫的工作是乡级部门要加强对各村免疫工作的监督，以确保其质量。

村级单位已经是也应该是实施免疫工作的地方。然而，很少有村级人员完全理解免疫程序中固有的科学原理。因此，他们可能会犯严重的错误，从而削弱整个预防工作的价值。例如，他们可能没有意识到年龄作为免疫标准的重要性，并为错误的年龄组成员接种了疫苗，或者他们可能不了解正确储存疫苗的重要性。联合国儿童基金会专门开发了将疫苗运送到村庄时使用的适温储存设备并将其分发，为第三世界的儿童健康做出了重大贡献。为充分利用这一概念，对疫苗接种项目科学基础了解更多的乡级人员必须要与村级人员密切合作。只有疫苗接种工作是持续的，其长期价值才不会丧失。

加强对公共卫生专家的教育是我国另一个需要进一步研究的问题。如前所述，目前以苏联体制为蓝本的公共卫生教育侧重专题论述，例如研究人类环境中的物理因素，以及关注实验室实验的进展情况，而不是将科学知识应用于常见的健康问题。在我看来，如果公共卫生领域能从理论转向更实用的方向，特别是如果现场培训得到更广泛的应用，将对国家有更大的好处，并且可能会吸引更高素质的学生加入公共卫生领域。

In moving our health care approach farther along the road toward a population-based system that combines curative and preventive procedures, we would be making an important step in providing more fieldwork to public health students. Work could be coordinated systematically with the health service organizations at the county, xiang, and village levels. Some of our health centers (antiepidemic stations) offer facilities that would be excellent field training sites, especially for communicable disease control, health education, and school health.

Public health education in medical colleges in China could be strengthened as well; as long as good teachers are in short supply, the organization of separate schools of public health within the universities of medical sciences may be unwise. In particular, public health teaching to medical students could be made more effective by building a field training capability into our medical service. As long as the faculty themselves have no field experience, the teaching of public health or community medicine is bound to be largely classroom work sprinkled with some simple, even trivial, laboratory exercises. Yet as long ago as in my preliberation work at Xiaozhuang, my experience taught me that medical students in public health benefit less by didactic instruction than by participation in practical field activities.

Clinical instruction cannot be satisfactory without a good teaching hospital; public health teaching cannot be successful without a good teaching field. In the rural areas, students become inspired by direct contact with people; they begin to try to apply what they have learned to the solution of social problems; they see how problems can be handled through skillful organization and resourceful use of available technology; and they learn how to assess health conditions from the multiple perspectives of medicine, economics, education, sociology, and politics. In sum, in the field, they reorient their interests to the real needs of the people.

A good teaching hospital cannot be organized without compassionate

为推动我们的卫生保健系统进一步朝着以人群为基础、防治结合的道路方向发展，我们将迈出重要一步，为主修公共卫生的学生提供更多参与现场工作的机会。可以协调县、乡、村三级的卫生服务机构开展工作。我们的一些卫生中心（抗疫站）提供的设施将是极好的现场培训场所，特别是在传染病控制、健康教育和学校卫生等方面。

我国医学院校的公共卫生教育也可以加强；如果缺乏优秀教师，在医科大学内组建独立的公共卫生学院可能是不明智的。特别是，如果我们的医疗工作具备现场培训的能力，就能更加有效地对医学生进行公共卫生教育。如果教师本身没有现场工作经验，那么公共卫生或者社区医学的教学就必然是以课堂作业为主，并点缀些简单甚至微不足道的实验室练习。然而，我在晓庄的经历告诉我，医学生在公共卫生领域从讲授中获得的收益比参与实践活动所获得的要少得多。

没有好的教学医院，临床教学的效果不可能令人满意；没有好的教学现场，公共卫生教学就不可能成功。在农村地区，学生可以从与村民的直接接触中获得灵感；他们开始尝试将所学应用于解决社会问题；他们观察如何通过巧妙的组织和对可用技术的灵活利用来解决问题；他们学习如何从医学、经济学、教育学、社会学和政治学等多个角度评估健康状况。总之，在现场，他们将自己的兴趣点重新定位到人群的真正需要上。

如果没有富有同情心的人员，不从所有患者的益处出发考虑

effort by the staff, who consider medical problems for the benefit of all patients. Likewise, a good teaching field for public health education cannot be created except by a dedicated faculty with creative ideas and high ideals.

Underlying all this is the urgent need to instill a more community-oriented mentality in the next generation of physicians in our country. In my view, it is critically important that we make a greater effort to nurture young physicians who are public health-minded, that is, whose professional perspective is oriented on the community as a whole or that at least combines concern both for individuals and for the community.

For two reasons, this is essential not only for us, in China, but for countries throughout the world. First, universally, there are far greater numbers of medical students than of public health students. Consequently, once they enter the health field, their collective influence will be greater, and they can contribute just as much, or more, to the protection of the public at large as can the public health specialists. Second, it is medical school graduates, certainly in our country if not elsewhere, rather than public health school graduates, who come to occupy most of the administrative positions in the health system. Thus, if we are interested in the organization of a good health system, we must not fail to imbue our future administrators with an understanding and appreciation of community medicine. So far in China we have not done very much in that regard, and that is why the preventive aspect of our health picture has received less attention than some persons might have hoped.

Public health as a general field, particularly public health education, is a subject that has not elicited great interest in our country in recent years. In this respect, however, China is no different from many countries in the West. In many countries around the world, few people understand or are concerned about the meaning of the concept of public health. This is perfectly reasonable since many are struggling simply to

医疗问题，就不能组建一个良好的教学医院。同样，如果没有一支具有创新思想和崇高理想的敬业教师队伍，就不能创建出良好的公共卫生教育教学现场。

在这一切的基础上，迫切需要在我国的下一代医生中传递更加以社区为导向的思想。在我看来，我们应该更加努力培养具有公共卫生意识的年轻医生，即其专业视角面向整个社区或至少兼顾考虑个人和社区问题的年轻医生，这一点至关重要。

这不仅对我们中国至关重要，而且对世界各国都至关重要，具体原因有两点。首先，普遍而言，医学生的数量远多于公共卫生专业的学生。因此，一旦他们进入卫生领域，他们的集体影响力就会更大，他们可以像公共卫生专家一样，为保护广大民众做出同样或更多的贡献。其次，在我们国家（其他国家或地区情况可能有所不同），卫生系统的大部分行政职位都是由医学毕业生担任，而不是由公共卫生学毕业生担任。因此，如果我们希望建设一个良好的卫生系统，就一定要让我们未来的管理者了解并认识社区医学。迄今为止，在中国，我们在这方面做得并不多，这就是为什么我们卫生领域中预防工作受到的关注比某些人希望的要少的原因。

公共卫生，作为一个综合领域，尤其是公共卫生教育，近年来在我国并没有引起很大关注。而在这方面，西方许多国家与中国并没有什么不同。在世界上许多国家，很少有人了解或关注公共卫生概念的意义。这是完全可以理解的，因为许多人只是为了

secure the essentials of life.

In the industrialized West, however, where the term "public health" was coined, the level of affluence and education should be sufficient to ensure a different situation. One would hope to find not only that the abstract meaning of public health was generally understood but also that the significance of efforts to promote it were recognized and respected. Such is not necessarily the case, however. Even in medical circles in the West, one often encounters a somewhat disparaging attitude toward physicians in the public health field. It will be a change for the better when community medicine and public health are as respected as the branches of medicine on which individual clinical practice is based.

确保获得生活必需品而奋斗。

在创造出"公共卫生"一词的西方工业化国家，富裕程度和教育水平本应足以保证出现不同的情况。人们希望不仅公共卫生的抽象含义能得到普遍理解，而且促进公共卫生工作的意义也应该得到承认和尊重。然而，情况却未必如此。即使在西方国家的医学界，在公共卫生领域工作的医生也时常会遭到轻视。如果社区医学和公共卫生像临床医学一样受到尊重，情况便会好转。

译者：王晓琪，丁旭虹

A CLOSING COMMENT

It may be that a scientifically based system of health care for an entire population can evolve only in stages as a public perception of social responsibility increases. In a progressive society, health care eventually becomes a function of collective concern about all circumstances and conditions that at all times affect the well-being of the entire group rather than of the concern of a single physician seeking a cure for an individual patient. Along with this, there is a shift away from reliance on curative measures alone and toward the use of both preventive and curative measures.

To my way of thinking, four stages can be identified in this process: individualized medicine, with attention only to curative measures; individualized medicine, with attention to both curative and preventive measures; community medicine; and, finally, public health.

Community medicine, the third and relatively advanced stage, and the one at which China is currently developing its health care approach, entails organized community efforts in medicine and health, using combined curative and preventive techniques. Because it is population-based, that is, based on the needs and conditions of communities as a whole, it encompasses almost by definition, the fields of vital statistics, epidemiology, and health administration.

结语

也许只有公众对社会责任的认识不断提高，科学的全民卫生保健体系才能分阶段发展。在一个进步的社会中，卫生保健最终将成为一项众所关切的，且在各种情况和条件下随时都会影响整个群体福祉的社会功能，而不仅是单个医生关注如何治疗单个患者。与此同时，卫生保健也将从单纯依赖于治疗手段，向防治结合转变。

在我看来，这个过程可以分为四个阶段：（1）只关注治疗的个体化医学；（2）注重治疗和预防的个体化医学；（3）社区医学；（4）公共卫生。

居第三阶段的社区医学是个相对高级的阶段，也是中国目前正在发展其卫生保健方法的阶段，需要社区使用防治结合技术，有组织地在医学和卫生领域开展工作。因为社区医学是以人群为基础的，即以社区的整体需求和条件为基础，所以从定义上来看，它几乎涵盖了生命统计、流行病学和卫生管理等领域。

Public health carries the scientific approach to health care to its ultimate point. As I define it, it is a field concerned with the entire range of circumstances and conditions that affect the health of an entire population. Preventive medicine is the stronger of its two components; in its curative component, the emphasis is on early diagnosis. Given the many circumstances that directly or indirectly impact the health and well-being of a population, public health is closely linked to many other scientific fields, particularly engineering and education.

These close linkages attest to the need to seek health care improvements in conjunction with other measures and programs to improve popular well-being. For this reason medicine and medical scientists, especially in developing countries, cannot afford to be absorbed in technology alone, least of all isolated in laboratory research efforts. The education of young physicians for our needs must be focused on, not detached from, reality.

In a medical school, all too often both teachers and students are interested in technology. In terms of its application and development for the benefit of the general population, however, not many are interested. Yet medicine, after all, deals with human beings. So, in a country where pioneer leadership in health is badly needed, an initial step may be to rely heavily on those medical students who are sensitive to social needs and who have had some training in the liberal arts and humanities, for it is they who are more likely to think in terms of social well-being in the broad sense.

Such persons can be relied on to find an appropriate means of bringing health care to less advantaged segments of Asian, African, and Latin American societies. Large-scale extension of health services, however, is perhaps best avoided until the model on which it is based has proved practical on a local scale. Local communities cannot be expected to progress in health care delivery, regardless of how good the model,

公共卫生将卫生保健的科学方法推向了极致。正如我所定义的，它是一个对影响全人群健康的所有情况和条件加以关注的领域。预防医学是其两个组成部分中较重要的一个；在治疗方面，公共卫生主要关注早期诊断。鉴于有许多相关问题直接或间接影响人群健康和福祉，公共卫生与许多其他科学领域密切相关，尤其是工程和教育领域。

这些密切的联系表明，需要结合其他改善大众福祉的措施和项目来提高卫生保健水平。出于这个原因，医学和医学科学家，特别是发展中国家的医学和医学科学家，不能只专注于技术，尤其不能只局限于实验室研究。对年轻医生的教育必须着眼于现实，不能脱离实际。

在医学院，教师和学生往往都只对技术感兴趣。然而，并没有多少人关注为造福大众而进行的技术应用和技术开发。但是，毕竟医学是处理人类相关的问题。因此，在一个亟需卫生先锋领导力的国家，首先可主要依赖那些对社会需求敏感并受过一些文科和人文学科培训的医学生，因为他们更可能从广义的社会福利角度思考问题。

可以依靠这些人为亚洲、非洲和拉丁美洲社会的弱势群体找到合适的提供卫生保健服务的方法。但是，在所基于的模式尚未在地区性的范围证明可行之前，最好避免大规模推广相关卫生照护。如果没有政府或其他外部机构的大力支持，无论模式多么好，

without strong support from government or other outside agencies; they are simply too fragile. Firm central government effort is probably needed in every situation.

Whatever the specific nature of the delivery system that evolves, it should be marked by strong organization and integration at every level. It needs good administration at the top and enthusiastic workers, including lay workers, at the bottom. Clearly delineated technical and professional distinctions contribute to the coherence of the system. The contribution of education and training programs in this regard is self-evident. In every country continuing education to all technical personnel is crucial. The competency of the teachers is essential, for their role has much to do with determining the educational outcome.

Much can be gained through international exchange and foreign assistance, provided the focus of this assistance is appropriate. Acceptance of scientific equipment from abroad that local personnel know neither how to operate nor to maintain may not be very helpful. It is better that international assistance be directed toward better training of medical personnel and toward the expansion of the scientific horizons of the national leadership, possibly through foreign-sponsored visits to other countries or through international conferences.

Centuries have passed since people first began to organize themselves into nations. Each nation has had its own particular concerns, but all have been concerned with medical and health care. Now, in 1988, concern with "Health for all by the year 2000" becomes an appeal on behalf of all humankind. The response must come from people in many fields of endeavor, across the entire spectrum of society. Yet, in helping nature to protect and promote human health, the medical profession must bear the primary responsibility.

All this may sound banal, but even ideas based in common sense are often difficult to realize. I shall look back satisfied if I see that the far-

都不能指望当地社区在提供卫生保健方面取得进步；他们实在是太脆弱了。在任何情况下，都需要中央政府的坚定努力。

无论卫生保健系统的具体性质如何演变，它应该在各个层级都具备强大的组织性和整体性。它需要顶层良好的管理者和底层热情的执行者，包括非专业的工作人员。清晰的技术性和专业性的区分有助于整个系统的连贯性。教育和培训项目的重要性不言而喻。在每个国家，对所有技术人员开展继续教育都是必不可少的。教师的能力至关重要，因为他们的角色与教育成果有很大关系。

只要援助的重点合适，国际交流和对外援助大有裨益。如果接收了国外科学设备但当地人员不知道其操作和维护方法，这可能不会有太大帮助。最好将国际援助用于开展医务人员培训项目，可以考虑通过外方支持访问其他国家或参加国际会议等形式进行。

自从人们开始建立国家以来，已经过去了几个世纪。每个国家虽有自己的特殊关切问题，但都关心医疗和卫生保健。现在是1988年，"2000年人人享有卫生保健"成为代表全人类的呼声。社会各行各业的人们都应该积极响应。但在帮助自然保护和促进人类健康，医学界必须承担首要责任。

所有这些听起来可能平淡无奇，但即使是基于常识的想法也往往难以实现。如果基于过去的有远见的教导能继续激发年轻同事和朋友作进一步思考，我会感到很满足。中国的大部分问题，

sighted teachings of the past continue to flourish in the minds of younger colleagues and friends. Most of China's problems, medical and social, and probably those of the rest of the world as well, can be understood from a historical point of view. I hope that the contemporary history of my own country will be a source of pride for future generations.

"Birth, aging, sickness, and death" constitutes a life cycle, a biological law that no one can resist. Everyone desires to live long and well. Nature aids us in this context, in both health and illness, and medicine, a body of knowledge accumulated by humankind, is there to assist. As the stewards of this knowledge, physicians have a special responsibility to persons struggling to realize their human rights in regard to health.

In many parts of the world, the vast majority of people are beset by poverty, ignorance, and illness. The medical profession must join the fight to combat these afflictions. When it does not, or worse still, even aggravates these circumstances (when some physicians take advantage of their special knowledge at the expense of such persons), something has gone wrong in that society. In a just society, medical care of good quality should be easily available to all the people.

包括医疗和社会问题，可能还有世界其他地方的问题，都可以从历史的角度来理解。我希望今天中国的历史能成为子孙后代引以为豪的源泉。

"生、老、病、死"是生命的循环，这是不可抗拒的生物法则。每一个人都希望活得美满和长寿。自然赋予我们的是健康和疾病；而在这一点上，医学作为人类长期积累起来的主要知识是会帮助我们的。医生作为这一知识的拥有者，在实现人类的健康权利的斗争中，负有特殊使命。

世界许多地方，大多数人被贫困、无知和疾病所困扰。医学界一定要与这些困扰作斗争。如果不这样做，或者，甚至使情况恶化（如某些医生利用他们的专业技术知识加重人们的经济负担），那么这个社会就走错了路。在一个公平的社会中，高质量的医疗保健应使所有的人受益。

译者：丁旭虹